Medicine at Your Feet: Healing Plants of the Hawaiian Kingdom Volume One

by David Bruce Leonard, L.Ac.

"*A weed is a plant whose virtues have not been discovered*"
Ralph Waldo Emerson

Just what you need... another
Roast Duck Producktion

"*A peasant must stand a long time on a hillside with his mouth open before a roast duck flies in.*"
- - Chinese proverb

This book is dedicated:

To the Hawaiian people *in their struggle for justice*
&
With infinite gratitude to Stacey Guss,
who, for twenty years, has shown me ways of healing
I never knew possible

And in memory of:

Nahi'ena'ena
whose love and turmoil, to this day, still smoulders in Hawai'i

WARNING

Caution: Many plants used as medicine are poisonous! They can kill you. *Never* attempt to use herbal medicine without the guidance of a traditional elder or a licensed healthcare provider. If you wish to act on some of the information in this book, you must consult with a professional. *Do not try to be your own doctor.*

Dear Reader,

Your purchase allows us to continue research on the healing properties of medicinal plants and the restoration of our native Hawaiian ecosystems. A percentage of the profits from this work are given to Hawaiian cultural and environmental restoration groups. More information can be found at http://www.davidbruceleonard.com.

Thank you for your kind support of this work and our 'āina. Aloha no kākou.

Mahalo,

David Bruce Leonard

ACKNOWLEDGMENTS

This work is possible only through the grace and kindness of my Hawaiian and Chinese teachers:

Auntie Helen 'Ahia Walrath our beloved Kupuna Hulu

Kahu Kawika Ka'alakea
Kaipo Kaneakua
Kumu Dane Kaohelani Silva
Uncle Bill Kanekoa
Uncle Joe Hamakua
Keoki Sousa
Auntie Alice Kuloloio
Auntie Rachel Kanekoa
Auntie Nani Saffrey
Shirfu Zhao Zhen-ping
Shirfu Pang Zhen-neng
Shirfu Feng Chien
Shirfu Liao Yang-tze
Shirfu Lucy Hu
Shirfu John Yeh
Lama Tarchin, Rinpoche
Lama Khardhi

I also wish to acknowledge the following people who were indispensable in compiling this mana'o.

Special thanks to: The hundreds of people who have made a commitment to give back to the 'Āina.
Art Medeiros, Uncle Rene Silva, and Fred Stone for doing what they do. They are the real heroes of Hawai'i nei.

Inspirations: Pat Bily, Ken Bouché, Mitch Brinks, David Clausnitzer, Jennifer Crummer, Tracy Erwin, Ed Lindsey, Puanani Lindsey, Dave Metz, Iokepa Nae'ole, Anna Palomino, and Jill Wagner.

The Big Island Forest Team Ecosaints: Talena Adams, Albert Cortes, Lono Dunn, Ben Ikeda, Jenny Johansen, Micah Oliva, Katrice Powell, Barbara Rowe, Amanda Spaur, and Anya Tagawa.

Other appreciations:
Bodhi Arends and Kianna Stupakoff for their shining light of curiosity and passion.
Landish Armitage for his gift of Noni and for knowing exactly where the eyeball goes.
Lee Baarslag for help above and beyond friendship.
Andrew Benson for getting me off my 'ōkole.
Gill Brooks for his absinthe, friendship, and website wisdom.
Carol Colbath, book designer, for unraveling the digital mess I sent her.
J.R. "Bob" Dobbs for showing me how to beat the slack-sellers out of the temple.
Stacy Domer and Kelly Frith for their long hours of research.
Virginia Doran for her gift of numerous valuable research materials.
Jim and Peggy Duke for their hospitality and Jim's kind help in obscure plant research.
Barbara Fahs for helping with the index.

Heather Gavey for the use of her home as a classroom.
Cheryl Ginter for her unwavering belief in this work.
Christopher Hobbs, Don Hemmes, Forest Starr, & Kim Starr for last minute photo-emergencies.
Quentin Holt for providing much needed sanctuary and support.
Betsy Jacobsen for her help obtaining a computer.
Monica Cunuema Junqueiria for her guidance in the Rio de Janeiro botanical garden.
Kit Gentry for the use of his incredible paintings.
Nancy Kahalewai for holding my hand and maintaining the tradition.
Amara Karuna for financial assistance and for figuring out the best uses for her naugahyde.
Michael Klaper for having compassion and integrity when others did not.
Darrell Lapulapu for his friendship and traditional knowledge.
Dean Lem for his help obtaining a digital camera.
Julia Leonard, my mother, for proofreading this manuscript and trying her damnest to keep me in line.
Curt Leonard, my brother, for his infinite support and encouragement.
Dennis McKenna for his encouragement, patience, and help pulling my Jeep out of the river.
Janet Meredith for proofreading the manuscript.
Mike Moriarty for keeping me supplied with weird medicinal plants, goat cheese, and unique perspectives.
Kihei Nahale-a for showing me how to laugh in Hawaiian.
Phillipe and Gloria Nault for the use of their garden.
Robert Newman for his irreplaceable translation skills and guidance in translating Chinese texts.
Bill Schoenbart for his damn-the-torpedoes feedback and demented sense of humor.
Kalei Tsuha for tactfully correcting my Hawaiian.
German Velasco for his driving skills in the Amazon rainforest, continued friendship, and poor taste in sweaters.
Janet Wakatsuki for her hard work and infinite patience.

Thanks to the following people who were kind enough to send plant books during their travels:
Lee Baarslag, Jennifer Chesworth, Sally Conolly, Virginia Doran, Jason Glover, Ishaka Greenwell, Rita Regale.

Thanks to the following people who went out of their way to send research information:
Kabba Anand, Stephen Barstow, Gerald D. Carr, Denise Collins, Mike Croan, Dennis E. Desjardin, Subhuti Dharmananda, James Duke, Trish Flaster, Richard Grossman, Kristina Groth, Christopher Hobbs, Kyle Holladay, Abdul Ghani Hussain, Aaron Ishigo, Stuart Kahan, Colleen Keena, K.S. Manilal, Leda S. Meredith, Cheri Miller, Mike Moriarty, Linnie O'Flanagan, Antoinette Pahia, Andrew Pengelly, Joe Pepping, Mike Reynolds, Nina Rwomushana, Aadrian Short, Tony Simons, John R. Stepp, Stephen Vail, German Velasco, Dove White, Mark P. Widrlechner.

Contents

Introduction

Medicine at Your Feet: The Plants

Medicine at Your Feet: The Plants continued...

Appendices

INTRODUCTION

"The hottest places in hell are reserved for those who, in time of great moral crisis, maintain their neutrality."
- - Dante Alighieri, poet (1265-1321)

The Hawaiian Islands are the most isolated island chain on earth, a string of jewels over the heart of the Pacific Ocean. More than 2000 miles from any significant landmass, the isolation of the Hawaiian Islands places them at the center of one of the most spectacular biological symphonies in global history.

The islands known as the Hawaiian Islands are actually the eastern-most peaks of an underwater mountain range that stretches for 1200 nautical miles from the Big Island in the east to Kure Atoll in the west. This is the largest mountain range in the world, less than 10% of which peers above the surface of the ocean. The 100 or so older islands and atolls to the west are sometimes called the "Kupuna Islands" or Ancestor Islands.

The Hawaiian archipelago is a vast time capsule stretching back millions of years from east to west. Like an immense conveyor belt, the Pacific plate slides six inches per year over a magma chamber that lies 40 miles deep in the earth. This chamber is called a "hot spot" and as each island is formed it slides over and makes room for the next. All the islands in the Hawaiian chain have arisen from this single hot spot.

Because of our isolation, Hawai'i is most likely the best place in the world to study evolution. Charles Darwin offered a reward for any collector who would gather him plant and animal samples in Hawai'i.

Hawai'i has the highest rate of "endemism" in the world. A species is endemic to the place in which it evolved. 90% of our native Hawaiian plants and 99% of our native Hawaiian land animals evolved here and exist only in Hawai'i.

Historically, 75% of all United States extinctions are native Hawaiian plants and animals. Almost half of the species currently on the U.S. Endangered Species list are native Hawaiian. Half of our native Hawaiian birds are extinct. Half of those left alive are endangered. Thirty percent of the fish in our Hawaiian coral reefs exist nowhere else on earth.

When these species are gone, they are gone forever.

The Hawaiian archipelago is over 70 million years old. Hawai'i became home to one new species every 50,000 years. This time frame gave each new species plenty of time to naturalize and evolve into a multitude of other different species. This unprecedented explosion of biodiversity is called 'adaptive radiation'. The Hawaiian biosphere could well be the crown jewel of biological creation on planet Earth.

It has been said that when the first Polynesians arrived from the Marqueses Islands to Hawai'i, each valley had it's own species of spider and each ridge had it's own species of snail, each descended from a few common ancestors.

We are now introducing new species into Hawai'i at the rate of 20-30 per year. This is 2 million times faster than the natural rate. The impact of humans on Hawai'i nei is systematically destroying our biodiversity. Hawai'i has become the extinction capital of the world. We now have 500,000 feral cats on Maui alone, not to mention hoofed weed-whackers like goats and pigs. We have highly aggressive bees, coqui frogs, stinging ants, 'stinging nettle' caterpillars, and psychopathic seaweeds - all brought here by *Homo sapiens.* This does not have to happen. We are simply unwilling to make the hard choices that are necessary to protect our home.

The current unprecedented destruction of native Hawaiian ecosystems must be factored into any decision regarding Hawai'i, including the gathering of herbal medicines. Given the rare nature of many Hawaiian plants, I've purposely excluded certain endangered native plants which I consider to be "at risk" for abuse.

There is a Hawai'i that exists beyond the coconut palms, umbrella drinks, and basted pink flesh. It is a place beautiful beyond description. To view a forest only as a "resource" is to never see the forest at all. How many dollars is a Palila (a native Hawaiian bird) worth? What is the value of a ten million year old ecosystem? The question is so transparent that we don't even see what it says about *us.*

NA WAO AKUA (HAWAIIAN FORESTS), NA'AU (KNOWLEDGE), A ME NA'AUAO (ILLUMINATED MIND)

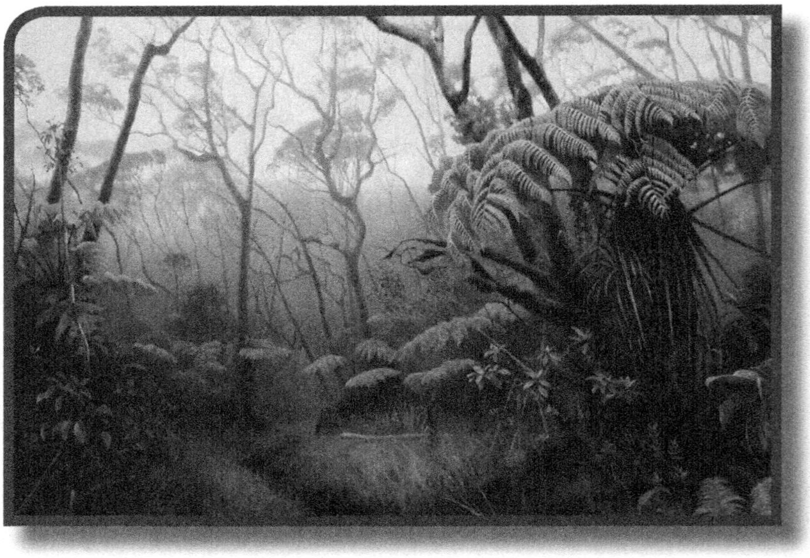

Artwork by Kit Gentry kitgentry.com

Your gods, your ghosts,
your demons & dreams bear witness
as you pull rich gifts from your darkness

May they return...
to hunt you,
to haunt you,
to heal you.

This darkness is my gift to you,
an anchor through time in the bones of your ancestors.
This darkness is my gift to you,
a rich compost to take root in.
This darkness is my gift to you,
a place in the earth... an anchor through time.

The forests in old Hawai'i were known as "Wao Akua" or "Lands of the Gods." The Wao Akua was a place untouched by the hand of man, a place where God could be experienced directly.

The best way to enter and move through the Wao Akua is to draw one's focus or awareness into the "na'au" (the area of the lower abdomen). This area is significant in many traditional medicine practices. It is known as the "dan tien" in traditional Chinese medicine and the "hara" in traditional Japanese medicine.

Na'au means literally "guts," however it also implies "knowledge" or "intuitive mind." From a Hawaiian perspective, viewing the world through our head or thinking mind can mislead us, but our na'au (intuition or gut feeling) will rarely lead us astray.

The word "ao" means "light" or "daylight," as well as "earth" and "world". Thus, when na'au is combined with ao it becomes "na'auao": The Hawaiian word for "spiritual wisdom" or "enlightenment". This is literally: "Illuminated Mind".

Walking in the forest while experiencing the world from the na'au adds remarkable depth to the gathering of medicine. The world is experienced through our skin and organs, not watched like television with our talking heads. The knees are bent, the center of gravity is low, the awareness is brought to the abdomen, and the attention is "focused" on the peripheral vision ("haka hele"). While gathering we feel for signs ("hō'ailona" or "naka") that give us direction in what we are doing. This practice can take years to master but it is well worth the effort. When we gather herbs we must be willing to *listen* to the forest, not just with our ears, but also with our bodies and our intuition. Rather than telling the forest what *it* is, we let the forest tell *us* what it is. We empty our minds and *pay attention.* Our thinking mind takes a back seat as we learn to pray with our bodies. These plants become our teachers.

This "body knowing" is used not only in the Wao Akua, but also while working with patients. When we pay attention with our bodies, our patients become our teachers.

The intellect, like science or technology, is a good servant but a poor master. It is not an end in itself. Like a cup that holds tea, the intellect is a vessel that can "hold" the intuition or spiritual connection. The cup without the tea is dry and unsatisfying. Tea without the cup is unfocused and is not held in a useful manner. When we "study" plants, the intellect is the "driver" and in control. While gathering medicine the intellect should move out of the way and allow the body to direct the process, interrupting only when necessary. This shift in perception is a critical part of gathering plant medicines.

HAWAIIAN PLANT GATHERING PROTOCOLS: BRINGING THE MEDICINE HOME

If we are to create a world suitable for human habitation, we must bring the sacred back into our medicine and into our lives. Without a genuine connection to the earth, we lose our medicine *and* the roots of our humanity.

While I am imparting one outline of a Hawaiian gathering protocol, it is only a brief description of a subject that can be quite complex. If you are interested in collecting medicines, you should receive further instruction from a teacher or Hulu Kupuna (Treasured Elder).

Experiencing herbs as live beings conveys *information* to us that is missing from our experiences with store-bought bottles of pills. Through our intent, we can become more deeply connected to the source and origins of the medicines we use. This can also help us understand their "energetics," which is the way they interact with their environment and with us. When we herbalists use local plants rather than using store-bought herbs, we are developing a different *relationship* to plants... *and* to the Earth. This relationship is at the heart of most traditional medicines and is missing from most modern medical practices, both Asian and Western.

I regard local plants as old friends. I am familiar with the neighborhoods where they live. I know if it has been rainy or dry in that area and the condition of the soil. I know who their neighbors are, and I know if they've been troubled lately. I can tell by looking at them if they are happy or not. We always understand our friends better if we know where they live and visit them there.

Please note that while I often refer to "Wao Akua" (the forest), it is not necessary to only gather plants in a forest. Medicines can be gathered from any place that is not contaminated by pollution or bad feelings.

In traditional Hawaiian culture there were likely as many gathering rituals as there were families. I have included one that was taught to me that I sometimes use while collecting medicine for a patient. There are many others. The order and sequence of any protocol will vary depending on the family and tradition. My focus while teaching is not so much that students use a "*correct*" protocol. For example, in Hawaiian medicine we will often use the left hand to gather for a female patient and the right hand to gather for a male. But other traditions may use a different protocol, and that is fine. I am more concerned that the student's approach is at least earth-centered. I believe that any protocol that is earth-sensitive will create a profound shift in our usual "feed the trash and take out the cat" mentality.

While gathering medicine we are taking lives, the lives of these plants. In order for us to live, many things must die each day. Some day we too will die and become food. It is important to remember this and honor the gifts we are given. It is also important to ask permission before we gather, sometimes days or weeks before we begin. Plants have an intelligence that we must strive to appreciate. This is where our work begins.

A specific gathering lei (garland) is sometimes worn and I often create a medicine bundle to house the herbs that have been gathered for the patient. Upon leaving the forest (Wao Akua), the gathering lei or a woven article is sometimes left as an offering (ho'okupu). The patient is then given the bundle. They can prepare the gathered ingredients as their medicine and the bundle itself can be replanted in their yard, where it will continue to grow. This can create a sense of healing continuity through time.

The plants, during gathering and preparation, may be consecrated with the Hā (breath) of the practitioner. As it was taught to me, I do this with breath from the nose.

Bright clothing, particularly bright yellow, is discouraged in Wao Akua, as it is considered loud or disrespectful behavior. Traditionally medicine is gathered fresh, for one person at a time, before sunrise, and while going toward the ocean ("makai"). At the very least, it is best to gather before the sun is high. When gathering for a male patient, the right hand is used to gather materials from the East side of a plant, and for a female patient the left hand is used to gather from the West side of a plant. Sometimes a "male" God such as Kāne, Kū, or Wākea is invoked for men, and a "female" deity such as Hina, Pele, Papa, or Laka is invoked for women. I almost always invoke Lono and Hi'iaka, regardless of the gender of the patient. Some Hawaiian practitioners gather with a specific knee bent for a male or female patient. Certain plants (such as *Solanum americanum* or *Cordyline terminalis*) have their own specific gathering and preparation "rules." Remember that these are only a few of many possibilities and that they will vary according to the plants being gathered, situation, family traditions, etc.

Sometimes a sacred space ("kapu" space) will be created before starting a journey through the forest. A kapu space is a place inside of us that is unaffected by the outside world. This can be done alone or collectively within a group. It is very powerful and can radically change both the experience and outcome of medicine gathering.

Omens (hō'ailona) both "positive" and "negative" are *always* acknowledged. If a gathering companion falls and stumbles repeatedly, or if there are "unexpected obstacles" to the process of gathering medicines, those involved should stop and pray or meditate together. If the disruptions continue, the gathering should be re-evaluated and done another time.

One gathering protocol I use is as follows:

1. *Gratitude, Meditation, and Prayer - Turning to Spirit, tuning into Spirit*
Gratitude is the only emotion that will never fail us, no matter what our circumstances. For those who are atheists or agnostics, please remember that one can turn to Spirit without "praying" to a bearded white-guy-in-the-sky with a radio voice. This gratitude or meditation can be expressed to the Earth, to the Universal mind, or to the "Great Spirit" as it is called in the Native American tradition. What is important is not who or what we pray to, but that we pray at all. It's not the prayer, but whom we become through praying that makes the difference. All things in Hawaiian culture begin and end in prayer. If we don't know what to do, we pray. And if we don't know why we're praying... we pray to find out.

2. *Offering a gift: A mele oli (a chant), a lei, etc.*
Just as one would never visit a respected elder ("Kupuna") empty handed, the same applies while visiting Wao Akua (Hawaiian forest). A gift of a chant, food, or lei is an appropriate expression of appreciation. (Whatever is left as the gift however, should be made of natural materials and should blend in reasonably well. Don't bring your childhood decoder ring or your favorite Nine Inch Nails CD as an offering)

3. *Permission: May I gather?*
A basic courtesy.

4. *Introduction: Who am I?*
Your name, or a nickname to protect you from "kolohe" or mischievous sprits is given.

5. *Where am I from?*
This is a description of your ethnic background, your family history. This is a Polynesian custom, based on the importance of family ('ohana) in interpersonal relations. Polynesian peoples "know" each other through family connections.

6. *Who am I gathering for?*
The patient you are gathering for is named.

7. *Why am I gathering, to what end?*
This is a statement of your intent to create the desired outcome for that specific patient. "I am gathering so that Auntie Alice can breath freely and share her Aloha with the world."

8. *Why am I really here?*
The answer to this question might go something like this: "I am here because I didn't feel like doing my income taxes this morning and needed an excuse to get out of the house." Or, "I am here because I want my patient to think I'm a good practitioner." Or perhaps, "I am here because I *really* do love Auntie Alice and I want her to live a long life."

This is a question that is answered in the depth of our self-honesty and is typically shared only with God. The answer to this question is an acknowledgement of the shadow of our psyche and our humanness. While saying this can be embarrassing (even when said silently) it is an important form of self-honesty. We do this as a gift to ourselves... to bring our unconscious forces into the light of the conscious mind. And, lest we get too impressed with ourselves as practitioners, it gives us humility.

9. *Giving thanks. Again, Gratitude.*

A typical protocol may be done out loud or silently and might go something like this:

• *Meditation, Prayer, Music, or Chant.*

• *Recognition of Ke Kuahiwi* (the mountain), *Ka 'Āina* (the land), *and Ke Kai* (the ocean) *as the source of who we are and from which we receive blessings.*

• *A gift is then given to the forest.*

• *May I gather plants from this forest?* (Wait for a sign / hō'ailona) *I am David Bruce Leonard, a student of Hawaiian medicine under Kahu Kawika Ka'alakea. I am descended from the Northern European families of Leonard, Lincoln, Rich, Heyndrickx, and DeNutte. I am here gathering for my patient* XXXX *so that she can heal the sores on her legs and stabilize her blood sugar.* (The patient is visualized throughout this process as having healthy legs, mobility, and vitality). *I am here also because I needed to get out of the house.*

• *Thank you. I vow to honor, sustain, and nourish this Wao Akua as my kuleana* (privilege / responsibility).

This is a simple and adaptable protocol that can be used in numerous kinds of situations. Done often enough, these steps will soon become unconscious habits. There are other detailed protocols involving very specific plant combinations and *kinolau* (divine physical manifestations), however they are beyond the scope of this book. The subject of traditional gathering protocols can be very complex. Again if you are interested in collecting herbs, you should receive further instruction from a teacher of traditional medicine.

And remember, (as my Hawaiian teachers never tire of telling me), there is no medicine in the plants per se; the plants are simply a vehicle. Our medicine is our relationship to God.

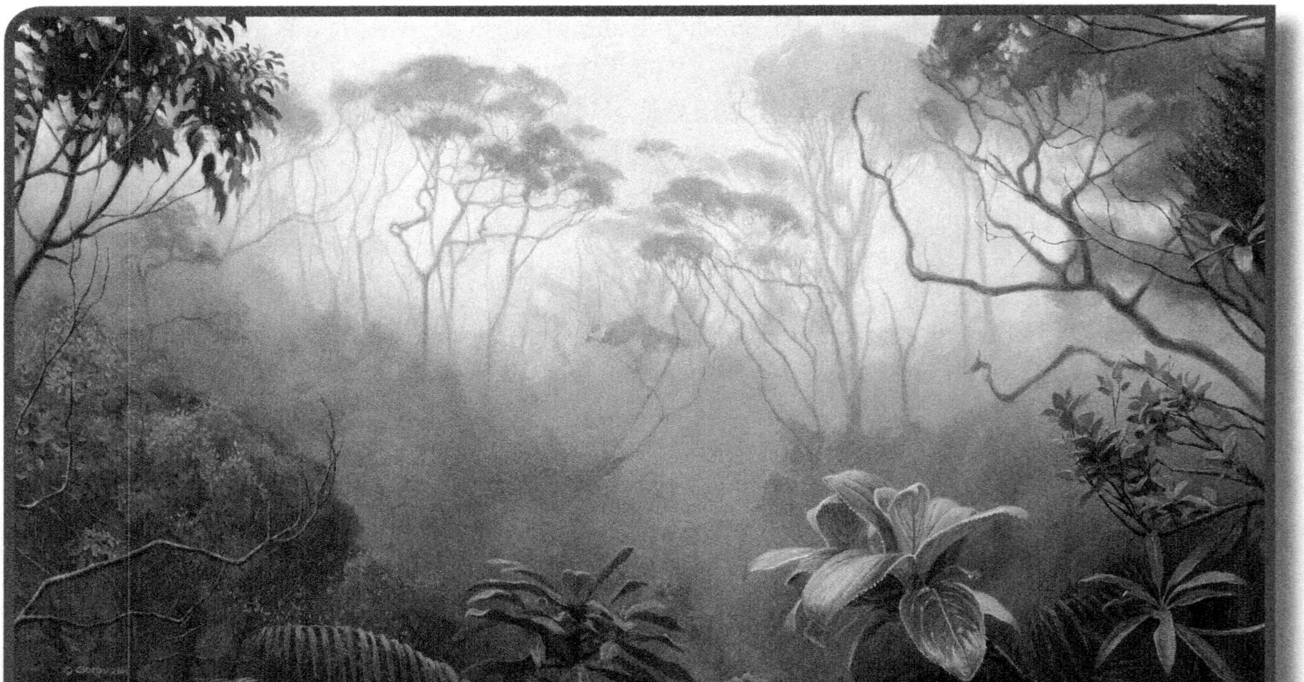

Artwork by Kit Gentry kitgentry.com

HOW PLANTS ARE ORGANIZED

All life forms are organized into categories. The most commonly used category for life is called a *species.* A number of species together forms a *genus.* A number of *genera* (the plural of genus) constitute a *family.* Families are combined to create an *order*, and so on. From a larger perspective it looks something like this:

Division
　Class
　　Subclass
　　　Order
　　　　Family
　　　　　Genus
　　　　　　Species (specific epithet)

The most common designator of an individual plant is the species name, which consists of the genus and the specific epithet. Thus the plant name for the common dandelion is *Taraxacum officinale. Taraxacum* is the genus and *officinale* is the specific epithet. Together, they make up the species name: *Taraxacum officinale.* However, there is another dandelion that grows in China and is sufficiently different from *Taraxacum officinale* to be classified as a separate species. That plant is called *Taraxacum mongolicum.* Thus, *Taraxacum officinale* and *Taraxacum mongolicum* are two species within the genus *Taraxacum.* The genus *Taraxacum* is one of the many genera that make up the family Asteraceae. Family names generally end in "aceae." The system looks something like this:

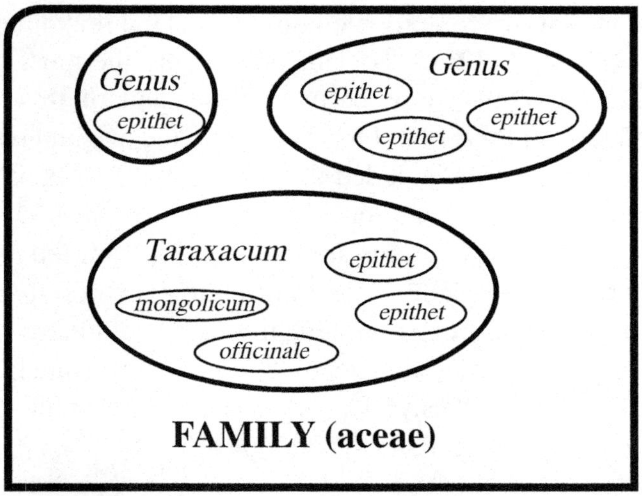

Each plant and flower has a specific "look" to it. That "look" more than likely indicates that a plant is in a certain family. Each family may have common chemical constituents that involve predictable pharmacological actions on the human body. The medicinal effects of plant families are a very important field of study for herbalists, but it is also a subject of too large a scope for this book.

HOW THE INFORMATION IN THIS BOOK IS ORGANIZED

PLANT NAME: The botanical name of the plant is given here, italicized, with the genus capitalized, and the specific epithet in lower case. In some cases the genus is given, and then "spp." is placed after it, which is an abbreviation for "species." This means that numerous species in the same genus are covered under that heading. The funny alphabet soup stuff after the italicized names are references to the beloved herb-nerd botanists who named the plant.

OTHER NAMES: These are botanical "synonyms," a different botanical name under which a plant is sometimes listed. I know... plants are *supposed* to have only *one* botannical name. It turns out that botany can be confusing even to botanists. But, because this confusion helps keep them employed, we are grateful.

SIMILARLY USED SPECIES: These are other herbs with similar uses, often listed under the same common name in TCM (traditional Chinese medicine).

COMMON NAMES: These are the common names used in various cultures and languages.

PHARMACEUTICAL NAME: A name sometimes used by professional herbalists.

NOMENCLATURE: This is information about the origins of the plant names.

FAMILY: This is the family the plant belongs to, ending in "aceae."

CATEGORY: The placement of herbs into Chinese "categories" is a somewhat subjective and historical venture, with many sources offering different points of view. I've often gone with my personal use and experience of a plant, but be aware that some sources may place these plants in different categories.

PROPERTIES: Properties include taste and energetic "temperature" from a TCM perspective. When there are conflicting Chinese opinions regarding energetic "temperature," I've gone with the one that makes the most sense in my experience. Conclusions that are mine alone are marked with a tilde (~).

PLANT PART USED: This is the part of the plant most often used as medicine. Part used may vary widely from culture to culture. The term "aerial parts" refers to any part of the plant not under ground. "Rhizome" refers to an underground stem, often confused with a root.

TOXICITY: This includes any known toxicity including the LD50 if available.

CAUTIONS AND CONTRAINDICATIONS: This is arguably the most important information about any plant, when not to use it. After you have properly identified a plant, this section along with "toxicity" should be the first places you look in this book. I have included the original research references here when possible. If these were not available, I've included the secondary sources in the bibliography, preferring to keep the caveat and to err on the side of caution.

ENERGETIC CAUTIONS: Energetic cautions are included for traditional Chinese medicine practitioners. These may not be included for all plants if the information is currently unavailable. Common sense should still hold true here, however. For example, practitioners should still take care with a cool or cold plant when a patient presents with spleen qi deficiency or cold liver channel.

PREPARATION OF MEDICINE & DOSAGE: These sections cover the various methods of preparing medicine, including decoction, infusion, tinctures, and topical uses.

Given the cross-cultural nature of this work, each herb may have a very different method of preparation than the one preceding it. However, should any confusion arise with a patient, I always default to traditional Chinese diagnosis and methodology, which is then tempered by experience. I use formulas of 5-15 herbs at a time, closer to 4-6 when using local plants, each herb weighing 8-20 grams. Dosages and preparation must always be modified to account for the individual patient, their condition, and their willingness to put disgusting things into their mouth.

Herbs are often prepared fresh, usually decocted (boiled for one half hour or more), but sometimes infused (steeped). Specific herbs may be added as tinctures, poultices, or prepared as food.

Most of my Hawaiian teachers used one to three herbs at a time for a patient or family member. They would typically use herbs by the "handful" and make preparations to color or taste. So a rule of thumb when making smaller formulas this way is 1-2 ounces (~ 28 - 52g) per herb.

For ease of use I have sometimes included dosages from Western herbal and Eclectic traditions for specific herbs.

STATUS IN HAWAI'I: This indicates whether the plant is native or alien. Native plants should be gathered with particular caution, if at all. The aliens can be carted away at your leisure, though be careful not to spread the seeds. I also have included a reference for each alien rating its potential "pest factor," typically low, moderate or high. This is a subjective assessment on my part and not quantified.

MERIDIAN AFFINITIES: This reference is for acupuncture-based TCM (traditional Chinese medicine) practitioners.

WESTERN FUNCTIONS REPORTED: These are the western actions reported from various sources, and I cannot vouch for their accuracy. This information may be useful for those approaching herbal medicine from a Western or Eclectic tradition.

TRADITIONAL CHINESE ENERGETIC FUNCTIONS (~ = extrapolated): These are TCM actions attributed to the plant. Hawai'i is filled with plants that, while not appearing in common Ben Caos (herb books), have been well delineated in obscure Chinese texts. I have included this information from China on Hawaiian plants, and, with help from Robert Newman, much of it is from the original Chinese sources. I've also included some of my own conclusions about the energetic functions of certain plants. These are marked with a tilde (~).

OTHER ENERGETIC FUNCTIONS: This lists energetic actions from other traditional medical systems such as Ayurveda.

COMMON MEDICINAL USES: These are the most common uses of the plant from my experience. Often, when looking at this book, people exclaim "But it looks like everything does everything!" Indeed, it does appear so at first; but everything does not do everything equally well. If you look deeper, interesting patterns of use will emerge. To make it easy, however, I've included this section as a "cheat-sheet."... a quick and dirty summary of how a plant is "really" used... or at least how I use it or see it used.

CROSS-CULTURAL MEDICINAL USES These are worldwide uses of this plant. What I've done is taken a cross-cultural "snapshot" of a specific medicine. Please remember, that just because a plant is used for a specific condition does *not* mean that it is *effective* for that condition!

The following physiological categories are somewhat arbitrary, as many ailments could be placed under more than one heading. Wherever possible I've used common language rather than "medicalese." Cross-cultural categories include:

BITES & STINGS - From insects, reptiles, attorneys, in-laws, etc.
COSMETIC - Uses that enhance appearance.
CARDIOVASCULAR - Including heart disease, high blood pressure, bleeding and vascular issues.
DERMATOLOGICAL - Uses ranging from herpes, eczema and psoriasis to boils and infected sores.
DIGESTIVE - Anything related to the GI tract, from nausea to hemorrhoids.
ENDOCRINE - Including diabetes.
HEAD AND THROAT - Uses relating to the eyes, ears, nose, and neck.
HEPATIC - Uses for liver and gall bladder health.
IMMUNITY - Uses affecting immune function.
INFECTION - Usually bacterial, but sometimes viral.
LYMPHATIC - Swollen glands, etc.
MUSCULOSKELETAL / TRAUMA - Including back pain, broken bones, sprains, and cuts.
NEUROLOGICAL - For nervous system disorders.
ONCOLOGY - Uses for various types of cancer.
PARASITES - Including malarial parasites.
PEDIATRIC - Use in the treatment of children.
PSYCHOSPIRITUAL - Covering emotional, spiritual, and ritualistic uses for the plant.
REPRODUCTIVE - Including menstrual disorders.

RESPIRATORY - Usually asthma, but also common cold, influenza, and bronchitis.
URINARY - Often bladder infections, but including kidney disorders.
VETERINARY - Uses in the treatment of animals.
OTHER MEDICINAL USES - Any medical uses not covered above.

USE AS FOOD: Food uses are listed here as well as some preparation information.
OTHER USES: Other uses for the plant such as fiber, building, dyes, etc.
ESSENTIAL OIL: Any information about the essential oil of the plant is listed here.
CONSTITUENTS: These are the known chemical constituents, usually in alphabetical order. This list of constituents is very likely not complete.
POSSIBLE DRUG INTERACTIONS: Patients taking pharmaceutical drugs should avoid taking any herbal substances (including common herb teas like chamomile and peppermint) unless properly supervised. This is particularly true (but not limited to) Coumadin (Warfarin) or any other anticoagulant including aspirin. Very little information is available in the literature on herb-drug interactions.
LOCAL COMBINATIONS: Combinations of plants that grow in Hawai'i for specific presentations, but not necessarily the best choices.
CROSS-CULTURAL COMBINATIONS: These are combinations of herbs from different traditions. ***I do not have experience with some of these combinations and cannot attest to their efficacy.***
RANGE: This refers to other places in the world where this plant is found. All, of course, grow in Hawai‘i, but you may be surprised at how globally widespread our local plants are. The locale where it evolved (from its native habitat) is also mentioned here.
HABITAT: This is the area, climate, and altitude in which a plant grows, its “neighborhood.”
GATHERING: Tips, pointers, and warnings on gathering, including some information on kinolau (Hawaiian deity correspondences).
PROPAGATION & CULTIVATION: Where applicable. Many of these little beasts (bad-boy aliens!) should not be propagated. Be sure you check the “Status in Hawai'i” section before planting anything. Or, locate H.E.A.R. (Hawaiian Eco-systems At Risk) on the World Wide Web at www.hear.org. The Nature Conservancy also has very good Hawaiian alien plant information on their website: http://www.nature.org/wherewework/northamerica/states/hawaii/
RESEARCH: This is scientific research related to each plant or to constituents in each plant. Left-brain research sources are cited for scientific types.
NOTES 'N QUOTES: A grab bag of fun stuff to amuse and confuse.

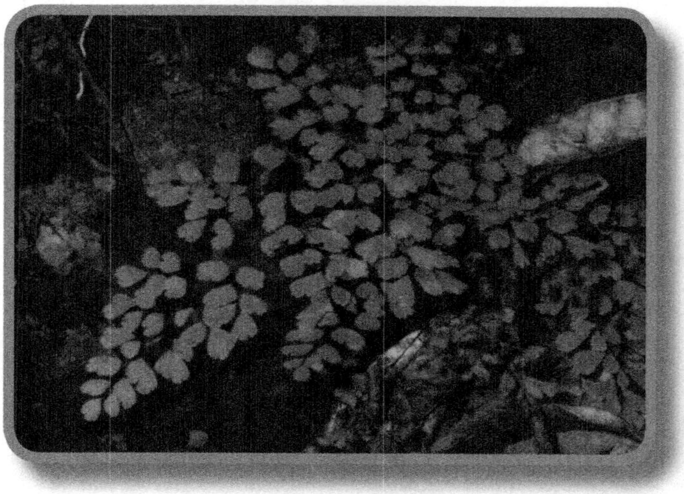

Adiantum spp. ('Iwa'iwa)

PLANT NAME: *Adiantum* spp.

SIMILARLY USED SPECIES: *A. aethiopicum; A. aleuticum; A. capillus-veneris; A. caudatum; A. concinnum; A. flabellatum; A. fragile; A. lunulatum; A. michelii; A. modestum; A. monochlamys; A. nigrum; A. pedatum; A. philippense; A. raddianum; A. radiatum; A. schaffneri; A. tenerum; A. trapeciforme; A. trapeziforme; A. venustum.*

Status: Some are native

Habitat: Wet Shady

COMMON NAMES: **'Iwa'iwa** [Hawai'i]; **maidenhair fern**, lady fern [USA]; culantrillo [Amazonia]; culantrillo de piedra [Panama]; avenca [Brazil].

NOMENCLATURE: The genus name is from the Greek "adiantos" (ou = not, and diano = wet), "not wet." This is a reference to the frond's ability to repel water.

FAMILY: Pteridaceae.

CATEGORY: Cool herbs that transform hot phlegm ~.

PROPERTIES: Cool to cold ~.

PLANT PART USED: Fronds, leaves and rhizomes.

TOXICITY: Although there are no reports of toxicity of *Adiantum* ferns, many ferns have a substance called thiaminase that can rob the body of B vitamins, so caution is advised. Thiaminase is destroyed by cooking or drying the plant.

CAUTIONS AND CONTRAINDICATIONS: Not in pregnancy. Use with caution and monitor blood sugar levels in diabetes. See *Possible Drug Interactions* below.

STATUS IN HAWAI'I: *Adiantum capillus-veneris* is indigenous.

MERIDIAN AFFINITIES: Lung, liver, kidney.

While going "holoholo" (wandering) up riverbeds one will often come across overhanging walls of delicate ferns glistening with moisture. If you are fortunate enough to come across a maidenhair leaf that looks a bit larger than the others and has deeper clefts in the leaves gently turn it over and look at the spore packets (sori) on the underside of the leaf. If they are rectangular rather than kidney shaped, ("boomers" may have to put on their reading glasses to do this), then you are viewing a living relic of Hawai'i's ancient past: This is a native Hawaiian maidenhair.

WESTERN FUNCTIONS REPORTED: **Analgesic** (*A. jordanii, A. pedatum*) [Costanoan, Iroquois]; **antiasthmatic**; **antibacterial**; **anticonvulsive** (*A. pedatum*) [Micmac]; **antidandruff**; **antidiarrheal** (*A. pedatum*) [Menominee]; **antidote**; **antifungal**; **antihemorrhagic** (*A. pedatum*) [Makah]; **antihyperglycemic**; **antimicrobial**; **antirheumatic** (internal and external) (*A. capillus-veneris, A. pedatum*) [Cherokee, Iroquois, Mahuna]; **antitussive** (*A. aethiopicum, A. capillus-veneris, A. pedatum*) [Egypt, Iraq]; **antiviral**; **astringent** (*A. capillus-veneris*) [Iraq, USA]; **demulcent** (*A. capillus-veneris, A. caudatum, A. pedatum, A. venustum*) [India, USA]; **depurative** (*A. capillus-veneris*) [Mexico]; **diaphoretic** (*A. capillus-veneris*) [Egypt]; **diuretic** (*A. capillus-veneris, A. pedatum,* A. philippense) [Egypt, Iraq, Iroquois, USA]; **emetic** (*A. pedatum*) [Cherokee, Iroquois]; **emmenagogue** (*A. capillus-veneris, A.* concinnum, *A.* philippense, *A.* tenerum) [Iraq, Mexico, USA, Venezuela]; **emollient** (*A. capillus-veneris, A. pedatum*) [Iraq, USA]; **expectorant** (*A. capillus-veneris, A. caudatum, A. pedatum, A. venustum*) [India, Iraq, USA]; **febrifuge** (*A. pedatum*) [Cherokee]; **galactogogue**; **laxative** (*A. capillus-veneris*) [Mexico]; **pectoral**; **promotes menstruation**

[China]; **refrigerant** (*A. monochlamys*) [China]; **stimulant** (*A. capillus-veneris, A. pedatum*) [Iraq, USA]; **sudorific** (*A. capillus-veneris*) [Iraq, USA]; **tonic** (*A. caudatum, A. capillus-veneris, A. pedatum, A. venustum*) [India, Iraq, USA]; **vermifuge**.

TRADITIONAL CHINESE ENERGETIC FUNCTIONS (~ = extrapolated):

1) Clears heat and transforms phlegm~.
2) Opens the chest~.
3) Resolves damp heat ~.

PREPARATION OF MEDICINE: Decocted, infused or used in syrup.

DOSAGE: 3 - 10 grams steeped.

'Iwa'iwa (Maidenhair) Cross-Cultural Medicinal Uses

COSMETIC

- **Hair wash** [Europe, Lummi, Makah, Navaho, Skokomish]; **balding** [Europe, Mexico, Peru]; **dandruff** [Europe].

CARDIOVASCULAR

- **Heart medicine** [Cherokee].

DERMATOLOGICAL

- **Skin problems** [China]; **eczema** [India].

DIGESTIVE

- **Digestive problems** [Costanoan, Makah]; **indigestion, "sour stomach"** [Amazonia]; **heartburn** [Amazonia].
- **Diarrhea** [Europe, India, Malaya, Menominee]; **dysentery**.
- **Used to induce vomiting** [Cherokee, Iroquois].

'Iwa'iwa (Maidenhair) Common Medicinal Uses

- Bronchitis
- Hepatitis and jaundice
- Sore throat
- Balding

ENDOCRINE

- **Diabetes** [Europe, India].

HEAD AND THROAT

- **Head and throat inflammation** [Egypt, Iraq, Spain, USA]; **sore throat** [Native American]; **hoarseness** [USA].

HEPATIC

- **Jaundice** [Eclectics, Europe, Peru]; **hepatitis** [Egypt (*A. capillus-veneris*)]; **liver problems** [Iroquois, Mexico], **alcoholism**.
- **Gallstones** [Peru].

INFECTION

- **Boils and sores** [Hawai'i, India, USA]; **fever** [Cherokee, China, India, Native American].

MUSCULOSKELETAL / TRAUMA

- **Pain** [Costanoan, Iroquois]; **joint pain** (internal and external) [Amazonia, Cherokee, Iroquois, Mahuna]; **muscle pain** [India]; **swelling** [Indonesia].
- **Bleeding from trauma** [Makah (leaves chewed and applied topically)]; **wounds** [India].
- Topical for **insect bites and stings** [Navaho]; **snake and spider bite** [Egypt, Iroquois].
- **Dogbite** [India].

NEUROLOGICAL

- **Convulsions** [Micmac].

PARASITES

- **Worms**.

PEDIATRIC

- **Colic** [Malaya].

PSYCHOSPIRITUAL

- **Smoked or infused for insanity** [Navaho].

REPRODUCTIVE

- **General menstrual problems** [Costanoan, Iroquois, Menominee, Potawatomi, Universal, USA]; **abnormal uterine bleeding** [Kickapoo-Mexico]; **excess menstrual flow** [Europe]; **menstrual discomfort**, **late menses** [Europe, India, Mexico, Spain, USA].
- **Genital warts** [Mexico].
- **"Morning-after" tea** [Kickapoo - Mexico].
- **Childbirth** [Spain].

RESPIRATORY

"It helps cure asthma, coughs, and shortness of breath. It is good against jaundice, diarrhea, spitting of blood and the biting of mad dogs. It also provokes urination and menstruation and breaks up stone in the bladder, spleen, and kidneys."

-- 'K'Eogh, 18th century herbalist.

- **General respiratory problems** [Brazil, Cherokee, USA]; **bronchitis**, **pertussis**, **cough with sticky phlegm**, **excess mucous**, **coughing blood** [Amazonia, Brazil, Egypt, Europe, India, Iraq, Lesotho. Mexico, Native American, Turkey, USA, Venezuela]; **pleurisy** [Eclectics].
- **Asthma** [Brazil, Egypt, Native American];
- **Chronic nasal congestion** [Native American];
- **Common cold** [Amazonia, China, Egypt, Haiti, Iraq, India, Lesotho, USA]; **chills** [Native American]; **influenza**, **sore throat** [Native American].

URINARY

- **Bladder problems** [Amazonia, Mexico]; **edema** [Egypt].

OTHER MEDICINAL USES

- **Degenerative wasting from chronic disease** [India].
- **Tumors** [India].
- **Rabies** [India].
- **Stings**.

USE AS FOOD: Used as a garnish on sweet dishes (fronds). Also made into a thick syrup using sugar and orange water.

OTHER USES: Maidenhair stems are used in basket designs in Karok.

CONSTITUENTS: Adiantone, adiantoxide, astragalin, beta-sitosterol, caffeic acids, caffeylgalactose, caffeylglucose, campesterol, carotenes, carotenoids, coumaric acids, coumarylglucoses, diplopterol, epoxyfilicane, fernadiene, fernene, filicanes, flavonoids, hopanone, hydroxy-adiantone, hydroxy-cinnamic acid, isoadiantone, isoquercetin, kaempferols, lutein, mutatoxanthin, naringin, neoxanthin, nicotiflorin, oleananes, phenylpropanoids, populnin, procyanidin, prodelphinidin, quercetins, querciturone, quinic acid, rhodoxanthin, rutin, shikimic acid, triterpenes, violaxanthin, zeaxanthin.

POSSIBLE DRUG INTERACTIONS: One source listed *Adiantum* as potentiating insulin or diabetes medications but I could not verify this in published studies.

'Iwa'iwa (Maidenhair) Local Combinations

Bronchitis, asthma: Add *Sonchus oleraceus* (pualele).
Hepatitis: Add *Zingiber officinale* ('awapuhi pākē / ginger).
Common cold: Add *Pandanus tectorius* (hala).
Irregular menses, cramps: Add *Cyperus rotundus* (xiang fu).

HABITAT: Likes it wet, cool, an' shady.

GATHERING: Hawai'i year round. Gathered in June in Europe.

RESEARCH: An extraction of *A. ceneatum* is anti-inflammatory in mice and a stronger analgesic than aspirin or acetaminophen [Bresciani 2003].

NOTES 'N QUOTES

"It consumeth and wasteth away the King's Evil and other hard swellings, and it maketh the haire of the head or beard to grow that is fallen and pulled off."

-- Gerard

"This and all other Maiden Hairs is a good remedy for coughs, asthmas, pleurisy, etc., and on account of its being a gentle diuretic also in jaundice, gravel and other impurities of the kidneys. All the Maidenhairs should be used green and in conjunction with other ingredients because their virtues are weak."

-- Nicholas Culpepper

- Maidenhair has been used since the time of Dioscorides and Pliny (Caius Plinius Secundus, A.*D.* 23-79)
- In France, Maidenhair fern was once made into "syrup de capillaire" and used for lung problems.

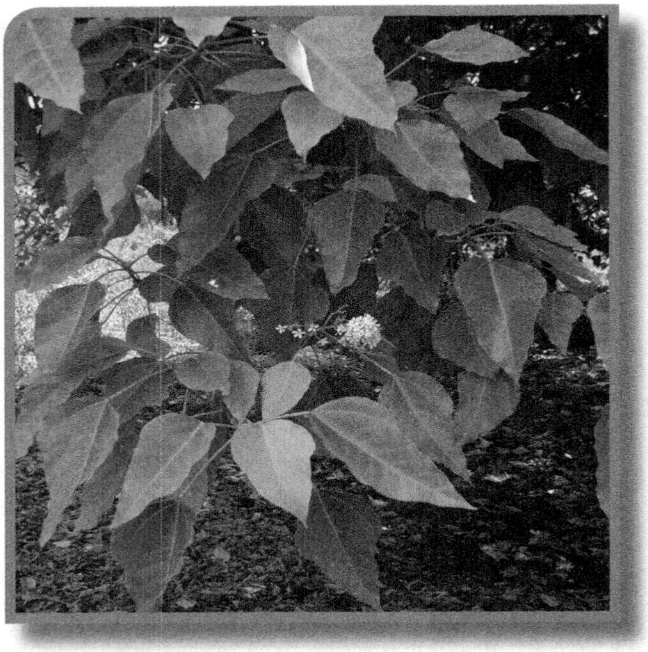

Aleurites moluccana (Kukui)

PLANT NAME: *Aleurites moluccana* (L.) Willd.

Status: Polynesian Introduction

Habitat: Moist Valleys

OTHER NAMES: *Aleurites triloba, Croton moluccanu*

COMMON NAMES: **Kukui** ("Light") [Hawai'i]; **candlenut** [USA]; tuitui [Cook Islands; Tonga]; lama [Samoa]; ti'a'iri [Tahiti]; 'ama [Marquesas]; tutu'i [Austral Islands]; shi li [China]; lauci [Fiji]; kurup [Papua New Guinea].

PHARMACEUTICAL NAME: Nope.

NOMENCLATURE: *Aleurites* comes from the Greek "aleuron" which means "covered with flour." This is a reference to the fine hairs of kukui that make it look as if it were dusted with flour. The word kukui means, "light" in Hawaiian. It is also a word for "lightbulb."

FAMILY: Euphorbiaceae (spurge family).

CATEGORY: Downward draining herbs - purgatives ~.

PROPERTIES: Astringent, bitter, cold.

PLANT PART USED: Whole plant.

TOXICITY: **TOXIC**. Kukui is used as a "poison" in Haiti and Turkey. If too much kukui was taken in old Hawai'i, and diarrhea resulted, specially prepared *Tacca leontopetaloides* (pia) root was given with poi.

CAUTIONS AND CONTRAINDICATIONS: Not in pregnancy. Not with diarrhea. (Please note: Kukui was once used for digestive infections such as dysentery to remove pathogens. This is NOT recommended.)

ENERGETIC CAUTIONS: Not with weak central Qi. ~

PREPARATION OF MEDICINE: For oil, use nuts that sink in water. Crack them with a hammer, take the meat out and place it in a baking pan. Heat oven to 450°. Bake for 15 minutes. Let cool, mash, and place in a glass jar. Place the glass jar in the sun. Add nuts and pour off oil as desired. Please note that kukui oil can go rancid. To preserve it, add 5 drops of grapefruit seed extract plus 2 drops of vitamin E per ounce of oil. You may have to experiment with different types of vitamin E oil until you find one that blends easily.
To obtain sap, young fruits are pulled from the tree and the sap is taken from where the stem meets the fruit. A dap on the tip of your tongue will show how it might be used for teething in babies... or even thrush. This sap from the green fruit is called waikea, and the juice of the green nut is called kohu kukui.

DOSAGE: For constipation, 1 roasted nut. Topical as needed.

STATUS IN HAWAI'I: Polynesian Introduction. Low to moderate pest factor. It is presumed that because kukui seeds were too heavy to be carried by birds that kukui is a Polynesian introduced plant, and not a native. Considering that kukui can create monostands, this might be the case. But it can also beg the question about the ancestors of our endemic heavy-seeded *Pritchardias*.

MERIDIAN AFFINITIES: Stomach, large intestine ~.

WESTERN FUNCTIONS REPORTED: **Anti-infective**; **anti-mycotic**; **aperient**; **aphrodisiac**; **emollient**; **laxative**; **purgative**; **stimulant**; **sudorific**.

TRADITIONAL CHINESE ENERGETIC FUNCTIONS (~ = extrapolated):

1) Drains downward and moves the bowels~.
2) Clears damp heat~.
3) Clears stomach heat and stomach fire~.
4) Mends the tissue, stops pain~.

Kukui (Candlenut)
Common Medicinal Uses

- Oil for massage
- Roasted nuts as a colon cleanser
- Sap for thrush

Kukui (Candlenut) Cross-Cultural Medicinal Uses

COSMETIC

- Oil is used topically **to stimulate hair growth** in Fiji.

DERMATOLOGICAL

- Oil topical for **burns**, **stretch marks**, **and "lump in stomach"**[Hawaii].
- Sap for **skin fungus** [Hawai'i].
- **Coral cuts** [Tahiti (bark infused)].
- **Septic wounds** [Samoa (bark, root); Tahiti (bark infused)]. A salve is made from the nuts for **external ulcers and sores** [Hawai'i, Malaya].

DIGESTIVE

- **Constipation or cleansing** [Costa Rica; Hawai'i (flowers/roasted nuts); Papua New Guinea (leaves)]. Raw Kukui nuts are more cathartic than cooked ones.
- **Diarrhea**, **dysentery** [Fiji, Java].
- **Sprue** (a tropical digestive disease) [Malaya]; **stomach ache** [Celebes]; **"lump in stomach"**[Hawaii (oil topical)]; **voracious appetite** [Hawai'i]; **stomach and abdominal problems** ("kahi") [Tonga (bark infused in combination)]; **bowel cramps** [Sumatra (charred nuts applied topically on navel)].
- **Food poisoning** [Papua New Guinea (leaves)].

HEAD AND THROAT

- Sap, flowers, and bark infusion for **thrush**, **sore throats**, **tonsillitis**, **toothache**, **canker sores**, **or bad breath** [Hawai'i].
- **Headache** [Cook Islands (oil topical); Malaya (boiled leaves topical)].
- **Conjunctivitis** [Fiji (fruit sap)].

INFECTION

- Sap topical, or salve made from nuts for **external ulcers**, **infections and sores** [Hawai'i, Malaya].
- **Fever** [Malaya].

MUSCULOSKELETAL / TRAUMA

- Young leaves topical (sometimes heated) for **broken bones**, **bruises**, **wounds**, **pain** [Hawai'i, Western Samoa (bark)]; **sciatica** [Malaya]; **swelling** [Hawai'i, Malaya].

ONCOLOGY

- **Tumors** (bark topical) [Japan].

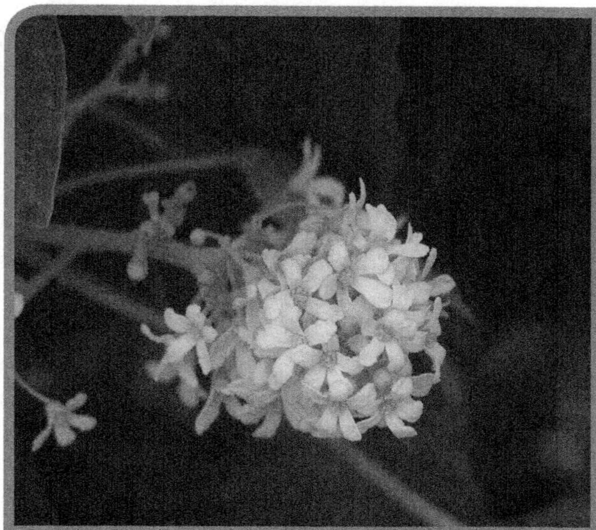

Aleurites moluccana: Kukui flowers

PEDIATRIC

- **Teething** (sap from nut) [Hawai'i]; **thrush** [Hawai'i (sap from nut); Polynesia (bark infused as a gargle)]. Dried flowers have been used in **childhood coma** [Hawai'i].
- **Pediatric mouth infections** [Tonga (leaves infused)].

PSYCHOSPIRITUAL

- In Hawaiian language, **the word kukui can imply "enlightenment."**
- In old Hawai'i, Kukui nuts were sometimes thrown into a fire and **used to place a curse upon a thief.**
- Kukui (especially the variety with long narrow leaves) is **kinolau** (the physical manifestation) **of the prankster Hawaiian pig-god Kamapua'a**, who throughout the millennia has seduced, annoyed, and intrigued the volcano goddess Pele.

REPRODUCTIVE

- **Groin swelling**, **"swollen womb"**. Sap used, and also smoke used **as a "douche"** [Hawai'i]; **gonorrhea** (boiled leaves topical) [Malaya]; **male contraceptive** [Papua New Guinea (seeds topical on the genitals)]; **post partum weakness and "bone pain"** [Fiji]; **infertility** in women [Tonga (bark decocted)].

- The oil was used topically **to prevent stretch marks** on a pregnant woman's belly.

> **Kukui is the state tree of Hawai'i and the flower of the island Moloka'i. Kukui leaves are used to make the "lei of Moloka'i." The polished seeds are also used in lei making.**

RESPIRATORY

- Bark and green fruit used for **asthma**, **wheezing** [Hawai'i]; **cough** [Fiji].

OTHER MEDICINAL USES

- **Weakness**, **debility** [Hawai'i]; **unconsciousness** [Fiji (bark decocted)], Hawai'i].
- **Hernia** [Fiji].
- **Chest pain** [Fiji].
- **Recurring illness** [Fiji (bark decocted)].
- **Neuralgia** [Fiji (fruit or bark boiled in seawater as a mouthwash)].

USE AS FOOD:
Kukui nut is roasted, mixed with Hawaiian sea salt (pa'akai) and made into a tasty condiment called 'inamona. 'Inamona was also traditionally eaten to help deliver a child. To make 'inamona, mix 12 roasted, shelled, and ground kukui nuts with 1 small *Capsicum frutescens* (chili pepper/nīoi), and 1 teaspoon of Hawaiian sea salt (pa'akai).

> ***"It is advisable for the visitor to partake sparingly of the inimona* [sic] *until he has observed how this dish agrees with him."***
>
> ***- - Otto Degener***

OTHER USES:

- In old Hawai'i soot from burning nuts were used for tattoos and fixed with the juice of *Plumbago zeylanica* ('ilie'e).
- The dried sap from a slashed kukui trunk was mixed with water and used to make an adhesive or "varnish" called "pīlali." It was used to protect kapa cloth, and the root-bark provided a copper-colored dye.
- Kukui nuts were chewed by fishermen and spat on the surface of the water to reduce ripples, reduce glare, and aid in locating fish. An inner bark infusion was used to season and dye fishnets for camouflage. They were treated every month or so. The wood was sometimes used to make fish net floats, and a type of fish bait was made with baked coconut meat.

> ***"Whenever anyone grows tired of the secondhand sort of existence that depends on purchased products, and wants to resume the intimate relationship with nature that man once enjoyed, the kukui-nut stands ready to furnish him with food, flavor, tannin, oil, paint, varnish, medicine, and magic."*** **- - Euell Gibbons**

Kukui oil

- Kukui nuts can contain up to 80% oil. This oil was once used for almost everything in old Hawai'i, but its primary function was to provide fuel for light. Numerous lamps, torches, and other devices were used to burn kukui oil as illumination. A kalikukui was a kind of "shishkabob" of kukui nuts skewered on a coconut midrib. Six to ten kalikukui were sometimes placed together to make a large torch called an 'aulama. A smaller torch called a lama was made from a piece of bamboo stuffed with kukui nuts. There were also stone oil lamps called poho kukui that used a strip of kapa as a wick.
- The oil can be used to protect wood in a similar way as linseed oil. To oil wood on a lathe, the roasted nuts can be placed in a piece of fabric and rubbed onto the wood. The oil was used to stain surfboards and the root was mixed with charcoal to dye canoes black. It was also used to make soap and as waterproofing for paper.

CONSTITUENTS: Moluccanin, moretenone, moretenol, alpha-amyrin, and beta-sitosterol. The oil contains linoleic acids. The fruit contains alkaloids. The nuts have 626 calories, 7 grams of water, 19 grams of protein, and 63 grams of fat. They also contain 8 grams of carbohydrates, 3 grams of ash, 80 milligrams of calcium, 200 milligrams of potassium, 2 milligrams of iron, and 0.06 milligrams of thiamine.

Kukui (Candlenut) Cross-Cultural Combinations

Warning: These traditional combinations are offered for informational purposes only and not recommended for use. Ingredients may be irritating, toxic, or both.

"Lumps": the green shells with *Artocarpus altilis* ('ulu / breadfruit) sap and powdered *Diospyros* spp. (lama) or powdered *Mariscus javanicus* ('ahu'awa) [Old Hawai'i].

"General debility": With *Christella cyantheoides* (kikawaiō) fern, *Bidens* spp. (ko'oko'olau), fish, and "'uala poi" (sweet potato poi) [Old Hawai'i].

Disturbed digestion: With weakness in children (6 months to two years) with *Peperomia* spp. ('ala'alawainui) stems, *Jambosa malaecensis* ('ōhi'a 'ai / mountain apple) bark, onion, *Morinda citrifolia* (noni), *Saccharum* spp. (kō / white sugar cane) [Old Hawai'i].

Asthma: With *Syzygium malaccensis* ('ōhi'a 'ai / mountain apple), *Acacia koa*, *Peperomia* spp. ('ala'alawainui), *Bidens pilosa* (kīnehi / spanish needle), kokohe (?), *Morinda citrifolia* (noni), *Waltheria americana* ('uhuloa), *Solanum nigrum* (pōpolo) [Old Hawai'i].

Severe headaches: Oil with *Phyllanthus virgatus* (moemoe) leaves. This may be a reference to headache due to meningitis [Tahiti].

Abscess: With *Bobea* spp. ('ahakea) juice and spring water, boiled, topical [Old Hawai'i].

Enema: With salt water, and juices of kukui, *Sida fallax* ('ilima), *Osteomeles anthyllidifolia* ('ūlei) bark and *Cordyline fruticosa* (lā'ī / ti) shoots [Old Hawai'i].

"Sprue" (a tropical disease): bark juice with *Cocos nucifera* (coconut) milk [Java].

RANGE: Pan tropical. Native to Malaysia.

HABITAT: Likes moist valleys. Up to 1200 meters.

GATHERING: Fruits twice per year. Gather fruits from trees or nuts from the ground. Throw away nuts that float in water. Kukui is kinolau of Lono or Kamapua'a.

PROPAGATION & CULTIVATION: From seed: Use nuts that sink. Soak in hot water 5 minutes before planting. Seeds take 3-4 months to germinate. To transplant seedling, keep soil surrounding the start intact.

RESEARCH:

- Methanol extract lowers cholesterol in rats [Pedrosa 2002].

- Constituents inhibit *Staphylococcus aureus* and *Pseudomonas aeruginosa* [Locher 1995].

NOTES 'N QUOTES

- A kukui tree can be one beeg buggah, up to 3 feet in diameter and 60 feet tall.
- Two useful fungi: *Auricularia auricula* (pepeaio) and *Trametes versicolor* (yun zhi) grow on rotting kukui logs. In the 1800s the Chinese grew a similar fungus, *Auricularia cornea*, on fallen kukui logs for export to China.
- In the early 1800s, up to 10,000 barrels of kukui oil per year were shipped to Russians living in Alaska. Today kukui oil is used in high performance racecars.
- Hawaiian valleys often glisten with the shiny leaves of the kukui tree, painting a reminder of the ancient land divisions called "ahupua'a" and land stewardship called "kuleana".
- Kukui flowers are monoecious, with both male and female flowers on the same plant.

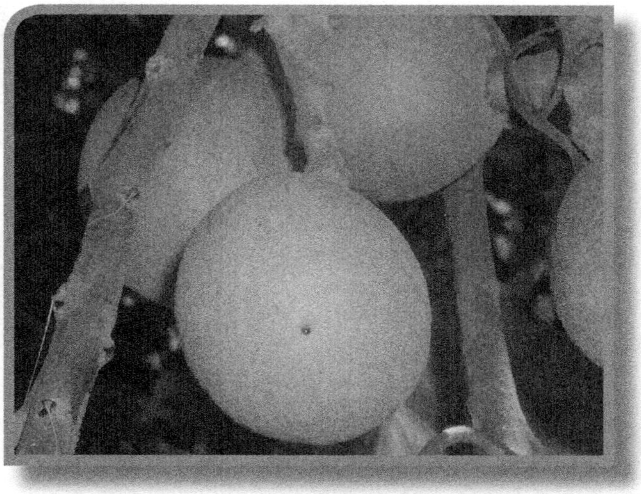

Aleurites moluccana: Kukui fruit

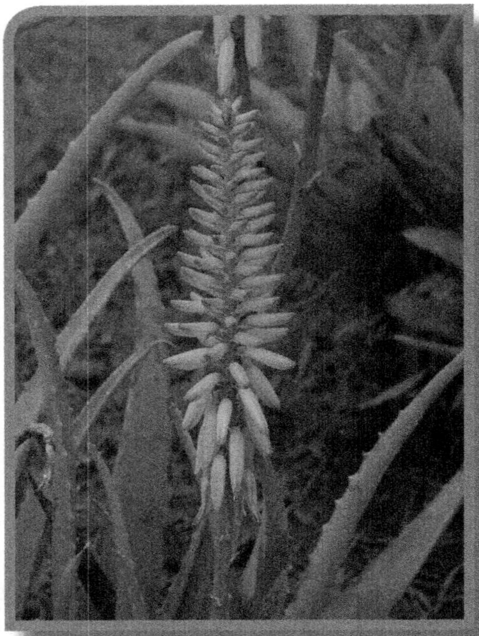

Aloe spp. (Aloi)

PLANT NAME: *Aloe spp.*

OTHER NAMES OR SIMILARLY USED SPECIES: *A. ferox, A. barbadensis, A. vulgaris, A. perfoliata, A. capensis, A. perryi, A. bainesii, A. saponaria*

Status:
Alien. No
pest factor.

Habitat:
In
gardens

COMMON NAMES: **Aloi**, **pānini 'awa'awa** [Hawai'i]; **aloe** [English]; **lu hui**, nu hui, no hui, xiang dan [China]; rokai [Japan]; rapahoe [Tahiti]; kumari, kattarvala [India]; ghui kumari [Nepal]; sink-am-bible [Creole].

PHARMACEUTICAL NAME: Herba Aloes

FAMILY: Liliaceae (Lily family).

CATEGORY: Downward draining herbs - purgatives.

PROPERTIES: Bitter cold [China]; Leaves: bitter hot (?) moist. Gel: salty, cool, moist. Bitter, cool [India].

PLANT PART USED: Different parts of *Aloe* have different effects on the body. The yellow sap that emerges from near the skin of a sliced *Aloe* plant is called "bitter aloes" (luhui). Energetically cold, it is dried, and used as an irritant laxative... a purgative. See *Cautions and Contraindications.*

The *Aloe* gel from the center of the leaf is much milder. The gel is used internally to soothe the digestive tract and topically for burns.

TOXICITY: Chronic long-term toxicity.

CAUTIONS AND CONTRAINDICATIONS:

Caution for internal long-term use

- Not during pregnancy, menstruation, with hemorrhoids or liver / gall bladder degeneration.
- Long-term use can lead to loss of electrolytes, especially potassium. Long-term use can (rarely) lead to hyperaldosteronism, heart arrhythmias, nephropathies, edemas, and accelerated bone deterioration, albuminuria and hematuria.

ENERGETIC CAUTIONS:
- Not in rectal bleeding from cold deficiency.
- Not with spleen qi deficiency ~.

PREPARATION OF MEDICINE:
- Pills powder or gel. Fresh or dried.
- Gel topical as needed.
- *Aloe vera* leaf of length 15-18 cm. Boil in water and add sugar for oral use [China].
- 1 leaf about 15 cm in length mashed and soaked in a cup of water for 20 minutes, then strained and drunk [Belize].

DOSAGE: **Bitter aloes** (luhui): 0.01-0.6 gram (laxative). 1.0 to 1.5 g (drastic). **Gel**: Topical as needed. **Gel internal**: 2-6 oz twice a day.

STATUS IN HAWAI'I: Alien. No pest factor.

MERIDIAN AFFINITIES: Large intestine, stomach, liver

WESTERN FUNCTIONS REPORTED:
Abortifacient (*A. barbadensis*) [Trinidad]; **alterative**; **analgesic**; **antiasthmatic**; **antibacterial**; **anticarcinogenic**; **antifertility**; **antifungal**; **antileukopenic**; **antipeptic ulcer**; **antipyretic**; **antiseptic** (*A. barbadensis*) [Trinidad]; **antithelmintic**; **antitumor**; **antiulceration**; **antiviral**; **aperient** [Japan, Malaya]; **aphrodisiac**; **bitter tonic**; **burn healing**; **cathartic** (*A. zebria*) [China]; **central nervous system depressant**; **decoagulant** (*A. barbadensis*) [Trinidad]; **demulcent** (*A. barbadensis*) [Panama]; **diuretic** (*A. barbadensis*) [Haiti]; **ecbolic** (*A. barbadensis*) [Egypt]; **embryotoxic**; **emmenagogue** (*A. barbadensis*) [China, Egypt, India, Turkey]; **emollient** (*A. barbadensis*) [Haiti, Trinidad]; **expels worms**; **hair stimulant**; **heals wounds**; **hypocholesterolemic**; **hypoglycemic**; **hypolipemic**; **insecticidal**; **larvicide** (*A. barbadensis*) [Haiti]; **laxative** (*A. barbadensis*) [Africa, Bahamas, China, Panama]; **liver sedative**; **liver stimulant**; **local anaesthetic**; **mitogenic**; **promotes bile flow**; **promotes menstruation**; **purgative** [Egypt, Haiti, India, Lesotho, Nepal, Trinidad, Turkey];

refrigerant; **rejuvenative**; **removes stagnation**; **sedative**; **stimulant** (*A. barbadensis*) [Haiti, Turkey]; **stimulates appetite**; **stomachic** [China, India, Spain]; **stops bleeding**; **teratogenic**; **tonic** (*A. barbadensis*) [Egypt]; **uterine stimulant**; **vulnerary**.

TRADITIONAL CHINESE ENERGETIC FUNCTIONS (~ = extrapolated):

1) Clears heat and moves the bowels.
2) Drains heat and fire.
3) Clears liver heat and damp heat.
4) Cools the blood ~.
5) Invigorates blood ~.
6) Promotes the menses ~.
7) Promotes healing and benefits the skin ~.
8) Benefits the digestion ~.
9) Kills parasites.

OTHER ENERGETIC FUNCTIONS: For pitta and kapha (The gel is a tonic for excess fire.). Will aggravate vatta in low doses [Ayurveda].

Aloi (Aloe)
Common Medicinal Uses

- **Burns**
- **Constipation**

Aloi (Aloe) Cross-Cultural Medicinal Uses

COSMETIC

- **Baldness** (topical) [Ancient Greece, Belize, India].

CARDIOVASCULAR

- **Anemia** [China]; **arteriosclerosis** [Europe]; **bleeding** [China, Dominican Republic, India]; **hemophilia** [India]; **varicose veins** [Europe].

DERMATOLOGICAL

- **Inflammatory skin conditions** [Haiti, India]; **skin disorders**, **skin diseases** [Europe, India, Native American]; **eczema** [China, Europe].
- **Burns**, **sunburn** (gel topical) [Universal]; **blisters** [Hawai'i]; **rashes**, **bed sores**, **diaper rash**, **boils**, **scars**, **to prevent scarring**;**"black skin spots"** [Belize].
- **Herpes** [Hawai'i, India].

DIGESTIVE

- **As a "purgative for the lazy and the weak"** [Belize]; **constipation** [Africa, Ancient Greece, Ancient Rome, Belize, China, India, Trinidad (rectal suppository)]; **irritability from constipation** [China]
- **Stomach disorders** [Ancient Greece, Europe, Native American]; **stomach ache** [Tonga]; **indigestion**, **gas** [Europe, Haiti (in rum), India].
- **Peptic ulcers and irritable bowel syndrome** [Europe, India]; **tenesmus** [Russia].
- **To promote appetite and digestion** [Caribbean]; **obesity** [India].
- **Hemorrhoids** [Ancient Greece, India].

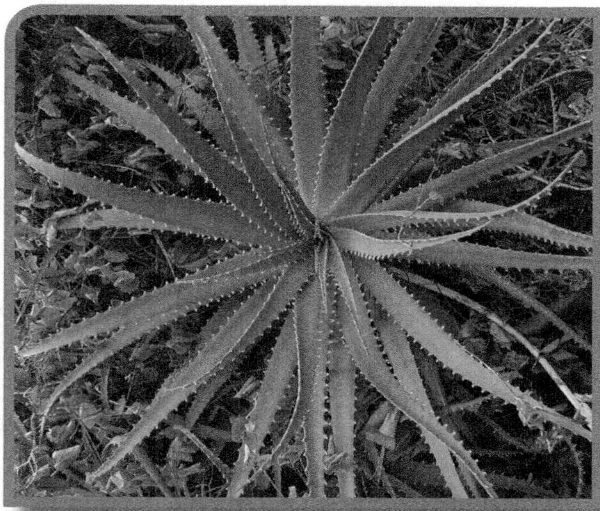

Aloe vera: Aloi leaves

ENDOCRINE

- **Diabetes** [Europe, Haiti (in rum)].

HEAD AND THROAT

- **Dental cavities** [China]; **mouth and gum disease** [Ancient Greece].
- **Nasal inflammation** [China].
- **Eye infections and inflammation** [Caribbean, Europe, India].
- **Headaches**, **migraine headaches** [Africa, Ancient Greece, China, Java, Native American].

HEPATIC

"Those who have jaundice should put aloe in cold water overnight and drink in the morning and before going to sleep. Repeat this three or four days and the person will be healed."

- - Hildegard of Bingen

- **Jaundice**, **hepatitis** [China, Dominican Republic, Egypt, India, Trinidad]; **headache and delerium from hepatitis** [China]; **gall bladder stimulant** [Egypt, Turkey].

INFECTION

- **Boils**, **carbuncles**, **sores** (*A. barbadensis*) [Bahamas, Guatemala, Haiti]; **infections** [Europe]; **fever** [China, Egypt, Haiti, India, Malaya].

LYMPHATIC

- **Scrofula** [China]; **enlarged spleen** [India]; **swollen glands** [India].

> **In India prepared aloe gel with honey and spices is called Kumaryasava and is used for anemia, poor digestion, and liver problems. Kumari means "young girl" or "virgin." Aloe is thought to bring the energy of youth and renewal to women.**

MUSCULOSKELETAL / TRAUMA

- **Bruises** [Bahamas, Mexico]; **bursitis** [India]; **swelling** [Africa, Bahamas, Malaya, Panama]; **burns** [Haiti, Malaya]; **extraction of thorns** (leaf topical, change bandage once per day for 3-5 days) [Belize]; **wounds** [Africa]; **sacral pain** [Russia].

NEUROLOGICAL

- **Convulsions** (adult and infantile) [China, India]; **irritability**, **dizziness** [China].

ONCOLOGY

- **Cancer** [India, Samoa]; **leukemia** [China]; **throat cancer** [USA].

PARASITES

- **Intestinal parasites** [China, Europe, India, Native American]; **malnutrition due to parasites** [China]; **ringworm** [Africa, China]; **roundworm** [China]; **threadworms** [Native American].

PEDIATRIC

- **Colic** [Europe]; **infantile malnutrition** [China]; extracts of leaves used **to stop children from biting fingernails** [Caribbean]; used by nursing mothers **to purge a child** [Europe]; put on the breasts during **weaning** [Caribbean]; **infantile convulsions** (adult and infantile) [China, India]; **irritability or dizziness** [China]; **pertussis** [China].

PSYCHOSPIRITUAL

- **Insomnia** [Ancient Greece].

REPRODUCTIVE

- **Bleeding** [India]; **late menstrual period** [Caribbean, Europe, India, Native American]; **late period with constipation** [USA]; **painful menses** [India]; **prolapsed uterus** [Russia]; **vaginitis** [India].
- **Post partum** [Bahamas, Lesotho].
- **Menopause** [India];
- **Prostatitis** [Russia];
- **Venereal diseases** [India]; **syphilis** [South Africa].

RESPIRATORY

- **Asthma** [Amboina, Curacao, Egypt, Haiti, India, Samoa]; **chest congestion** [Java]; **cough** [Egypt, Java].
- **Common cold** [Bahamas, Barbados, Curacao, Haiti, India, Jamaica, Lesotho]; **influenza** (*A. saponaria*) [Lesotho].

URINARY

- **Painful urination** [India]; **edema** [Bahamas].

VETERINARY

- Topical for **cuts on dogs' paws** (Wrap sliced leaf around wound and bandage. Change daily) [USA].

OTHER MEDICINAL USES

- **General debility** [India].

> **In the African Congo Slukari hunters rub *Aloe* over their bodies to hide their scent. Related species are used as an antidote to poison arrow wounds.**

CONSTITUENTS:

1,8-dehydroxyanthraquinone, acemannan, aldopentose, aloe peptides, aloe-emodin, aloeferon, aloin (also called barbaloin), aloin derivatives, amino acids, aminoacids. anthranols, anthraquinones, anthrol, anthrones, barbaloin, benzothiazolone, calcium oxalate. campesterol, cholesterol, chrysophanic acid, cyclohexane derivatives, dehydro-abietal, emodin, enzymes, glucomannan, glucose, isocitric acid, lipids, lupeol, methyl esther of dehydro-abietic acid, organic acids, para-coumaric acid, stigmasterol, sugars.

POSSIBLE DRUG INTERACTIONS:

- Can cause potassium deficiency when used with thiazide diuretics, licorice, and corticosteroids [Brinker 2001]. This can increase toxicity of digoxin [Brinker 2001; Chen 2004].
- Potentiates the hypoglycemic effects of gliben-

clamide, and (topically in mice) the anti-inflammatory effects of topical hydrocortisone [Okyar 2001].
- Can cause a strong odor when used for radiation burns [Leonard 2003].

Aloi (Aloe) Cross-Cultural Combinations

Headaches, irritability, and flank pain ("heat in the liver meridian"): With *Gentiana scabra* (long dan cao) and *Scutellaria baicalensis* (huang qin) [China].
Worms: With *Quisqualis indica* [China].
Eczema: With *Glycyrrhiza uralensis* (gan cao / licorice), topical [China].
Radiation exposure: With *Eucalyptus* spp. (nuholani) or castor oil topical [Hutchens 1983].
To prevent intestinal irritation: With *Hyoscyamus* spp., *Humulus* spp. (hops), or *Ipecacuanha* spp. [Europe].
Colds, asthma, and for bruises: Beaten with egg whites and taken internally [Trinidad].
Stomach ulcers: Juice with seawater [Trinidad].

HABITAT: In a pot on your windowsill.

GATHERING: Can be smelly and messy.

RESEARCH:

Dermatology

- Accelerates wound healing in humans [Visuthikosol 1995, Davis 1989(c)], and in rats [Somboonwong 2000; Chithra 1998; Heggers], possibly due to the glycoprotein content [Choi 2001]. In another study of wound healing, 100mg / kg was given to mice for 2 months with no mention of toxicity but a reported decrease in wound diameter of 62.5% [Davis 1989].
- Useful for burns [Visuthikosol 1995]. May reduce inflammation in burns via reduction of cytokines and leukocyte adhesion [Duansak 2003], and increases microcirculation [Somboonwong 2000].

Inflammation

- Anthraquinones are anti-inflammatory (inhibiting arachidonic acid) [Vazquez 1996; Davis 1989(a); Davis 1989(b)].
- Anti-oxidant [Malterud 1993; Yagi 2002; Saada 2003].

Oncology

- Antineoplastic. Acemannan, a substance in aloe, increases immunity in mice whose immune systems had been damaged by radiation [Shimpo 2000, 2002; Saada 2003]. Some constituents are anti-mutagenic against leukemia & neuroectodermal tumors [Lee / Hong 2000(a); Lee / Kim 2000(b); Pecere 2000], inhibit chemical hepatocarcinogenesis [Shamaan 1998], and pancreatic cancer in lab animals [Furukawa 2002].

Immunity

- Extract is immunoregulatory [Qiu 2000; Womble 1988].
- May prevent ultraviolet radiation (UBV) induced immune suppression in the pancreas and in the skin [Lee / Han 1997].

Endocrine

- May prevent pancreatic tissue damage in lab animals [Beppu 2003; Furukawa 2002; Lee / Han 1997]. The leaves (but not gel) lower blood sugar in IDDM and NIDDM rats [Okyar 2001]. *Aloes* (the concentrated sap) also lowers blood glucose [Ghannam 1986].

Other

- *Aloe* inhibits hepatotoxicity, [Norikura 2002; Corsi 1998] and lowers hepatic cholesterol in rats [Lim 2003].
- Antiviral for Herpes 1 & 2 [Arvigo 2001].
- *Aloe* gel is being researched as a battlefield blood substitute to prevent hemorrhagic shock in wounded soldiers. The results in lab animal studies look promising [Macias 2004].

> ***"Aloes are one of the most sovereign agents we have among the herbal medicine being cleansing to the morbid matter of the stomach, liver, spleen, kidney and bladder. Does not gripe and is very healing and soothing to all the tissue it obliges."*** **- - Alma Hutchens**

NOTES 'N QUOTES

"*I have perfumed my bed with myrrh, aloes, and cinnamon.*"

- - Proverbs 7:17.

- Greek physician Dioscorides wrote of *Aloe* for constipation, burns and kidney ailments. Pliny (Caius Plinius Secundus, A.D. 23-79) recommended rubbing the leaves on male genital ulcers [Greece].
- Mentioned in the New Testament as a purgative (John 19:39).

- Napoleon's wife Josephine used a milk / aloe gel lotion for her skin. It was used by Cleopatra for the same reason, and also used in Egyptian embalming processes [Egypt].
- Indigenous to the Sudan. *Aloe ferox* is indigenous to South Africa.

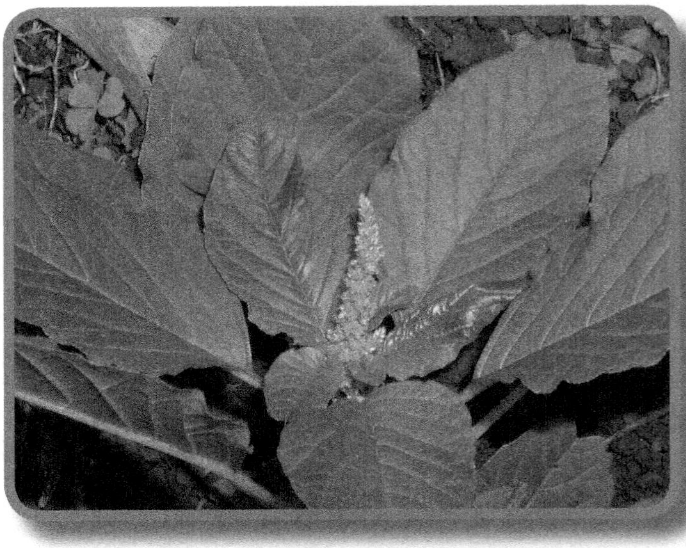

Amaranthus spp. (Pakai)

PLANT NAME: *Amaranthus* spp.

SIMILARLY USED SPECIES: *A. blitus; A. caudatus; A. dubius; A. edulis; A. hibridus; A. hypochondriacus; A. viridus.* Please note that for all practical purposes, *A. viridus* can be used as a substitiute for *A. spinosus.* A lot easier on the hands, too, as *A. viridus* has no spines.

Status: Alien bad boy

Habitat: Low elevation, disturbed areas

COMMON NAMES: **Pakai** (*Amaranthus* spp.), **pakai kūkū** (*A. spinosus*) [Hawai'i]; zhi xian, tz'u hsien-ts'ai, [China]; tan-duliyah [India] ban lunde [Nepal]; **amaranth**, **spiny amaranth** (*A. spinosus*), red cockscomb, love-lies-bleeding, pigweed [USA]; chiori con espinas [Bolivia]; khichka jat'aqo [Quechua]; mullu keerai, neer keerai, tanduliuyah [India]; gansam lodut, surindi [Borneo]; ntungu [Tanzania].

NOMENCLATURE: *Amaranthus* is from the Greek "amarantos" which means "unfading", a reference to the persisting color of certain amaranth flowers. Or.... the name Amara means "bitter." Take your pick. Spinosus means "spiny," as does kūkū.

FAMILY: Amaranthaceae.

CATEGORY: Herbs that stop bleeding~.

PROPERTIES: Sweet and bland tasting, astringent, cool.

PLANT PART USED: Aerial parts.

TOXICITY: *Amaranthus retroflexus* (not known to

grow in Hawai'i) is reportedly nephrotoxic to large domestic animals [Oladosu 1979], although not to rabbits [Schamber 1985]. In China, the roots are said to be mildly toxic and overdose can cause dizziness, nausea, and vomiting.

CAUTIONS AND CONTRAINDICATIONS: Never treat bleeding without first determining its cause.
Not during pregnancy or normal menstruation. Caution with osteoporosis or calcium imbalances~ [Larsen 2003]. See *Use As Food* below. The genus has been reported to cause dermatitis and photosensitivity. The pollen has been reported to cause keratitis of the eye.

PREPARATION OF MEDICINE: Usually decocted or poulticed.

DOSAGE: 10 grams in formula, 30 – 60 grams as a single herb. Up to 300 grams of the fresh root is used in China for duodenal and gastric ulcers. (I would not consider using such a dose).

WESTERN FUNCTIONS REPORTED: **Antiemetic; anti-inflammatory; astringent; blood purifier; carminative; diaphoretic; diuretic; emmenagogue; emollient; expectorant; febrifuge; galactogogue; hemostatic; improves digestion; lactogogue; laxative; mucilaginous; promotes appetite; purgative; sudorific.**

TRADITIONAL CHINESE ENERGETIC FUNCTIONS (~ = extrapolated):

1) Clears heat and poison.
2) Improves digestion.
3) Stops bleeding.

OTHER ENERGETIC FUNCTIONS: Benefits pitta and kapha.

Pakai (Amaranth) Common Medicinal Uses

- Excessive menstruation
- GI bleeding

Pakai (Amaranth) Cross-Cultural Medicinal Uses

BITES & STINGS

- **Insect bites** [Philippines (leaves)]; **scorpion sting** [India (root)]; **snakebite** (root internal) [Ghana, India, Philippines].

CARDIOVASCULAR

- **Mild internal bleeding** [China, India].
- **Hemophilia** [India].

DERMATOLOGICAL

- Topical for **eczema** (leaves & root) [China, India, Nepal, Philippines]; **psoriasis** [Philippines (leaves)].
- **Rashes** [Philippines (leaves)].
- **Sunburn** [Philippines (leaves)].
- **Burns** (leaves poulticed) [Nepal, Philippines].

DIGESTIVE

- **Enteritis**, **dysentery** [Borneo, China]; **mild diarrhea** [USA].
- **Gastric or duodenal ulcer** [China].
- **Indigestion** [India]; **nausea** [India].
- **Enema** [Ghana].
- **Hemorrhoids** [China, Ghana, India].

HEAD AND THROAT

- **Nose bleeds** (topical).
- **Mouth ulcers** (topical).
- **Toothache** [India (root chewed with salt)].

HEPATIC

- **Gall bladder inflammation**, **gall stones** [China].

INFECTION

- Topical for **boils**, **abscesses** (leaves or root poulticed) [China, India, Nepal]; **foot sores** (stem decocted, topical) [India].
- **Fever** [China, Philippines].

MUSCULOSKELETAL / TRAUMA

- **Broken bones** (seeds poulticed).
- **Bruises** [Malaysia (leaves poulticed)]; **wounds** (topical).

ONCOLOGY

- **Tumors** (poulticed) [Mauritius, Java, South East Asia].
- **Uterine tumor** [Cambodia].

PEDIATRIC

- **Colic** (root) [India, Nepal].
- **Laxative for children** [Nepal (leaves and roots boiled)].

PSYCHOSPIRITUAL

- The Lodha of West Bengal, India, reportedly make **a hallucinogenic smoking powder** from the root

of *A. spinosus.* (Sounds like "banana peels")
- **Ceremonial medicine** in a type of ceremony called "Green Corn Medicine" [Cherokee].

REPRODUCTIVE
- **Excess menstrual bleeding** (leaves, roots) [Cherokee, India, Nepal]; **abnormal uterine bleeding**.
- **Edema during pregnancy** [India (young leaves internal)].
- **Vaginal discharge** (topical),
- **Gonorrhea**, **genital discharge** [India, Nepal].

RESPIRATORY
- **Cough**, **coughing up blood** [India (seed)],
- **Bronchitis** [Malaya]; **wheezing** [Malaya].

URINARY
- **Edema** (in bath or leaves as a vegetable) [Ghana, India].
- **Bladder infections** [India].

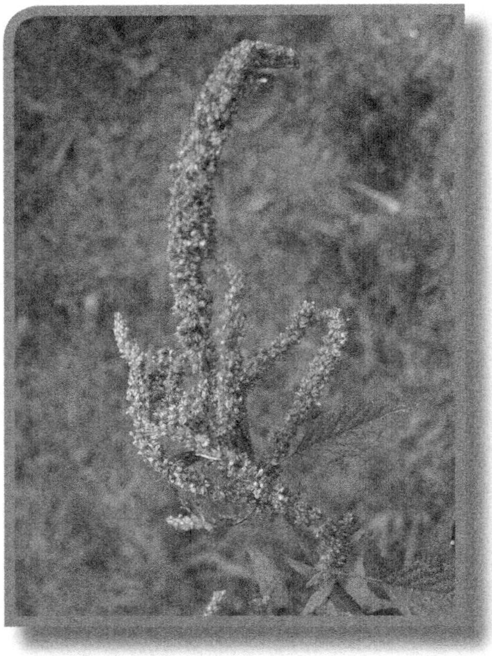

Amaranthus spp.: Pakai tops

OTHER MEDICINAL USES
- **Burning sensations**, **"heat in the body"** [India (seed)].
- **Inflammation** [Java].
- **"Poisonous afflictions"** [India].

USE AS FOOD: High in protein and calcium. It is used as a food crop by the Aztec Indians of Mexico, as a spinach substitute in Australia, and as a vegetable in China. The seeds can be boiled into a hot cereal. Cook for at least an hour.

The young shoots make a very tasty potherb or in salads. While high in calcium, however, amaranth that also contains large amounts of oxalates may actually inhibit calcium absorption [Larsen 2003]. Because it may absorb nitrates from the soil and form oxalate crystals in the leaves, only organic pakai should be used [Elpel 2000].

OTHER USES: In Swaziland the ash of the whole plant is used as a snuff, sometimes alone and sometimes with tobacco.

A red dye made from pakai kūkū is used to color food and medicine. A green and yellow dye can be made from the whole plant.

Pakai (Amaranth) Local Combinations

Bleeding: Add *Erigeron canadensis* (fleabane), *Eclipta prostrata* (han lian cao), and *Capsella rubella* (shepherds purse).

Pakai (Amaranth) Cross-Cultural Combinations

Warning: These traditional combinations are offered for informational purposes only and not recommended for use. Ingredients may be irritating, toxic, or both.

Hemorrhoidal bleeding, **dysentery**, **enteritis**: Decocted with *Eclipta prostrata* (han lian cao) & *Pteris ensiformis.* [China]

Juvenile vomiting or colic: With *Lavendula officinalis* (lavender) or *Matricaria camomilla* (chamomile)

Post partum: Stem pulp with castor oil [India].

To cause abortion: With *Carica papaya* (hē'ī / papaya), *Tamarindus indica, Plumbago zeylanica* ('ilie'e) & *Capsicum annum* (nīoi / cayenne) [India].

RANGE: Southeast Asia, Malaysia, Southern Africa. Native to tropical Americas. Accidentally brought into Hawai'i in 1900.

HABITAT: Found in the sun almost everywhere in Hawai'i

GATHERING: Use the young ones… or use gloves. When gathering as food, take the young shoots. Can cause hay fever.

PROPAGATION & CULTIVATION: Don't. Seeds

are dispersed by water & have long viability.

RESEARCH:

- The essential oil of *Amaranthus* spp. lowers cholesterol in hamsters and the seeds of *Amaranthus esculantus* lowers cholesterol in rats [Berger 2003; Chaturvedi 1993].
- *A. caudatus* and *A. paniculatus* seeds are antioxidant [Klimczak 2002].

NOTES 'N QUOTES

"*The redder the stem, the stronger the effects.*"
- - Michael Moore

- The family amaranthaceae includes more than 900 species in 60 genera.
- Most amaranths photosynthesize using a different method than some other plants. Called the "C4 carbon-fixation pathway," it is a mechanism best suited for sunny areas.
- *A. spinosus* and *A. viridus* are used almost interchangeably, with *A. viridus* preferred as it has no spines.
- Astringent for the mucous membranes
- Up to 66% of weed species are said to be edible. While "edible" and "digestible" may not always be the same thing, young *A. viridus* and *A. spinosus* are definitely both.

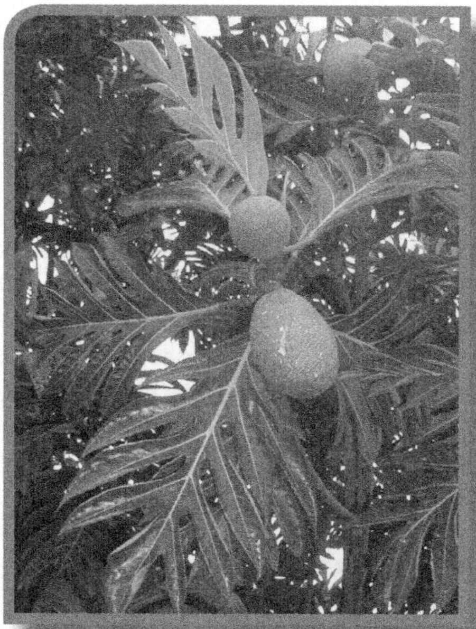

Artocarpus communis ('Ulu)

PLANT NAME: *Artocarpus communis*

OTHER NAMES: *A. altilis, A. incisa*

Status: Polynesian introduction

Habitat: Likes it hot and moist

SIMILARLY USED SPECIES: *A. odoratissinus, A. elasticus, A. elastica, A. mariannensis, A. integer, A. cumingiana, A. lakoocha, A. elastica, A. vrieseanus.*

COMMON NAMES: **'Ulu** [Hawai'i]; **breadfruit** [English]; fruit a pain [French]; fruta pao, pao de massa [Portuguese]; broodvrucht, broodboom [Holland]; pan de ano, pan de palo, topan [Venezuela]; mazapan (seedless), castana (with seeds) [Guatemala, Honduras]; marure [Peru]; castano de malabar (with seeds) [Yucatan]; panapen (seedless), pana de pepitas (with seeds) [Puerto Rico]; timadang, kadazan, dusun (*A.* odoratissinus) [Borneo]; suku (seedless), kulur (with seeds) [Malaya & Java]; sa-ke, [Thailand]; rimas (seedless) [Philippines].

NOMENCLATURE: It doesn't resemble bread, nor does it taste like a fruit.

FAMILY: Moraceae (Mulberry family).

PLANT PART USED: All of it. The male flowers are called ule'ulu (breadfruit penis), and the female flowers are called 'ulupua (breadfruit flower).

TOXICITY: None noted

CAUTIONS AND CONTRAINDICATIONS: Some varieties of 'ulu are purgative if eaten raw.

PREPARATION OF MEDICINE: I have used 'ulu almost exclusively as food, and have little clinical experience with it as medicine, but I have included it because others seem to have found many uses for it.

WESTERN FUNCTIONS REPORTED: **Anodyne** (*A. altilis*) [Trinidad]; **antibacterial** (root bark); **antitumor**; **aperient** (*A. elastica*) [Malaya]; **astringent** (root) [Pacific Islands]; **contraceptive** (*A. elastica*) [Java]; **hemolytic** (leaves); **laxative** (*A. altilis*) [Dominican Republic]; **masticatory** (*A. cumingiana*); **purgative** (root) [Pacific Islands]; **styptic** (*A. cumingiana*); **vermifuge** (*A. communis*) [Samoa].

'Ulu (Breadfruit) Cross-Cultural Medicinal Uses

CARDIOVASCULAR

- **High blood pressure** (yellow leaf decocted) (*A. altilis*) [Bahamas, Haiti, Trinidad, West Indies].
- **Chest pain and vomiting from heart problems** [South Pacific].

DERMATOLOGICAL

- **Boils, abscess, and skin infection** (*Artocarpus* spp. sap topical) [Dominican Republic, Haiti, Hawai'i, Malaya, Java, Samoa, Tahiti & Tonga (leaf ash, macerated root, or latex topical)].
- **Cracked-skin & dermatosis** (*A. communis*) [Hawai'i, Java].
- **Burns** (*A. altilis*) [Haiti].
- **Rashes** (sap topical) [Tahiti, Tonga].

DIGESTIVE

- **Stomach pain** (*Artocarpus* spp. diluted latex internal) [Samoa (bark), Solomon Islands, Tonga (bark)]; **diarrhea or dysentery** (diluted latex or roots boiled internal) [Borneo, Java, Pacific Islands, Samoa]; **vomiting blood** [South Pacific (juice from young fruit)].
- **Fish poisoning** [South Pacific (leaf sprouts), Micronesia (sap from the shoots)].

ENDOCRINE

- **Diabetes** (yellow leaf as tea) [Trinidad, West Indies].

HEAD AND THROAT

- **Headache** (*A. communis*) [Bahamas (leaves poulticed on head for headache); Samoa (bark), Pacific Islands (bark)].
- **Toothache** (toasted flowers topical on gums) (*A. communis*, *A.* integra) [Java, Malaya]; **thrush** (crushed leaf buds & latex topical on tongue) [Bahamas, Trinidad, Pacific Islands]; **tonsillitis** [Tahiti].
- **Eye problems** (*A. communis* leaf or petiole juiced, topical) [Futuna, Samoa]; **puncture wounds to the eyes** [Micronesia (sap)].
- **Ear infections** (leaves juiced or diluted latex topical) [Pacific Islands].

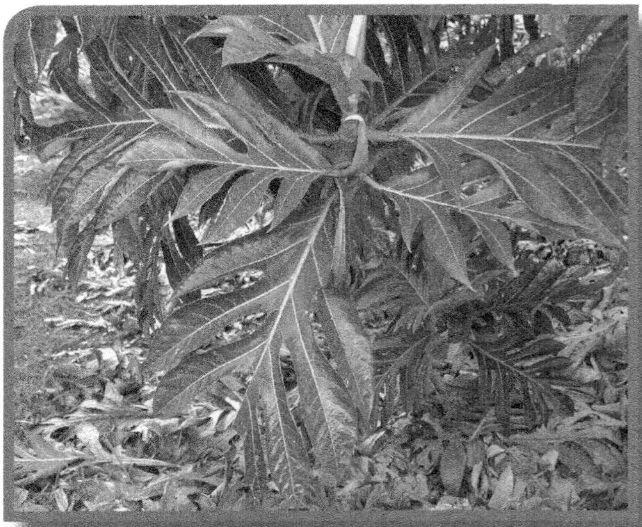

Artocarpus communis: 'Ulu leaves

INFECTION

- **Herpes** (*A. communis*) [Amboina]; **fever** [Bahamas, Malaya, Samoa, Sumatra]; ashes of leaves topical for **infection** [Hawai'i].

HEPATIC

- **Liver disease** [Taiwan].

LYMPHATIC

- **Enlarged spleen** (*A. communis*) [Java]; **inflammed spleen** (*A. lakoocha*) [India];

MUSCULOSKELETAL / TRAUMA

- **Wounds** [Hawaii, Java, Samoa, Tahiti (sap topical), Tonga (sap topical)]; **fractures**, **broken bones** [Fiji (*A. altilis*); Pacific Islands (latex topical)]; **bone pain** [South Pacific (stem bark juice)]; **sprains**, **contusions**, **swelling** [Samoa (*A. communis*), Tahiti (sap)]; **spasms** [South Pacific (leaf sprouts)].
- **Back pain & sciatica** (latex topical) [Pacific Islands, Samoa (*A. communis*) Java (*A. elastica*)]; **rheumatism** (*A. altilis*) [Haiti]; **gout** (*A. altilis*) [Haiti].

ONCOLOGY

- **Tumor** (fruit crushed topical) (*A. altilis*) [Brazil].

PEDIATRICS

- Crushed leaves for **thrush** [Hawai'i].
- **Pediatric anal thrush** (smoke from a burning branch, topical) [Samoa, Tonga].
- **Cough in children** [Polynesia].
- **Childrens facial rash** (bark infused topical) [Tonga].

PSYCHOSPIRITUAL

- In old Hawai'i, 'ulu was considered a symbol of creation and the generosity of the Creator.
- The volcano goddess Pele, said to be angry with King Kamehameha I for not making offerings to her, destroyed his 'ulu orchard in a volcanic eruption.
- Near Moanalua Gardens in Honolulu grew an 'ulu tree from which the spirits of the dead leaped into the afterlife.
- A Hawaiian hero named Niheu was said to have stolen a breadfruit from a god who had used it to roll across the underworld causing thunder.
- Both *Cocos nucifera* (niu / coconut) and *Artocarpus communis* ('ulu / breadfruit) are kinolau (physical manifestation) of Kūka'ilimoku (Kū), the war god. It is said that Kū was married to a Hawaiian woman and had a family with her. One year there was a drought and they were without food. Kū placed his head in the earth and his body became an 'ulu tree (or a niu palm, depending on who you ask). The tears of his wife watered the plant and gave it life. Thus he sacrificed himself and bore food for his family to eat. Unlike other kinolau of Kū, 'ulu was not kapu for women.
- 'Ulu is also said sometimes to represent the goddess Haumea.

REPRODUCTIVE

- **Post partum infections** [South Pacific (stem bark juice)]; **post partum weakness** [South Pacific (roots)]; **to help expel afterbirth** [Polynesia].

RESPIRATORY

- **Asthma** (yellow leaf decocted) [West Indies, Trinidad, Bahamas]; **cough** [Tahiti]; **difficult or painful breathing** [South Pacific (root juice or young fruit juice)].
- **Tuberculosis** (*A. elastica*) [Java].

URINARY

- **Decreased urination** [Trinidad (*A. altilis*)].
- **Blood in the urine** [Tahiti].
- **Urinary problems** [Samoa (root or bark infused)].

VETERINARY

- The leaves and uncooked fruit are **fed to livestock** and fruit peelings are used **to fatten pigs** [Hawai'i]. **Fractured bones in animals** (*A. lakoocha*) [India].

OTHER MEDICINAL USES

- **Recurring illness** [Tonga (bark)].
- **Abdominal pain** [Cook Islands (crushed stem tips internal)].

Coming across a breadfruit tree while hiking is always a gift. Some of my most memorable meals have included 'ulu as the main entrée. It is said that when a Marquesan child was born, the family would plant one coconut palm and one breadfruit tree, and that would supply enough food for that person for life.

USE AS FOOD:

- The uses of breadfruit as food are unlimited, although in old Hawai'i it was not a primary food but a secondary one. It was made into poi, baked in an imu (underground "oven"), and over ripe 'ulu was also made into a pudding called pepeie'e 'ulu. This could be dried and if put in the sun occasionally it could last for months.
- 'Ulu may be eaten ripe as a fruit or unripe as a vegetable, although (caveat emptor) some varieties can cause vomiting if eaten raw.
- Ripe pulp is mixed with coconut milk, salt and sugar to make a pudding.
- In Melanesia and New Guinea, 'ulu seeds are called "breadnut" and are roasted or boiled like a chestnut.
- It was possibly used as baby food. The fallen male flower spikes are sometimes candied.
- In other parts of Polynesia, 'ulu was specially prepared by a young male and stored in pits (called mā) and lined with *Cordyline* spp. (lā'ī) leaves as a hedge against famine. The breadfruit would ferment and could last years. The young man who would mash the breadfruit with his feet had to be specially circumcised and abstain from sex.
- A delicious use of breadfruit is to steam it, marinate it in coconut water or coconut milk and orange juice, and then lightly sauté it.
- In Barbados and Brazil highly nutritious breadfruit flour is mixed with wheat flour and made into bread. In Jamaica the flour is made into breakfast porridge.

OTHER USES:

Arrow poison (?) (*A. bracteata*) [Malacca].
Breadfruit leaf designs are often used in Hawaiian quilt patterns.

Starch

In Central and South America, the starch has been explored for use in textile manufacturing.

Wood

The wood of *Artocarpus communis* has uses as timber for houses, canoes, drums, surfboards, furniture, statues (ki'i), firewood, & poi boards (papa ku'i ai). It is resistant to termites and marine worms. It was used in canoes (wa'a) for gunwales and bows.
'Ulu surfboards (papa he'e nalu) were stained black. After use, they were dried in the sun and oiled with coconut oil (this helped waterproof the board). They were then wrapped in kapa and hung in a dry place for storage.

Sap

The sticky sap is used as an adhesive and caulk for catching birds, sealing canoes, and joining gourds into a drum. In Kosrae the sap is mixed with coconut oil to make a kind of "flypaper" and used as "chewing gum" in the Caribbean and Hawai'i.

Bark

The bark is used for cordage and the inner bark was made into a coarse kapa cloth called pō'ulu.
The cordage has been used for shark nets and Water Buffalo harnesses.

Leaves

Used to wrap food and as livestock feed. The dried leaves have been used as fishing kites. The sheath of the leaf (malo 'ulu) was used as a type of "sandpaper" for finishing wooden bowls.

Male flowers

Used as mosquito repellent [Vanuatu (dried flowers burned)]. The male flower was mixed with *Broussonetia papyrifera* (wauke) fiber to make elegant malo (loincloths). The flowers were used as a yellow to brown dye [Hawai'i].

CONSTITUENTS: Alpha amyrin, artocarpin, artocarpine, beta amyrin acetate, cycloaltilisin, cycloartenol, cycloartenone, cycloartenyl acetate, cyclomorusin, flavonoids, folic acid, hydrocyanic acid, lectin, linoleic acid (seed oil), linolenic acid (seed oil), oleic acid (seed oil), papayotin (enzymes), pectins, starch, vitamin C.

'Ulu (Breadfruit) Cross-Cultural Combinations

Skin ulcerations or mouth sores: The sap with powdered *Cyperus laevigata* (makaloa) and powdered wood of *Diospyros* spp. (lama) [Old Hawai'i].
Skin disease and boils: The sap with *Cassia occidentalis* and tobacco ashes [Old Hawai'i].
Shingles: Leaf ashes with banana sap [Cook Island Maoris].
Post partum weakness: The bark with *Citrus sinensis* (moli kai) leaves [Tonga].
Thrush: The leaf buds were mixed with 'alaea (iron oxide), and put in the mouth topically. A small fish called aeāea was then eaten [Old Hawai'i].

RANGE: Global distribution near the equator. Probably native to Java

HABITAT: Likes it hot and moist: temperature of 60° to 100°F, rainfall around 80 to 100 inches per year with humidity of 60 - 80%. Likes fertile, deep, and well drained soil, but some seedless varieties do well in sandy areas.

GATHERING:
- Sticky. Gather when the fruit begins to "weep." There is an old Hawaiian proverb: He has become a breadfruit that oozes gum. (He has become wealthy) Breadfruit sap can stain, and will often spew forth its "wealth" on your brand new seat covers, so cover your covers. Cooking oil rubbed on the hands before handling may prevent staining of the skin.
- Do not climb breadfruit trees to gather 'ulu, the branches are known for breaking off.
- Gather in the summer: June, July and August. Some trees have a brief winter season.

PROPAGATION & CULTIVATION: Propagate by root cuttings. Will bear fruit within 5-7 years.

RESEARCH:
- Flower inhibits arachidonic acid-induced ear edema in rats [Koshihara Y 1988].

NOTES 'N QUOTES:
- Legend has it that the first breadfruit trees were brought in the 1100s by chief Kahai from an island in Samoa called Upolu. They were then planted at Kualoa on O'ahu for another Mō'ī (chief).
- In old Hawai'i there was a special class of Kahuna (experts) called "Kia Manu" (bird catchers). They would catch specific birds whose feathers were then sewn into the cloaks of the Ali'i (royalty). They would use either the sap from the 'ulu tree or the pāpala kēpau (*Pisonia* spp.) to catch the birds on a long stick. After a few feathers were plucked from the birds, it is said that (by order of Kamehameha I) these Kahuna would then use kukui oil to release the birds' feet from the sticky sap, freeing them.
- The first 'ulu was seen by Europeans in the Marque-

sas in 1595.

- Captain Cook's botanist, Solander, was introduced to breadfruit in Tahiti in 1769 and raved about it back in England. As a result, King George III sent Captain Bligh to the Pacific to propagate and collect breadfruit. H.M.S. Bounty was filled with breadfruit during the ill-fated voyage when officer Fletcher Christian and the crew mutinied in 1788. Bligh survived, and within four years of the mutiny, he had returned to Polynesia and then delivered 1200 breadfruit trees to Jamaica.
- 'Ulu is technically not a fruit but a "collective" fruit, similar to noni or pineapple.
- 'Ulu trees are thought be native to the East Indies, although speculation ranges from Western Micronesia to New Guinea. They can grow to 30 - 80 (?) feet tall, with up to three-foot leaves and ten-pound fruits. Trees can produce 25 - 200 fruits per year.
- A close relative of the breadfruit is called jackfruit (*Artocarpus heterophyllus*) and it is native to India.
- Kahanu Gardens in Hana, Maui, grows nearly 100 varieties of breadfruit.
- A long pole with a hook on the end called a lou was used to pick 'ulu fruit.
- Legend has it that on Kauai some breadfruit trees were planted by a bow-legged menehune with a deep voice. (Quite an image...)
- In old Lāhainā there was a young man named Kaulā'au who was the son of the ruling chief of Maui. Being kolohe (mischievous), he would spend his time uprooting breadfruit trees. As a punishment he was sent to the island of Lāna'i. Lāna'i was uninhabited at the time because it was believed to be haunted with evil spirits. Not to be outdone, Kaulā'au, hid from these spirits in 'ulu trees and used 'ulu sap to blind them. Eventually he was allowed to return to Lāhainā.

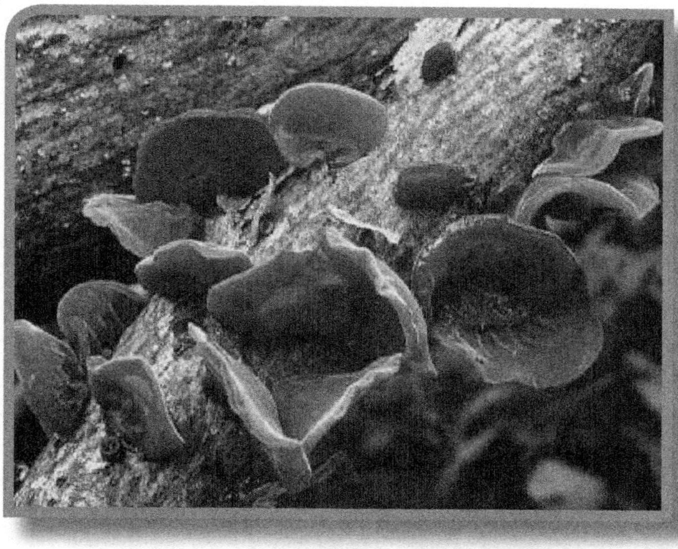

Photograph by Christopher Hobbs

Auricularia spp. (Pepeiao)

PLANT NAME: *Auricularia* spp.

SIMILARLY USED SPECIES: *A. auricula-judae, A polytrich, A. sambucina, A. mesenterica, Hirneeola auricula-judae, Tremella auricula,* and *T. cythiformis.* The species found in Hawai'i is *Auricularia cornea.*

Status: Unknown. Low pest factor.

Habitat: Wet and low.

COMMON NAMES: **Pepeiao** ("ear") [Hawai'i]; **mu er** ("wood ear"), hei mu er ("black wood ear") [China], yun erh (cloud ear) [China]; kikurage (edible fungus) [Japan].

NOMENCLATURE: *Auricularia*, Er, and Pepeiao all mean "ear" in their respective languages.
The specific epithet "*auricula-judae*" means "*ear of Judas*", and is a reference to Judas Iscariot. Both Judas and *Auricularia* have been known to hang from Elder trees. Jew's ear is a contraction of Judas' ear

PROPERTIES: Sweet, neutral.

PLANT PART USED: The fruiting body (ear).

TOXICITY: No significant toxicity.

CAUTIONS AND CONTRAINDICATIONS: DO NOT EAT WILD MUSHROOMS OR FUNGI UNLESS YOU ARE 100% POSITIVE IN YOUR IDENTIFICATION. Do not use *Auricularia* spp. during pregnancy, lactation, or for women trying to conceive. Not with pharmaceutical blood thinners. Not with gout.

PREPARATION OF MEDICINE: Steamed and eaten, or added in formulas.

DOSAGE: 10-30 grams. Up to 60 grams in soup.

STATUS IN HAWAI'I: Unknown. Low pest factor.

WESTERN FUNCTIONS REPORTED: **Antibacterial**; **antiparasitic**; **antitumor**; **antiviral**; **astringent** [Linnaeus]; **drying** [Linnaeus]; **hypoglycemic**; **immunomodulatory**; **laxative**; **lipid lowering**; **painkiller**; **reduces mucous**; **refrigerant** [Linnaeus].

TRADITIONAL CHINESE ENERGETIC FUNCTIONS (from various sources):

1) Tonifies qi, tonifies the stomach, refreshes the brain, strengthens the stomach.
2) Nourishes the yin and blood, moistens the lung, promoting production of the body fluid.
3) Invigorates blood, cools the blood.
4) Strengthens the will.
5) Invigorates blood, stops pain, strengthens the lungs.

Pepeiao (Auricularia) Common Medicinal Uses

- Cancer
- Fatigue and low energy
- Compromised immune system
- Cardiovascular disease

Pepeiao (Auricularia) Cross-Cultural Medicinal Uses

CARDIOVASCULAR

- **Angina**, **vascular sclerosis**, **arterial and vascular obstructions**, **poor circulation** [China].
- **Hypertension** [China].
- **Anemia** [China].

DIGESTIVE

- **Gastric or intestinal inflammation**, **dysentery with blood** [China].
- **Vomiting blood**; **nausea with phlegm**.
- **Bleeding hemorrhoids** [China].
- **Gas** [China].
- **Constipation** [China].
- **Abdominal pain** [China].
- **Nausea** [China].

GERIONTOLOGY

- **Chronic wounds in the elderly** [China].

HEAD AND THROAT

- **Conjunctivitis**, **ophthalmic bleeding**.
- Used with other materials topically for **eye irritations** [Ancient China].
- **Inflammation of the mouth or throat** [Europe].
- **Tooth pain** [China].

INFECTIONS

- **Bloody dysentery** [China].

MUSCULOSKELETAL / TRAUMA

- **Low back pain** [China]. **rheumatic pain**; **muscle spasms** [China], **cramps**
- **Traumatic injuries** [China].
- **Tetany**.

ONCOLOGY

- **Cancer**.

PSYCHOSPIRITUAL

- In old China, mu er was said to **make the body strong and light and to strengthen the will**. The properties of *Auricularia auricula-judae* were said to absorb the properties of the media on which it was grown.

REPRODUCTIVE

- **Vaginal discharge** [China].
- **Abnormal uterine bleeding** (specific); **excessive menses**; **spotting** [China].
- **Post partum weakness** [China].

RESPIRATORY

- **"Lung deficiency" cough** [China]; **dry cough with little sputum**; **coughing blood due to dry lungs** [China].

URINARY

- **Urinary tract diseases** [China].

OTHER MEDICINAL USES

- **General weakness**, **compromised immune response**.
- **Numbness**.
- **Excess mucous** [China].

USE AS FOOD: In soups or stir-fries with chicken or tofu. They can then be dried at home and later reconstituted with water. Cook well when using as food.

OTHER USES: Because of its ability to absorb copper, *Auricularia polytricha* has been studied as a possible way to detoxify environmental pollution.

CONSTITUENTS: Calcium, carotene, iron, phosphorus, polysaccharides (beta-D-glucans), protein.

The medicinal compounds found in pepeiao are called "HDP" or "Host Defense Potentiators." Comprised mainly of polysaccharides, they regulate immune responses, possibly through cytokine production. Cytokines include interferon, interleukins and materials that stimulate the natural killer T cells of the immune system. Polysaccharides such as beta-D-glucan are used in the treatment of cancer.

POSSIBLE DRUG INTERACTIONS: Not with Coumadin or other anticoagulants ~ [Agarwal 1982].

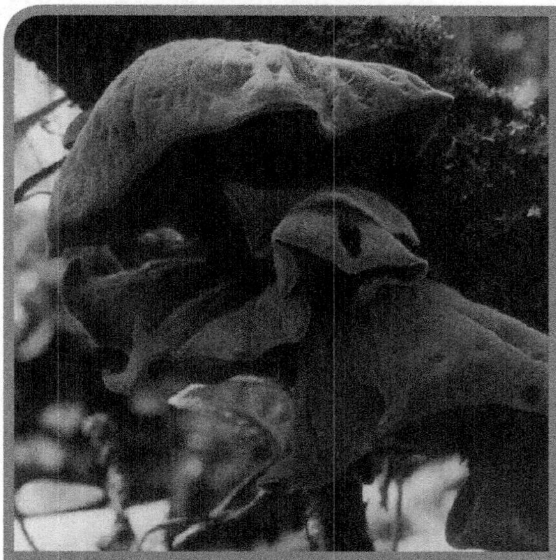

Photograph by Don Hemmes

Auricularia spp.: Pepeiao fungus

Pepeiao (Auricularia) Local Combinations

Compromised immunity: Add *Trametes versicolor* (yun zhi) and *Centella asiatica* (pohe kula).

Low energy: Add *Morinda citrifolia* (noni) and *Trametes versicolor* (yun zhi).

Cardiovascular disease: Add *Centella asiatica* (pohe kula), and *Leonorus sibiricus* (motherwort).

Pepeiao (Auricularia) Cross-Cultural Combinations

Bleeding hemorrhoids with constipation: 6 grams of Pepeiao with 28 grams of *Diospyros kaki* (persimmon calyx). Baked and eaten as food. [China]

Anemia: With *Zizyphus jujuba* (da zao) fruit [China].

High blood pressure and dry cough: With *Apium graveolens* (celery) in soup.

Throat inflammation: Boiled in vinegar, beer, or milk [Europe].

HABITAT: Likes it on wet rotting logs.

GATHERING: Can be gathered year round, even on the mainland. The color can range from pale tan when young to brown / purple as they age. The texture is always rubbery, never brittle.

Approximately half of the 5 million metric tons of cultivated edible fungi produced annually have medicinal properties. The most frequently cultivated species of medicinal mushroom is *Lentinus* spp. (shitake), followed by *Peurotus* spp. (oyster mushrooms), *Auricularia* spp. (pepeiao / mu er), and *Tremella* spp. (bai mu er). In 1994, the world's supply of cultivated *Auricularia* spp. (pepeiao / mu er), was 420 tons, which accounted for 8.5% of mushrooms.

RESEARCH:

- In three randomized, double blind, placebo-controlled clinical trials, patients receiving beta-glucan had significantly lower frequency of postoperative infections [Babineau 1994].
- Polysaccharides improved glucose tolerance in mice [Yuan 1999].
- Some constituents strongly inhibit Sarcoma 180 solid tumors in mice [Misaki 1981].
- *Auricularia auricula* (pepeiao) inhibits platelet aggregation in both rats and humans. While they contain adenosine (a substance that inhibits platelet aggregation) they also seem to work through some other mechanism [Agarwal 1982].

NOTES 'N QUOTES

Medicinal mushrooms were often more popular in China than in Europe: "*... they grow amongst rusty nails or rotten rags, or ye holes of serpents, or amongst trees properly bearing harmful fruits.*"

- - Dioscorides

- Hippocrates (455 B.C.), the father of medicine described fungus as being used as "moxa" (the smoke of the burning herb was used topically) for kidney problems or back pain.

- *Auricularia* is a microrhizal fungus. Microrhiza create symbiotic (mutually beneficial relationships) with many plant, fern, and lichen members of Hawaiian ecosystems.

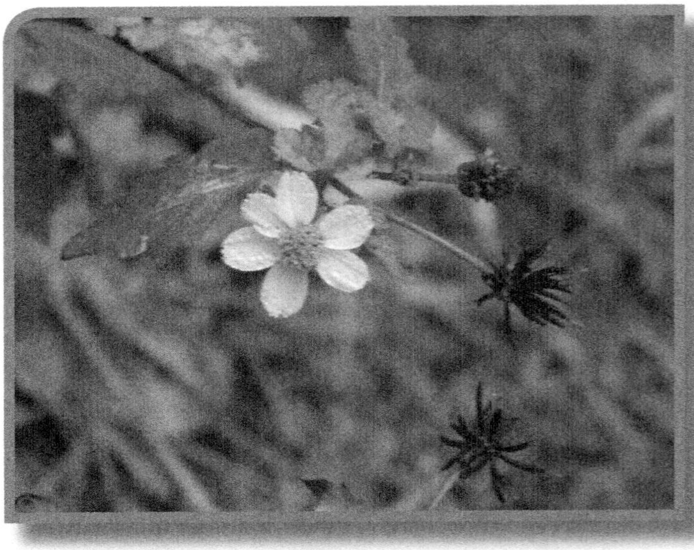

Bidens spp. (Kīnehi)

PLANT NAME: *Bidens* spp.

OTHER NAMES: *Adenolepis* spp., *Campylotheca* spp.

SIMILARLY USED SPECIES: *Bidens pilosa, B. bipinnata* (gui zhen cao, nian shen cao) *B. biternata, B. chinensis, B. parviflora* (xiao hua gui zhen cao), *B. tripartite, B. chilensis.*

Status:
Bad boy weed

Habitat:
All over your socks

COMMON NAMES: **Kīnehi** (*Bidens pilosa*) , **ko'oko'olau** (native *Bidens* species) [Hawai'i]; **xian feng cao** ("abundant weed"), gui zhen cao ("demon spike grass" or "ghost needle weed") [China]; aceitilla [Spanish]; amor seco (*Desmodium adscendens* is also called "amor seco") [Peru]; beggars tick / **spanish needle** / needle grass [USA]; black jack [South Africa]; cobblers peg [Australia]; fisi 'uli [Tonga]; has kung chia, han feng cao [Taiwan]; muni [Aymara, Quechua]; ottrancedi [India]; picao preto, cuamba [Brazil]; piripiri [Cook Islands]; saetilla, sillk'iwa [Quechua]; sanana vinillo, saytilla, natilluna [Bolivia]; spanish needle, needle grass [Barbados, St. Thomas]; te de coral [Mexico]; z'herbe zedruite [Caribbean]; fisi'uli [Tonga]; uqadolo [Southern Africa]; z'herbe zedruite, z'herbe z'aiguille [Dominica, Martinique].

NOMENCLATURE:

- From a Western perspective, *Bidens* (meaning "two teeth") is a reference to hairy calyx (pappus) of some species. The name "*pilosa*" means "hairy."
- In China the many species and varieties of *Bidens* are often lumped under the names xian feng cao ("abundant weed") or gui zhen cao ("demon spike

grass" / "ghost needle weed"), but each species (see "similarly used species" above) will sometimes have a different Chinese common name. In Taiwan *Bidens* species are called "ham hong chho."

- Many common names of *Bidens* are a reference to the fruits that are aggravating hitchhikers. Hence the names "demon spike grass" and "ghost needle weed." Beggars tick is a reference to the fact that hobos would gather these on their clothing as they walked along railroad tracks.
- Some Chinese will use *Bidens* interchangeably with *Desmodium* spp, as they are thought to be almost therapeutically identical. In China they even share the same name: "nian shen cao." In South America *Bidens* is also used interchangeably with *Desmodium* spp. and there they also share a local common name: "amor seco."
- On a clinical note, current research has shown both plants to be liver protective.

FAMILY: Asteraceae

CATEGORY: Clear Heat and Toxins

PROPERTIES: Bitter, bland, sweet, neutral to cool [China].

PLANT PART USED: Whole plant.

TOXICITY: See *Cautions and Contraindications.*

CAUTIONS AND CONTRAINDICATIONS: Can irritate the bladder and kidney in high doses. Some constituents may be weak esophageal carcinogens [Mirvish 1979].

PREPARATION OF MEDICINE: Prepare as decoction or tincture 1:5 40-50%. A good way to use kīnehi is to pull it out by the roots (gathering with prayer) while it is still flowering. Some Hawaiians prefer to gather only those without white ray florets. After pule (prayer), the roots are scalded in boiling water and the plant is hung upside down to dry. This allows the mana (power) of the plant to penetrate into the flowers and leaves. The tops are then cut and stored.

DOSAGE: 15-60 grams per day. 15-30 grams in combination. Some Chinese sources list doses as high as 120 grams per day for acute appendicitis. Because kīnehi is photo-activated, there is some speculation as to polyacetylines being activated even in the capillary bed by strong sunlight. Ingest during daylight hours for maximum effect.

STATUS IN HAWAI'I: *Bidens pilosa* is a bad boy weed. The native *Bidens* spp. are endemic. Learn the differences before you gather.

WESTERN FUNCTIONS REPORTED: **"Blood purifier" (infused); antibacterial; "antibiotic"; antidote; antidysenteric; antihemorrhagic; anti-inflammatory; antimalarial; antimicrobial; antipyretic; astringent; carminative; circulation promoting; diuretic; emmenagogue; emollient; hepatoprotective; hypotensive; intoxicant; lactogogue; liver protective; mucous membrane tonic; prevents flu & colds; sialogogue; stagnant blood dispelling; stimulates childbirth; styptic; urogenital system tonic; vulnerary**.

TRADITIONAL CHINESE ENERGETIC FUNCTIONS (~ = extrapolated):

1) Cools and resolves the surface.
2) Clears heat and toxins, removes toxins, removes stagnation.
3) Invigorates blood.
4) Clears damp heat from the lower jiao.
5) Removes wind dampness.
6) Purges fire.
7) Reduces swelling [Taiwan].

Kīnehi (Spanish Needle) Common Medicinal Uses

- **Colds and flu**
- **Acute or chronic hepatitis**
- **General bacterial infections**
- **Inflammatory conditions**
- **Urinary tract infections**

Kīnehi (Spanish Needle) Cross-Cultural Medicinal Uses

CARDIOVASCULAR

- **To prevent stroke** [Hawai'i].
- **To "cool the blood"** [Bahamas].
- **Angina** [Amazonia, Haiti, Peru, Research]; **cardiac spasm** [China (decocted)].

DERMATOLOGICAL

- **Skin disorders** [Hawai'i, India]; **eczema** (topical); **itching** [Bahamas, China]; **ringworm**; **heat rash**

[Bahamas], **hives** [Ghana]; **frostbite** [China].

- **Boils**, **abscess**; **sores**; **chronic ulcers** [Bahamas, China, Cook Islands, Exuma, India (leaf), Java, Peru, Philippines].

DIGESTIVE

Indigestion

- **Stomach ache**, **nausea & vomiting** [Amazonia, China, Hawai'i, Tonga (flowers infused)]; "**sick stomach**" [Bahamas]; **food poisoning** (flowers infused) [Tonga].

Digestive inflammation

- **Heartburn** [Hawai'i]; **stomatitis** [Haiti]; **ulcers** [India]; **gastroenteritis** [China, Peru]; **appendicitis** [China, Peru]; **intestinal problems** [Upper Volta]; **colitis** [China (decocted)]; **irritable bowel syndrome**; **intestinal carbuncle** [China]; **hemorrhoids** [China (decocted)].

Diarrhea

- **Diarrhea** [Africa, Burkina Faso, China, India (flower), Upper Volta].
- **Dysentery** [Amazonia, China, Bolivia, Peru, Tanzania, Venezuela].

Other

- **To stimulate appetite** [native species, Hawai'i]; **difficulty swallowing** [China (decocted)].
- **Weight loss** [Peru].

ENDOCRINE

- **Diabetes** [Amazonia, Brazil, Haiti, Mexico, Peru, Trinidad].

HEAD AND THROAT

- **Headache** [Amazonia, India, Peru, Zulu].
- **Eye problems**, **inflammation**, **conjunctivitis** (leaves juiced, topical) [Caribbean, Dominica, Ghana, Hawai'i, Malaya, Peru, S.E. Asia, Tonga, West Africa].
- **Ear complaints**, **earache** [Ghana, India (leaf & flower)].
- **Chronic nasal discharge**.
- **Toothache** [Amazonia (leaf topical), Dominican Republic, India (root), Java, New Zealand (shoots, flowers, or roots chewed), Peru].
- **Mouth ulcers**.
- **Promotes saliva** [Dominican Republic].
- **Sore or irritated throat**, **tonsillitis** [Amazonia, Bahamas, Brazil, China, Hawai'i, Martinique].
- **Inflammation of the amygdala** [Bolivia (decocted), Haiti].
- **Esophageal enlargement** [China (decocted)].
- **Laryngitis** [Amazonia, Peru].

HEPATIC

- **Jaundice**; **acute or chronic infectious hepatitis** [Amazonia, Bolivia, Brazil, China, Peru].
- **Alcoholic hepatitis** [Amazonia].
- **Biliary colic** [Bolivia (decocted)].
- **Malaria** [Brazil, China, Research, Peru].

INFECTION

- **Boils**, **abscess** [Exuma, China, Cook Islands, Java, Peru, Philippines]; **infections** [Amazonia, Bahamas, Brazil, China, Hawai'i, Martinique, Peru].
- **Fever**, **chills**, **common cold**, **flu** [Amazonia, Bahamas, Brazil, China, Hawai'i, Martinique].
- **Fungal infection** [Peru].

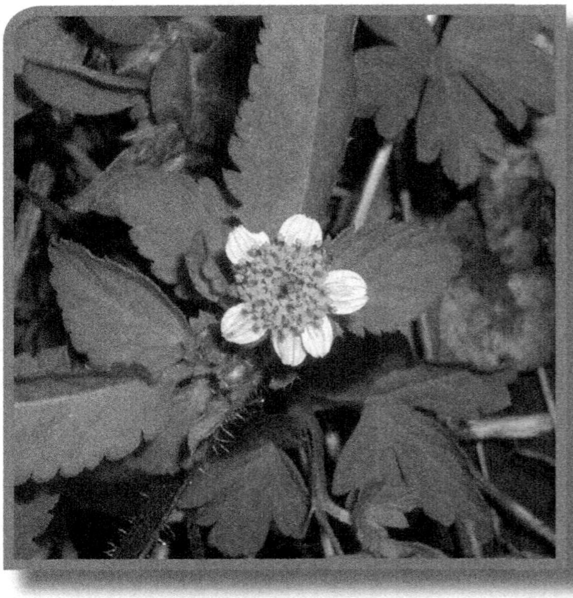

Bidens spp.: Kīnehi flower

LYMPHATIC

- **Glandular sclerosis** [Brazil].

MUSCULOSKELETAL / TRAUMA

- **Joint pain** [China, Hawai'i, Peru, Zulu (young shoots chewed)].
- **Traumatic injury**, **sprains**, **swelling**, **contusions** [China].
- **Rheumatoid arthritis** [China].
- **Gout** [USA].
- **Cuts** (leaves juiced, topical) [Africa, India, Marquesas, Rapa, Tonga]; **wounds** [Amazonia, India].

ONCOLOGY

- **Cancer** [Bahamas].
- **Gastric or esophageal cancer** [China (decocted)].

PARASITES

- **Worms** [Amazonia (root decocted)].

PEDIATRIC

- In old Hawai'i, ko'oko'olau (the native *Bidens* spp.) were much used for **digestion** in children and young adults. For children 10-50 days old, the buds were chewed and given to infants followed by milk. For children age 50 days to 8 months, the buds and flowers were given as tea. As the children grew they gradually were given leaves rather than buds or flowers. Sometimes the tea for the children was brewed with coconut water. The upper parts of many species in the genus, both (native and non-native), are useful for people of all ages and for an assortment of conditions.
- **Colic** [Burkina Faso, Hawai'i Upper Volta].
- **Constipation** [Hawai'i (native *Bidens* spp.)].
- **Epilepsy in children**, **infantile fever with convulsions** [China].
- **Malnutrition in infants** [China].
- **Thrush** [Hawai'i (native *Bidens* spp.)].
- **Worms in children** (infused, every day for 9 days) [Bahamas].

PSYCHOSPIRITUAL

- In Tonga this plant is used for **eye ailments caused by evil spirits**, and the Dani tribe of New Guinea uses it for **magick**.
- **Sedative**, **intoxicant.** "*To quiet down a smart-aleck.*" [Hawai'i, Philippines].

REPRODUCTIVE

- **Vaginal infections**, **discharge** [Brazil, Amazonia].
- **Lack of menses** [Caribbean]; **irregular or painful menses** [Amazonia, Bolivia (infused)]; **spotting**, **excessive menstrual bleeding**, **uterine hemorrhage**.
- **Stimulate childbirth** [Peru].
- **Stimulates breast milk** [Dominican Republic, Haiti].
- **For repeated miscarriages** [Hawai'i (douche)].
- **Benign prostatic hypertrophy** [USA]; **difficult urination** [Caribbean, Martinique].

RESPIRATORY

- **Respiratory problems** [Dominican Republic, Mexico].
- **Fever**, **common cold**, **flu** [Amazonia; Bahamas; Brazil; China; Costa Rica (flowers decocted and sugar added); Hawai'i; Martinique].
- **Asthma** [Hawai'i].
- **Bronchitis**, **chest congestion** [Burkina Faso; China; Dominican Republic; Haiti; Mexico; Upper Volta].
- **Cough** [Burkina Faso, India (leaf), Malaya, Southeast Asia, Upper Volta]; **spitting blood due to excess coughing**.
- **Sinus headaches**, **allergies**, **lung irritation from cigarettes**, **yelling**, **smog**, **vog**.
- **Pneumonia** [China].
- **Tuberculosis** [Hawai'i].

URINARY

- **Urinary tract infections**, **urinary discharge** [Amazonia, Peru, Brazil, Bahamas, Dominican Republic, Peru; USA]; **urinary abscess** [Brazil]; **cloudy or bloody urine**.
- **Edema** [Amazonia].
- **Urinary retention** (decocted) [Bolivia].
- **Acute nephritis**, **kidney stones**.

VETERINARY

- **Foot and mouth disease** [Amazonia, Haiti].

OTHER MEDICINAL USES

- **Allergies**, **hives** [Ghana].
- **Fatigue and weakness** [Hawai'i]; **general debility** [Hawai'i].
- **Needles used to puncture sores** [New Guinea].
- **Inflammation** [Africa (strong decoction), India (leaf), Zulu].
- **Insect bites and scorpion sting** (topical) [China]; **snake bite** [Burkina Faso, China, India, Upper Volta].
- **Leprosy** [India].
- **"Prickly heat"** (flowers and leaves)

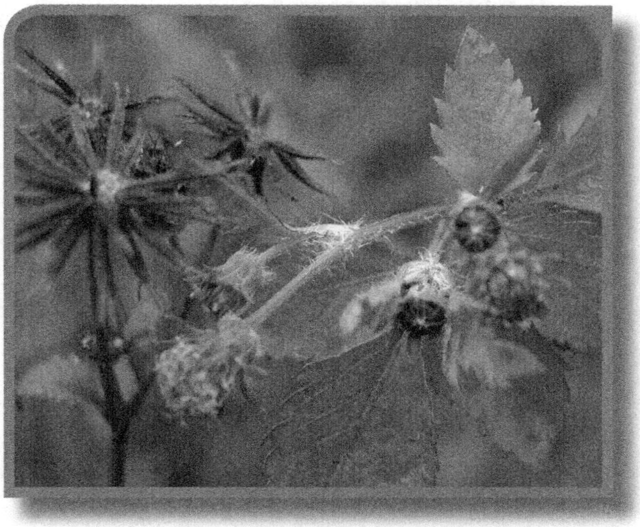

Bidens spp.: Kīnehi flowers and seeds

USE AS FOOD: Young leaves sometimes eaten raw or steamed, but the taste can be a bit strong. In Zimbabwe the leaves are boiled with peanut butter and eaten. *Bidens pilosa* is eaten in Africa as a vegetable. Fermented with rice to make "sake."

OTHER USES: Because *Bidens pilosa* secretes chemicals that attack fungi and nematodes it is sometimes used in a controlled way to increase corn yields.

CONSTITUENTS: Acetylenes; aurone glycosides; aylated okanin glycosides; b-amyrin; b-sitosterol; chalcone glycosides; esculetin; flavonoids; friedelin; gallic and oxalic acids; limonene; linolenic acid; linolic acid; lupeol; luteolin, (a flavonoid); phenylheptatriyne (PHT or PHY: polyacetylenes); phytosterin-b; polyacetylenes; sterols; tannins; volatile oils; xanthophylis; & "*some peculiar phenolic astringents*" [Michael Moore].

Kīnehi (Spanish Needle) Local Combinations

Asthma: *Bidens* (native) with *Waltheria americana* ('uhaloa) leaf buds and flowers, *Metrosideros polymorpha* ('ōhi'a) leaf buds and red flowers, and *Saccharum* spp. (kō honua'ula / sugarcane). 3 times a day for 5 days [Old Hawai'i].

Asthma: *Bidens* (native) with *Peperomia* spp. ('ala 'ala wai nui), *Syzygium malaccense* ('ōhi'a 'ai / mountain apple) bark, *Metrosideros polymorpha* ('ōhi'a) leaves, *Aleurites moluccana* (kukui) flowers and nuts, *Psilotum triquetrum* (moa), *Cocos nucifera* (niu / coconut) fruit, *Morinda citrifolia* (noni) fruit, *Portulaca oleracea* ('ākulikuli / purslane), & *Ipomoea dissecta* (koali / morning glory) [Old Hawai'i]

Boils: Topical (juiced or as tea) with *Plantago* spp. (laukahi / plantain).

Bronchitis: Add *Waltheria indica* ('uhaloa).

Common cold: With *Aleurites moluccana* (kukui) and *Piper methysticum* ('awa / kava). Used to potentiate the effects of 'awa.

Fatigue and weakness: *Bidens* (native) with sweet potatoes and coconut cooked in coconut milk [Old Hawai'i].

Fatigue and weakness: *Bidens* (native) with *Metrosideros polymorpha* ('ōhi'a) (leaf buds) and *Saccharum* spp. (kō honua'ula / sugarcane) [Old Hawai'i]

General debility: *Bidens* (native) with *Waltheria americana* ('uhaloa) root cortex, *Syzygium malaccense* ('ōhi'a 'ai / mountain apple) bark, *Peperomia* spp. ('ala 'ala wai nui), *Morinda citrifolia* (noni) fruit, *Musa* spp. (mai'a / banana) fruit, *Saccharum officinarum* (kō / sugar cane), & *Ipomoea dissecta* (koali) [Old Hawai'i].

General debility: *Bidens* (native) with *Waltheria americana* ('uhaloa), *Peperomia* spp. ('ala 'ala wai nui), *Saccharum officinarum* (ko / sugar cane). *Metrosideros polymorpha* (lehua) flowers [Old Hawai'i].

Gout: Add *Capsella rubella* (shepherds purse), *Vaccinium* spp. ('ōhelo / blueberries).

Hepatitis: Add *Desmodium* spp. (pua pilipili), *Eclipta prostrata* (han lian cao).

To induce lactation: *Bidens* (native) with *Sida* fallax ('ilima) flowers and *Hibiscus tiliaceus* (hau) flowers [Old Hawai'i].

Tuberculosis: With *Peperomia* spp. ('ala 'ala wai nui pehu) (leaves and buds), *Syzygium malaccense* ('ōhi'a 'ai / mountain apple) bark, *Metrosideros polymorpha* ('ōhi'a) (leaf buds and red flowers), *Aleurites moluccana* (kukui) flowers and burned nuts, *Morinda citrifolia* (noni) ripe fruit, *Oxalis corniculata* ('ihi mākole / sorrel) [Old Hawai'i].

Urinary tract infections: Add *Taraxacum officinale* (laulele / dandelion).

Kīnehi (Spanish Needle) Cross-Cultural Combinations

Please note some of the ingredients in the following combinations are toxic! Do not self-administer without the supervision of a licensed practitioner or an experienced Elder.

Angina, sore throat, water retention, hepatitis, and dropsy: With lemon juice [Amazonia].

Tuberculosis: *Bidens* spp. with *Chrysanthemum morifolium* (ju hua) and *Houttuynia cordata* (yu xing cao) [China].

Gout: With *Oplopanax horridus* (devil's club), *Arcticum lappa* (burdock) root, *Tribulus terrestris* (bai ji li).

Gout: With *Urtica dioica* (nettles).

Prostatitis: With *Salvia apiana* [Michael Moore].

Sores and lacerations: Dried leaves topical mixed with olive oil. [Exuma tribe].

RANGE: *Bidens pilosa* is native to South America, the Caribbean, Africa, and the Philippines. There are 60 native species of *Bidens* in Hawai'i, and 19 of those are endemic.

GATHERING: You don't have to... it gathers you. Gather before the achenes (hitchhikers) appear on the flower heads. In China it is gathered late summer - fall.

Note: Do Not gather native *Bidens* species. The introduced varieties work very well and are not endangered... not by a long shot. The rule of thumb is: If the *Bidens* gathers you (produces hitchhikers), then you can gather the *Bidens*. Native species do not produce hitchhikers.

PROPAGATION & CULTIVATION:

Native species: By seed.
Alien species: Not in Hawai'i.

RESEARCH:

Polyacetylenes

- The polyacetylenes in kīnehi are anti-pathogenic. Because polyacetylenes are also photoactivated (their medicinal properties are enhanced by daylight), kīnehi makes a particularly good topical poultice for infectious skin conditions [Wat 1980]. One of the active polyacetylenes in kīnehi is phenylheptatriyne. Unlike other photo activated plant chemicals (such as furanocoumarins), phenylheptatriyne does not alter DNA, [Wat 1979] but is one of the few plant chemicals that inhibit cytomegalovirus [Hudson 1986].

Oncology

- Interestingly, polyacetylenes in another genus, *Panax ginseng* (ren shen), have been shown to strongly inhibit growth in cancer cells, but not in normal cells.

Antimicrobial

- Phenylheptatriyne, linolic acid and linolenic acid are antimicrobial [Geissberger 1991].
- Constituents are antibacterial against gram-positive bacteria (methanol extracts) [Rabe 1997].
- Aliphatic acetylenes appear to inhibit *Plasmodium falciparum* (malaria) growth in vitro and in vivo [Brandao 1997].

Hepatic

- Protects the liver from hepatotoxins, a broad-spectrum liver protectant [Chin 1996].

Anti-inflammatory

- Anti-inflammatory effect: water and ethanol extracts are a prostaglandin-synthesis inhibitor (triggers of headaches & inflammatory disease) [Jāger 1996]. Flavonoids friedelin and friedelan-3 beta-ol are anti-inflammatory, inhibiting cyclooxygenase (an enzyme that stimulates pro-inflammatory prostaglandins) [Geissberger 1991].
- Methanol extracts of polyacetylenes are anti-inflammatory (immunosuppressive) in vitro [Pereira 1999].

Cardiovascular

- Methanol extract is hypotensive in rats, possibly due to vasodialation [Dimo 1999], but effect on cholesterol on lab animals is inconclusive [Dimo 1999; Li Qingdong 1989].
- Inhibits platelet aggregation & thrombosis in rats [Li Qingdong 1989].

NOTES 'N QUOTES

"*Bidens may be our best herb for benign prostatic hypertrophy*" - - Michael Moore

"*... probably the best herbal therapy we have for irritation, inflammation, pain, and bleeding of the urinary tract mucosa.*" - - Michael Moore

"*Bidens with Arctium and blended with pig fat can cure finger cut.*"

Prescriptions Worth a Thousand Gold
(Qian Jin Yao Fang)
- - Sun Si Miao, 581 - 682.

- *Bidens* spp. are used widely as a folk medicine in China and have a long history of use (particularly in Taiwan) for common cold, dysentery, and hepatitis. Two types of *Bidens* are mentioned in the Chinese classic, the Ben Cao Gang Mu (1596 A.D.)
- Kīnehi flowers are hermaphroditic, they have both male and female sex organs.
- An ingredient in the Chinese patent Gan Mao Qing.
- Please note that some of the above actions and indications are taken from old Hawaiian material may refer to native endemic species of *Bidens*, not to *Bidens pilosa.* Almost all other information (non-Hawaiian) contained here is a reference to *Bidens pilosa.* My experience is that the endemic species are more effective for digestion and the alien species is more effective with infections and inflammation. Do not use an endemic species of *Bidens* as medicine unless you are absolutely sure that it is not rare or endangered.
- Both a poignant blessing and an abominable curse, most herbalists in Hawai'i have a love-and-loathing relationship with kīnehi. Like a dysfunctional romance, it can make us joyous or crazy depending on the circumstances.

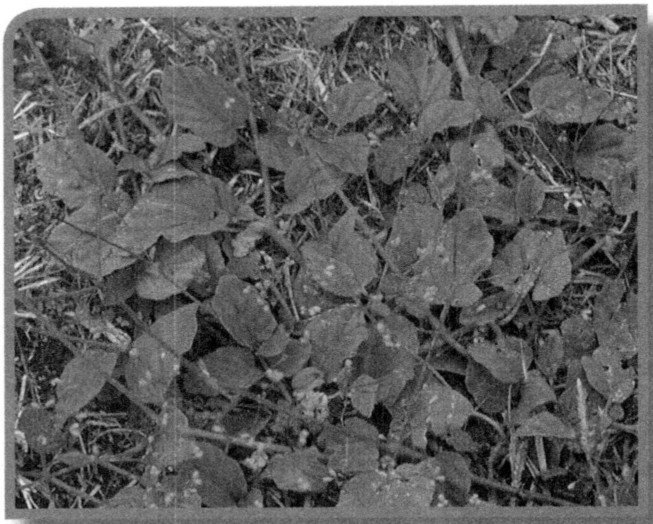

Boerhavia spp. (Alena)

PLANT NAME: *Boerhavia* spp.

SIMILARLY USED SPECIES: *B. diffusa, B. procumbens, B. repens, B. coccinea, B. glabrata, B. adscendens, B. caribaea, B. erecta, B. paniculata, B.viscosa, B. hirsuta.*

Status: Some alien, some native

Habitat: Sun and sandy soil

COMMON NAMES: **Alena** [Hawai'i]; huang xi xin (*B. repens, B. diffusa*), zhi li huang xi xin (*B.* erecta), zhou bo huang xi xin (*B.* crispa) [China]; a'atasi [American Samoa (*B. repens*)]; bashkhira [Pakistan (*B. procutribens*)]; erva tostão [Brazil (*B. hirsuta*)]; hog weed [Barbados (*B. coccinea*)]; patagon rouge [French West Indies (*B. coccinea*)]; puka k'ullu [Quechua (*B. coccinea*)]; punarnava [Nepal (*B. diffusa*)]; raiz de la china [Bolivia (*B. coccinea*)]; raktapunarnava [India (*B. diffusa*)]; ufi viole [Samoa (*B. repens*)]; urpa, tar vine [Australia (*B. coccinea*)]; wila k'ullu [Aymara (*B. coccinea*)].

NOMENCLATURE:
- Linnaeus named *Boerhavia* after his friend Hermann Boerhaave (1668 - 1738), a Danish botany professor.
- The specific epithet *diffusa* means "spreading" and coccinea means "dark red."
- The Chinese name for the genus *Boerhavia* is huang xi xin, which means "yellow thin heart." Another Chinese name for *B. diffusa* is huang shou dan, which means "yellow long life pill." The character "dan" implies a "long life" substance.

FAMILY: Nyctaginaceae.

CATEGORY: Invigorate blood (*B. diffusa* / *B. repens*).

PROPERTIES: Bitter, cool~.

PLANT PART USED: The whole plant.

TOXICITY: The toxicity of *Boerhavia* spp. in mammals is inconclusive. One study reported the LD50 of root extract injected into mice to be 1 g/kg [Taylor 1988]. Other studies reported no toxicity in orally in mice at 2-5 g / kg [Chandan 1991; Hiruma-Lima 2000]. Yet another study reported renal tubular karyomegaly and myocardial degeneration in mice after injection with constituents from *B. diffusa* [Wrench 1999].

CAUTIONS AND CONTRAINDICATIONS: Numerous unreferenced sources report that the roots contain punarnavine, an alkaloid that reportedly increases urination and blood pressure, but this could not be confirmed through published papers.

PREPARATION OF MEDICINE: Infused, decocted, poulticed.

DOSAGE: 10 grams in combination.

STATUS IN HAWAI'I: *B. coccinea* is alien in Hawai'i. *B. glabrata* and *B. repens* (*B. diffusa*) are indigenous, and *B. herbstii* is endemic.

WESTERN FUNCTIONS REPORTED: **Abortifacient; alterative; analgesic; anthelmintic; antiamoebic; antibacterial; anticonvulsant; antidiuretic; antifibrinolytic; anti-inflammatory; antispasmodic; antiviral; aphrodisiac; appetite stimulant; appetizer; cholagogue; choleretic; depurative; diaphoretic; diuretic; emetic in large doses; emmenagogue; expectorant; febrifuge; hemostatic; hepatoprotective; hepatotonic; hypotensive; immunomodulator; lactagogue; laxative; menstrual regulator; promotes vomiting; purgative; purifies the blood; rejuvenative; stomachic; tonic; vermifuge.**

TRADITIONAL CHINESE ENERGETIC FUNCTIONS:

B. diffusa (*B. repens*):

1) Moves blood and breaks up stasis.
2) Strengthens tendons and bones.
3) Regulates menses.
4) Clears out infantile malnutrition.

OTHER ENERGETIC FUNCTIONS: Some sources state that punarnava (*B. diffusa*) is tonic (rasayana) for all organs and tissues, calming for all three doshas. Others claim it is rejuvenating for kapha.

Alena Common Medicinal Uses

- Musculoskeletal or trauma pain
- Liver disorders
- Kidney, bladder problems
- Menstrual pain

Alena Cross-Cultural Medicinal Uses

BITES & STINGS

- **Rat bites** [India (root)].
- **Scorpion sting** [Pakistan (*B. procutribens*)].
- **Snake bite** (*B. diffusa*) [Brazil, India, Nepal (root)].

CARDIOVASCULAR

- **Albuminuria** [Brazil (*B. diffusa*)].
- **Anemia** [India (*B. diffusa* roots), Nepal (*B. diffusa* root), Pakistan (*B. procutribens*)].
- **Congestive heart failure**, **heart disease** [India (*B. diffusa*)]; **chest pain** [Nepal (*B. diffusa* root & leaves), India (root decocted)].
- **Hypertension** [Brazil (*B. diffusa*)].

DERMATOLOGICAL

- **Boils** [Nigeria (*B. diffusa*)].
- **Erysipelas** [Guatemala (*B. diffusa*)]; **skin diseases** [India (root)].

DIGESTIVE

- **Constipation** [India (*B. diffusa*), Nigeria (*B. diffusa*)].
- **Flatulence** [Iran (*B. diffusa*)].
- **Hemorrhoids** [India (*B. diffusa* root decocted), Nepal (*B. diffusa* root & leaves)].
- **Indigestion** [India (*B. diffusa*), Pakistan (*B. procutribens*)].
- **Low appetite** [China (*B. diffusa* root), Iran (*B. diffusa*)].
- **Stomach ache** [Pakistan (*B. procutribens*)].

ENDOCRINE

- **Kidney damage from chronic diabetes** [India (*B. diffusa*)].

HEAD AND THROAT

- **Cataracts**, **eye diseases** [India (*B. diffusa*)].
- **Toothache** [Hawai'i (*B. repens*)].

HEPATIC

" *(B. hirsuta)... a plant medicine of great importance, extraordinarily beneficial in the treatment of liver disorders.*"

-- G. L. Cruz

- **Jaundice** [Brazil (*B. diffusa* roots), India (*B. diffusa* roots), Iran (*B. diffusa*), Nepal (*B. diffusa* root), Pakistan (*B. diffusa*, *B. procutribens*)]; **liver cirrhosis** [Brazil (*B. diffusa*)]; **hepatitis** [Brazil (*B. diffusa* roots)].
- **Gall stones** [Brazil (*B. diffusa* roots)].
- **Chronic alcoholism** [India (root)].

IMMUNITY

- **Hives** [Iran (*B. diffusa*)].

INFECTION

- **Abscess** [Nigeria (*B. diffusa*)].
- **Fever** [India (*B. diffusa*), Nigeria (*B. diffusa*)].

LYMPHATIC

- **Enlarged spleen** [Brazil (*B. diffusa*), India (*B. diffusa*), Pakistan (*B. procutribens*)].

MUSCULOSKELETAL / TRAUMA

- **Gout** [Nepal (*B. diffusa*)].
- **Pain and soreness** [China (*B. diffusa* root), Pakistan (*B. procutribens*)]; **joint pain** [Bolivia (*B. coccinea* infused), India (*B. diffusa* roots decocted), Iran (*B. diffusa*), Nepal (*B. diffusa* root & leaves)]; **low back / leg pain**[China (*B. diffusa* root), Iran (*B. diffusa*)].
- **External swellings** [India (root decocted), Pakistan (*B. procutribens*)].

NEUROLOGICAL

- **Epilepsy**, **convulsions** [Nigeria (*B. diffusa*)].
- **Nervous system disorders** [India (root)].

ONCOLOGY

- **Abdominal cancer** [India (*B. diffusa*)].
- **Malignant tumors** [Pakistan (*B. procutribens*), Sri Lanka (*B. diffusa*)].

PARASITES

- **Parasites** [India (*B. diffusa*)].
- **Cholera** [India (*B. diffusa*)].
- **Guinea worms** [Brazil (*B. diffusa*), Guatemala (*B. diffusa*), India (*B. diffusa*), Nigeria (*B. diffusa*), Tropics (*B. diffusa* boiled roots poulticed), West Africa (*B. diffusa*)].
- **Round worms** [Nepal (*B. diffusa* root)].

- **Scabies** [Pakistan (*B. procutribens*)].

Numerous unreferenced sources report that the roots of Alena contain punarnavine, an alkaloid that reportedly increases urination and blood pressure, but this could not be confirmed through published papers.

PEDIATRIC

- **Childhood diseases** [Samoa (*B. repens*)].
- **Infantile malnutrition** [China (*B. diffusa* root)].

PSYCHOSPIRITUAL

- **Insomnia** [India (root)].
- **Hysterical paralysis** [Bolivia (infused) (*B. coccinea*)].

REPRODUCTIVE

- **Anemia in pregnancy** [India]; **childbirth** [India (*B. diffusa*)]; **hastens delivery** [Pakistan (*B. procutribens*)]; **hemorrhage due to childbirth** [India (*B. diffusa*)].
- **Pain from venereal disease** [Bolivia (infused) (*B. coccinea*)]; **gonorrhea** [India (*B. diffusa* roots decocted), Iran (*B. diffusa*)].
- **Menstrual problems** [India (*B. diffusa* roots)]; **irregular menstruation** [West Africa (*B. diffusa*)]; **excessive menstrual bleeding** (red stems) [Nepal (*B. diffusa*), West Africa (*B. diffusa*)]; **painful menses** [China (*B. diffusa* root)].
- **Low sex drive** [West Africa (*B. diffusa*)].
- **Vaginal discharge** [China (*B. diffusa* root)].

RESPIRATORY

- **Asthma** [India (*B. diffusa* root decocted), Nepal (*B. diffusa* root & leaves), Nigeria (*B. diffusa*), Pakistan (*B. procutribens*)].
- **Cough** [India (*B. diffusa* root), Nepal (*B. diffusa* root & leaves)]; **coughing blood** (red stems) [Nepal (*B. diffusa*)].

URINARY

- **Bladder infections** [Brazil (*B. diffusa* roots)]; **scanty urine** [Nepal (*B. diffusa* root)]; **urethritis** [India (*B. diffusa* root)]; **urinary abscess** [Brazil (*B. diffusa*)].
- **Edema** [Brazil (*B. diffusa*), India (*B. diffusa* root decocted), Iran (*B. diffusa* root), Nepal (*B. diffusa* root & leaves)]; **ascites** [India (*B. diffusa*), Nepal (*B. diffusa* root)].
- **Nephritis** [Brazil (*B. diffusa* roots), Iran (*B. diffusa*)]; **kidney stones** [Brazil (*B. diffusa* roots), India (*B. diffusa* roots), Nepal (*B. diffusa*)].

VETERINARY

- *B. diffusa* **may cause trunk paralysis in elephants**.

OTHER MEDICINAL USES

- **Abdominal pain** [India (*B. diffusa*)]; **internal pain & inflammation** [India (*B. diffusa* roots decocted), Nepal (*B. diffusa* root), Pakistan (*B. procutribens*)].
- **Debility**, **wasting diseases** [India (*B. diffusa* root)].
- **Hernia** [India (root decocted), Nepal (*B. diffusa* root & leaves)].
- **"Impure blood"** [India (root decocted), Nepal (*B. diffusa* root & leaves)].
- **Sequelae** (aftermath) **of polio** [China (*B. diffusa* root)].
- **Vitamin B1 deficiency** (beri-beri) [Brazil (*B. diffusa*)].

USE AS FOOD:

- Because of the possibility of calcium oxalate crystals in *Boerhavia* spp., alena should always be cooked before any use.
- The seeds can be ground and added to baked goods.
- The roots of *B. diffusa* are baked, skinned, and eaten in Australia and Fiji.

OTHER USES:
Sticky leaves used as flypaper [Hopi (*B. erecta*)].

CONSTITUENTS: (in some species of *Boerhavia*)
Alanine, arachidic acid, aspartic acid, behenic acid, boeravinone, boerhavic acid, borhavine, borhavone, calcium oxalate crystals (roots of *B. diffusa* & *B. erecta*), campesterol, daucosterol, ecdysone, flavones, galactose, glutamic acid, glutamine, glycine, hentriacontane, heptadecyclic acid, histidine, hypoxanthine, liriodendrin, oleaic acid, oxalic acid, palmitic acid, phlobaphens, potassium nitrate, proline, punarnavine (diuretic), reducing sugars, saponins (*B. coccinea*, *B. diffusa*, *B. erecta*), serine, sitosterols, stearic acid, stigmasterol, syringaresinol, tannins (*B. coccinea*, *B. diffusa*, *B. erecta*), threonine, triacontan, ursolic acid, valine.

POSSIBLE DRUG INTERACTIONS: One source listed possible potentiation with ACE inhibitors, alpha adrenergic, or cardiac depressant medications [Taylor 1998], but this could not be confirmed through published papers.

Alena
Local Combinations

Menstrual / musculoskeletal pain: Add *Piper methysticum* ('awa / kava).
Edema or bladder infection: Add *Taraxacum officinale* (dandelion / laulele).

Alena
Cross-Cultural Combinations

Febrile dysentery: With anise [Bolivia (*B. coccinea*)].
Digestive problems: *B. diffusa* (alena) with *Morinda citrifolia* (noni) fruit [Hawai'i].

RANGE: Africa, Asia, Central America. *B. coccinea* is native to the Caribbean. *B. diffusa* is native to Hawai'i and Brazil.

GATHERING: When gathering alena, the seeds stick to everything.

RESEARCH (all on *B. diffusa*):
- *Boerhavia* has no abortive or teratogenic effects in rats [Singh 1991].
- Reduces pain in mice [Hiruma-Lima 2000].
- Antiamoebic in rats [Sohni 1995].
- Alcohol and water extracts are liver protective in lab animals [Chandan 1991; Rawat 1997].
- Ethanol extract of roots may be immunosupressive [Mehrotra 2002].

NOTES 'N QUOTES
- In India, the roots of *Boerhavia diffusa* are considered to increase longevity ("Rasayana").

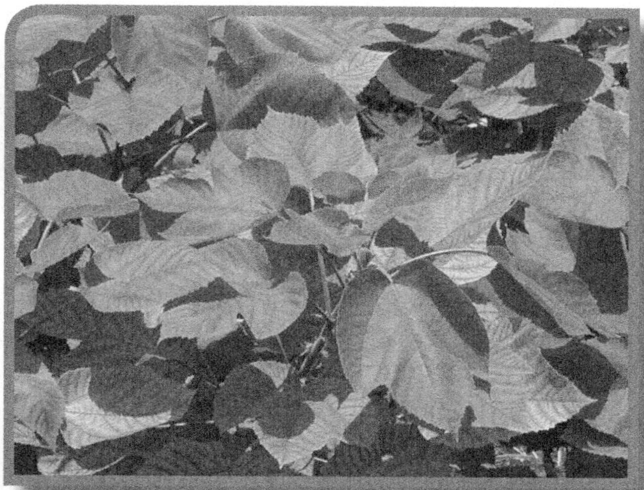

Broussonetia papyrifera (Wauke)

PLANT NAME: *Broussonetia papyrifera* (L.) Venten.

COMMON NAMES: **Wauke**, po'a'aha [Hawai'i]; paper mulberry [USA]; u'a [Samoa]; chu (whole plant), chu shi zi (fruit), gu shi (fruit), chu tao (fruit) [China]; kajinoki [Japan].

Status: Polynesian introduction

Habitat: Wet and sunny

NOMENCLATURE: The genus is named after P. M. Auguste Broussonet (1761-1807), a French naturalist. The epithet "*papyrifera*" means "paper bearing."

FAMILY: Moraceae (Fig family).

CATEGORY: Cool the blood ~ (leaves).

PROPERTIES: **Fruit**: sweet and cold. **Leaves**: sweet and cool. **Root cortex**: sweet and neutral.

PLANT PART USED: Fruit, leaves, bark, cortex, sap, stems. In China, the fruit is primarily used as medicine. **In Hawai'i this plant does not fruit.**

CAUTIONS AND CONTRAINDICATIONS: Prolonged use is reported to weaken the bones.

DOSAGE: Use 9-15 grams.

STATUS IN HAWAI'I: Polynesian introduction ("politically correct" alien). An aggressive pest in more than ten countries, including the US, wauke has minimal pest factor in Hawai'i. It has rich significance as a heritage plant in Polynesian societies.

MERIDIAN AFFINITIES: Spleen, liver, kidneys ~.

WESTERN FUNCTIONS REPORTED: **Antidiarrheal** (leaves); **anti-swelling** (sap); **astringent**; **diaphoretic** (leaf **juice**); **diuretic** (fruit); **galactogogue**; **hemostatic** (leaves, stembark); **insecticidal** (sap); **lactogogue** (root); **laxative** (leaf juice); **ophthalmic** (fruit); **reduces swelling** [China]; **stimulant** (fruit); **stomachic** (fruit); **tonic** (fruit); **vulnerary** (latex).

TRADITIONAL CHINESE ENERGETIC FUNCTIONS (~ = extrapolated):

Plant

1) Clears heat and cools the blood.
2) Drains dampness.
3) Clears damp heat in the middle and lower burners.
4) Stops diarrhea.
5) Nourishes the Liver and Kidneys.

Fruit

1) Strengthens joints.
2) Promotes absorption.
3) Drains damp.
4) Nourishing to the eyes.

Wauke Common Medicinal Uses

- **Skin problems**
- **Reproductive problems**

Wauke Cross-Cultural Medicinal Uses

CARDIOVASCULAR

- **Blood deficiency**, **vertigo** [China (fruit)]; leaves for **blood in sputum**, **vomiting blood**, **wound bleeding** [China].

DERMATOLOGICAL

- Stems used for **skin eruptions**, **neurodermatitis**, **tinea infection**, **eczema** [China (latex)].

DIGESTIVE

- Stops **diarrhea**, **abdominal distention** [China]; leaves also used for **dysentery, enteritis** [China].
- Leaves infused for **stomach and abdominal pain** [Samoa].
- Sap as a **laxative** [Hawai'i].

HEAD AND THROAT

- **Weak vision, nourishing to the eyes** [China (fruit)].

INFECTION

- Sap **removes pus** [China].

MUSCULOSKELETAL / TRAUMA

- **Weakness of joints and muscle** [China (cortex)].

PEDIATRIC

- The ashes of burned kapa were used in treating **thrush** [Hawai'i].

PSYCHOSPIRITUAL

- Wauke was believed to have **psychic or magical powers**.
- The Apache used wauke **as a narcotic** and **wore the seeds around their neck during ceremonies**.

REPRODUCTIVE

- **Impotence** [China (fruit)] "Leaves are astringent in "**fluxes**" and **gonorrhea**." [China]; **uterine bleeding, excess menstrual bleeding** [China].
- Kapa was worn around the neck of nursing mothers to **induce the flow of milk** [Hawai'i].

URINARY

- Bark decocted for **ascites** [China]; **edema** [China (fruit or cortex)]; juice used for **lack of urination** [China].

OTHER MEDICINAL USES

- **Debility of the loins and knees**, [China (fruit)]; **bee sting** [China (latex)]; **insect bites** [China (latex)].

USE AS FOOD: Edible fruit, but none in Hawai'i. Flowers and leaves are also said to be edible.

OTHER USES:

- "Wauke" is the name of the plant *Broussonetia papyrifera*, and "kapa" is the traditional cloth that is made from it.
- The leaves of wauke (called kaijioki in Japan) are used as paper on which poems are written during the summer Tanabata festival.
- The juice is used as glue.
- Sometimes used as cordage in Hawai'i.
- Wood is sometimes used for cups and bowls.

CONSTITUENTS: Benzofurans, biphenylpropanoids, coumarins, flavonoids (chalcones, flavans, flavanones, and flavones).

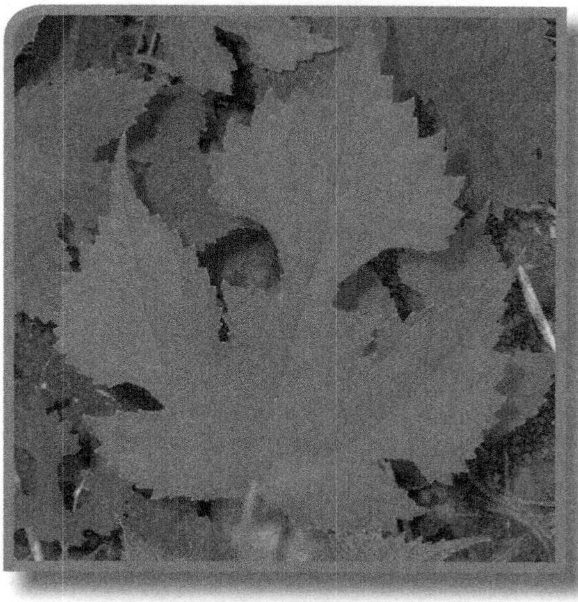

Broussonetia papyrifera: Wauke
young leaves

Wauke
Local Combinations

Skin eruptions: Add *Morus alba* (sang ye / mulberry) leaves, *Trifolium pratense* (red clover) and *Plantago* spp. (laukahi / plantain).
Excess menstrual bleeding: Add *Eclipta prostrata* (han lian cao).

RANGE: Native to China and Japan. The historical spread of *Broussonetia papyrifera* can be traced along known migration routes.

HABITAT: Edge of stream and lo'i (taro fields). Wet and sunny. Can tolerate partial shade.

GATHERING: In Asia, the plant flowers in May. Ripe fruit is collected and washed in fall. Cortex, latex, and bark are gathered all year round. Leaves are gathered fall and summer. The serrated lobed leaves are easily identifiable and have a coarse "sand-paper" texture.

PROPAGATION & CULTIVATION: By seed in China, by cuttings or root cutting in Hawai'i. *Broussonetia papyrifera* is a dioecious (each plant is an individual gender) shrub or tree. In Hawai'i it appears mostly as a tall shrub, but in Asia there are wauke plants up to 50' high. Germination 2 - 3 weeks.

RESEARCH: Broussochalcone A, a constituent of *Broussonetia papyrifera* is a potent antioxidant [Cheng 2001].

NOTES 'N QUOTES

- In 105 A.D., a man named Ts'ai Lun made the first paper from *Broussonetia papyrifera* in China.
- According to Li Zishen the character "chu" originallly meant "to make a textile from the skin."
- In Hawaiian mythology, the moon goddess Hina was unable to dry her kapa because the Sun moved too quickly across the sky. So her son, the demigod Māui, climbed to the top of Haleakalā and captured the Sun with rope made from his grandmother's hair. Māui refused to release the Sun until he agreed to move more slowly across the heavens.
- The best kapa in Hawai'i was considered "Po'a'aha" which had a softer texture than others. Since Hawaiian malo (loincloths) were made from kapa and kapa can be notoriously abrasive, I imagine this was a popular item.
- Although tapa (kapa) production thrives in Samoa, in Hawai'i it almost became extinct. Hawaiian kapa making was at one time the best in the Pacific, but the details of the Hawaiians' superlative kapa skills were lost to antiquity. The kapa-making process was single handedly revived by a remarkable and tenacious woman named Pua Van-Dorpe. Working with only the slimmest fragments of ancient information, she did experiments for years involving countless hours of trial and error, and succeeded in rediscovering the lost art of kapa making which she now shares with others.

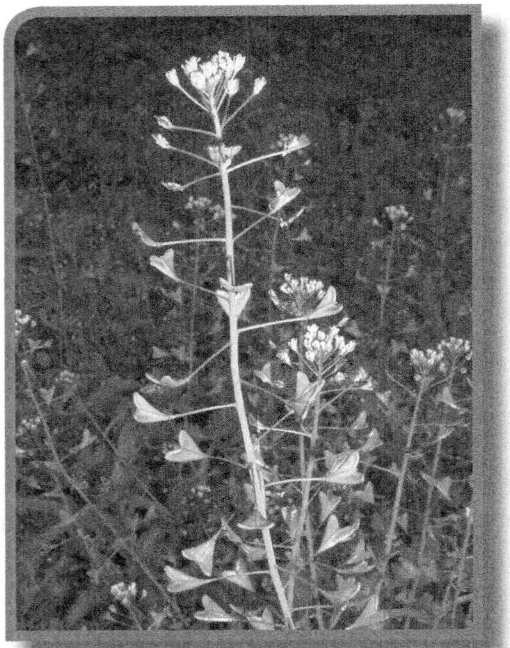

Capsella rubella (Shepherds Purse)

PLANT NAME: *Capsella rubella* Reut.

SIMILARLY USED SPECIES: *Bursa bursa-pastoris; Bursa gracilis; Bursa rubella; Capsella bursa pastoris; Thlaspi bursa-pastoris; Sanguinaria.*

Status: Alien. Low pest factor

Habitat: Everywhere

COMMON NAMES: **Shepherds purse** [USA]; **di mi cai**, ji cai, hu sheng cao ("life-protecting grass") [China]; borsa de pastor [Spanish]; borsa a pastore [Italy]; bourse de pasteur [France]; clappedepouch [Ireland]; hirtentasche, hirtenfaschel [Germany]; mother's heart [Scotland]; pastushya sumka [Russia].

NOMENCLATURE: *Brassica*, the root of the family name, is the Latin name for "cabbage." *Capsella* means, "little box" in Latin, a reference to the fruit. The common name "shepherds purse" derives from the appearance of its flat seed pouch, which resembles a leather purse once carried by shepherds.
The Irish name "clappedepouch" is a reference to the begging habits of Irish victims of Hansen's disease (leprosy). The seedpods are said to resemble the bags that they would hang at the end of a long begging pole. They could be seen begging along the road while ringing their bell or "clapper".

FAMILY: Brassicaceae (mustard family).

CATEGORY: Stop bleeding~.

PROPERTIES: Sweet bland neutral.

PLANT PART USED: All of it, but especially aerial parts.

TOXICITY: Unknown.

CAUTIONS AND CONTRAINDICATIONS:
- Never treat bleeding without first determining its cause.
- Not in thromboembolism, history of stroke, phlebitis.
- Not for children under 2 years old.
- Not during pregnancy or while nursing. In Western medicine, oxytocin is used to induce labor, and *Capsella* is an oxytocin synergist [Michael Moore].
- Use under supervision with acute kidney inflammation or high blood pressure.
- Topical use of seeds can cause skin blistering.
- May cause heart palpitations in large doses.

PREPARATION OF MEDICINE: It is better to be prepared fresh, but can be frozen or tinctured for later use. While some tinctures have a shelf life lasting (possibly) decades, some practitioners tincture *Capsella* fresh every year. **Tincture**: (Whole fresh plant, 1:2, recently dried plant, 1:5, 50% alcohol). **Juiced**: 1:1 in 25% alcohol (enough to keep it stable).

DOSAGE: **Infusion**: 1-2 teaspoonfuls of the dried or fresh herb in a cup of water, 3 - 5 times a day. (Or, if you are Chinese, 1-2 ounces decocted). For menstrual problems, it should be taken just prior to the onset of menses, every 2-3 hours. **Tincture**: 1/2 teaspoon, 3 - 5 times a day.

WESTERN FUNCTIONS REPORTED: **Abortifacient**; **analgesic**; **anthelmintic** (seed pods infused); **antidiarrheal** (infused or decocted); **anti-hemorrhagic**; **antihypertensive**; **anti-inflammatory**; **antineoplastic**; **antipyretic**; **antiscorbutic**; **antiseptic**; **astringent**; **blood cleanser**; **bradycardic**; **cardiotonic**; **central nervous system-depressant**; **coagulant**; **contraceptive**; **dermatological aid**; **detergent**; **diuretic**; **emmenagogue**; **expectorant**; **eye problems**; **febrifuge**; **flux**; **gastrointestinal aid**; **hemostatic**; **hypotensive**; **improves the vision**; **insect repellant**; **kidney**; **laxative**; **liver**; **oxytocic**; **parasiticide**; **pile**; **post-partum**; **reduces swellings**; **refrigerant**; **rubefacient** (seeds); **sedative**; **smooth-muscle stimulant**; **stimulant**; **stops vomiting**; **styptic**; **tonic**; **urinary antiseptic**; **uterine stimulant**; **vasoconstrictor & vasodilator** (regulates blood presssure); **vermifuge**; **vesicant** (seeds); **vulnerary**… and it washes your car….

TRADITIONAL CHINESE ENERGETIC FUNCTIONS (~ = extrapolated):

1) Cools the blood, stop bleeding.
2) Clears damp heat.
3) Harmonizes the spleen.
4) Drains damp.
5) Brightens the eyes.

Shepherds Purse Common Medicinal Uses

- **Menstrual and urinary bleeding**
- **Labor**
- **Gout**
- **Urinary tract infection**

Shepherds Purse Cross-Cultural Medicinal Uses

COSMETIC

- **Varicose veins** [USA].

CARDIOVASCULAR

- **General bleeding**, (including passive bleeding from mucous membranes) [China, Iraq, Scotland, Scotland, USA]; **any bloody diarrhea or dysentery** [China, Chippewa, Costanoan, Eclectic, Russia].
- **General digestive problems or stomach pain** (infused or decocted) [China, Chippewa (decocted), Mohegan (seed pods infused), Russia]; **weak digestion with discomfort** [Eclectic].
- **Gastritis, gastric or duodenal inflammation** [China, Russia]; **bleeding ulcers** [Russia (with vodka)]; **vomiting blood** [China].
- **Small intestine inflammation** [China].
- **Hemorrhoids**, **bleeding hemorrhoids** [Eclectics, USA (decocted fresh)].
- **Scurvy** [Turkey].

HEAD AND THROAT

"*The juice dropped into ears, heals the pains, noise and matterings thereof. A good ointment may be made of it for all wounds, especially wounds in the head.*"

- - Nicholas Culpepper

- **Eye problems** [China]; **ophthalmia or sore eyes** [China].
- **Ear ache**; **ringing in the ears**.
- The juice can be put on cotton and applied topically for **nose bleeds** or the plant can be brewed and taken as a tea [Eclectic].
- **Headache** [Cheyenne (cold infusion), Chippewa (leaves and stems infused)].

HEPATIC

" *… being bound to the wrists of the hands, and the soles of the feet, it helps the yellow jaundice.*"

- - Nicholas Culpepper

- **Liver problems** [China].
- **Jaundice** [Scotland].

INFECTION

- **Fevers, including malarial fever** [China, Russia]; **infections**; **sores** [China].

MUSCULOSKELETAL / TRAUMA

- **Gout** (for uric acid elevation); **arthritis or rheumatic joint pain** (topical) [Eclectic];
- **Bruises and strains** (topically) [Eclectic]; **swelling** [Asia]; **wounds and burns.**

ONCOLOGY

- **Cancer** [Italy, Poland].

PARASITES

- **Worms** (seed pods or flowers infused) [Mohegan, China].
- Shepherds Purse has been used as a **quinine substitute for malaria**.

PEDIATRIC

- **Bedwetting** [Native American].

PSYCHOSPIRITUAL

"*It is under the dominion of Saturn, and of a cold, dry, and binding nature, like to him.*"

- - Nicholas Culpepper

REPRODUCTIVE

"*It helps all fluxes (discharges) of blood, either caused by inward or outward wounds; as also flux of the belly, and bloody flux, spitting blood, and bloody urine, stops the terms in women.*"

- - Nicholas Culpepper

- As a menstrual regulator, it calms **excessive menstrual flow** and brings on suppressed menstruation.
- Traditionally **used before birth** (after the cervix is dilated). It **promotes uterine contractions** and can

address **bleeding after childbirth** [China, Europe, USA]. **Spotting during pregnancy**.

- **PMS**; **menstrual pain** [China, Eclectic, Spain]; **inflammed uterus** [China].
- **Abnormal uterine bleeding**, **excess menstrual bleeding** (too frequent or too long) [China, Eclectic]; **uterine hemorrhage**; **spotting** [China].
- **Constant**, **clear discharge** [Eclectic]; **venereal disease** [Russia]... although probably not your first choice in treatment options.
- **Vicarious menses** (a discharge of blood from a place other than the uterus, usually caused by endometriosis)
- Used as a **contraceptive** (*not* recommended).

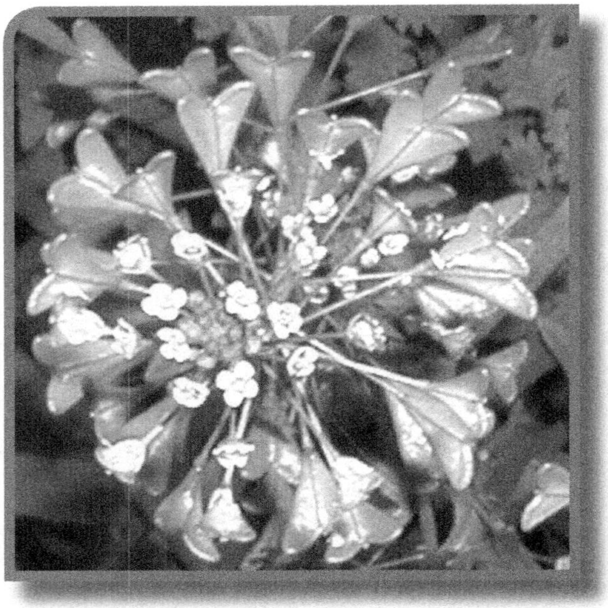

Capsella rubella
Shepherds Purse flowering tops

RESPIRATORY

- **Common cold** [China].
- **Chest congestion**
- **Coughing blood** (including tuberculosis) [China, Russia, USA].

URINARY

"*In urinary derangements of renal or cystic origin, and in hematuria, an infusion, and especially a tincture of the herb, will be found very efficient.*"

- - Kings Dispensatory

- **Acute bladder infections** (with or without blood in urine), **painful urination** (decocted fresh) [China, Eclectic, Scotland, USA]; **urinary tract infections with bladder abscess or phosphates in the urine** [Eclectic]; **"sandy sediment" or fat in the urine** [China]; **"honeymoon cystitis."**
- Shepherds Purse is used as a specific for **blood in urine** due to kidney tuberculosis [China].
- **Edema, water retention due to kidney problems, kidney inflammation** [China, Eclectics, Russia].

VETERINARY

- Decocted with milk to stop **diarrhea in calves** [England].
- Shepherds purse reportedly can be tasted in the milk of cows that eat it. When hens eat the herb freely their eggs develop a stronger flavor and the yolks take on an olive green hue.
- The seeds are used as bird food.

OTHER MEDICINAL USES

- **Typhus** (in vodka) [Russia].
- **Scurvy** [Scotland].

USE AS FOOD:

- Humans have used Shepherds Purse as a food for at least 8000 years. Seeds have been recovered from "Catal Huyuk" in Turkey (ca. 5950 B.C.E.) and from the stomach of the "Tollund Man" (ca. 500 B.C.E.–400 B.C.E.).
- The young leaves, with their peppery flavor, can be used in salads or cooked like spinach. The leaves should be gathered before the plant flowers. They get spicier with age. Native American tribes used Shepherds Purse as a potherb or cooked it with meat. The Apache and Mescalero ground the seeds into flour and made them into bread, or just used the ground seeds as a condiment. They are actually quite tasty. The seedpods add a nice touch when used in soups.
- Poor people of ancient China and Russia ate the seeds as food. The roots can be used as a "ginger substitute" (fresh or dried).

OTHER USES:

- Used in soil reclamation and as an insecticide. Shepherds purse was called "life protect plant" in China because it was thought to drive away mosquitoes. Indeed, the seeds (when placed in water) are reported to act as a sort of "fly-paper" for mosquitoes, reputedly attracting and trapping them. They are also said to secrete a substance toxic to mosquito larvae. A kilo of *Capsella* seeds is said to be capable of killing 10 million mosquito larvae.
- Shepherds Purse may one day be used as a "canary" to monitor heavy metal pollution in urban areas, as it absorbs pollution. Because of this, it is important not to wild-craft plants that may be contaminated.

ESSENTIAL OIL: An edible oil similar to mustard oil can be extracted. The seed is 35% oil.

CONSTITUENTS: Acetylcholine, amines, bursic acid, calcium, camphor, choline, citric acid, fumaric &

bursic acids, glucosinolates (sinigrin), histamine, iron, luteolin 7-galactoside, luteolin-7-rutinoside & quercitin-3-rutinoside, mustard oil, niacin, phosphorus, polypeptides, potassium salts, proline, quercetin 7-rutinosides, riboflavin, saponins, tannin, thiamine, tyramine, vitamin A, vitamin C, volatile oils (including camphor).

- A peptide (proline) may be responsible for Shepherds Purse's use in bleeding.
- Acetylcholine, tyramine, and choline have also been shown to stop bleeding and lower blood pressure.
- The flavonoids have an anti-inflammatory action and the tannins are astringent.
- The polypeptides may stimulate uterine contractions.

POSSIBLE DRUG INTERACTIONS: May antagonize anti-coagulants such as Coumadin or Dicoumarol. (Speculative).

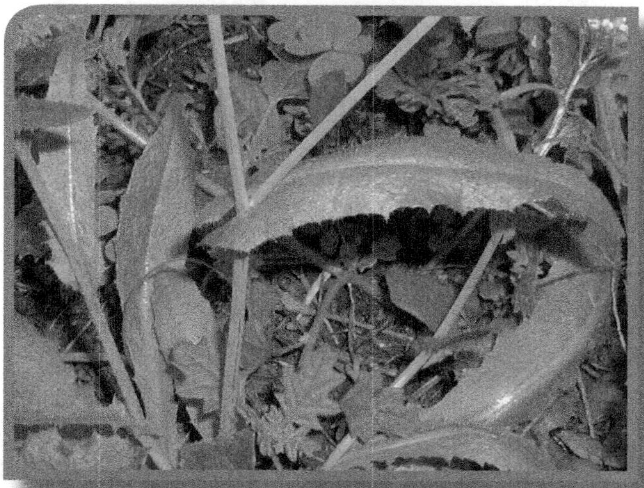

Capsella rubella
Shepherds Purse leaf attachment

Shepherds Purse Local Combinations

Varicose veins: Add *Centella asiatica* (pohe kula / gotu kola).
Gout: Add *Bidens pilosa* (kīnehi / spanish needle).
GI bleeding: Add *Erigeron canadensis* (fleabane).

Shepherds Purse Cross-Cultural Combinations

For bleeding: With agrimony or cranesbill.
For painful menses or spotting: With *Hydrastis* (goldenseal).
For abnormal uterine bleeding: With *Geranium maculatum* (astringent) and *Senecio aureus* (uterine tonic) [David Hoffman].
During labor: With *Gossypium* spp. (cotton root bark tincture) during labor (taken after the cervix is mostly dialated). 1 part *Capsella* to 2 parts *Gossypium*) [USA].
For kidney tuberculosis: Decocted with egg [China].
For urinary infections and edema: With couch grass [Eclectics].
For bedwetting: With agrimony [Native American].

RANGE: Native to Europe. Globally pandemic. The Pilgrims introduced Shepherds Purse to the New World.

GATHERING: Gather when seedpods are visible.

PROPAGATION & CULTIVATION: Sometimes cultivated in India. Please do not cultivate in Hawai'i, help us restore our native ecosystems. Flowers are hermaphrodite (have both male and female organs). When cultivating, the leaves can be harvested repeatedly and the plants will go to seed rapidly.

RESEARCH:
- Contains vitamin K [HerbMed].
- Contains fumaric acid that reduces cancerous tumors in mice [Kuroda 1976].
- Oxytocin synergist [Michael Moore] and causes uterine contractions [Shipochliev 1981]. In China, Shepherds purse has been ranked 7th amongst 250 potential birth control plants [Duke 1985].
- Liver protective in rats with chemically induced hepatocarcinoma [Kuroda 1975; Kuroda 1976].
- Extracts of *Capsella* are antibacterial and antifungal [El-Abyad1990].
- Clinical trials have been inconclusive. It has been theorized that a white fungus that sometimes grows on the plant is perhaps a medically active ingredient.

NOTES 'N QUOTES

And again, from old "Saint Nick" (Nicholas Culpepper): "*Few plants possess greater virtues than this, and yet it is utterly disregarded.*"

"*Widespread, common... and always hard to find when you want some.*"
- - Michael Moore

- Grown on salt marshes to reclaim the soil.

- In Japan *Capsella* is included in a ceremonial rice and barley dish that is eaten on January 7th.
- Shepherds purse is reputed to be the main herb in a mysterious blue "Electric Fluid" used by "Count Matthei" for bleeding.
- *Capsella bursa-pastoris* has been found to be a useful bio-monitor of heavy metal pollution in urban areas.
- Do not store the dried herb for longer than one year, as it loses its' potency. Because it warrants wild crafting and ideally should be dropped fresh into combination with other herbs, I don't use it as much as I might like.

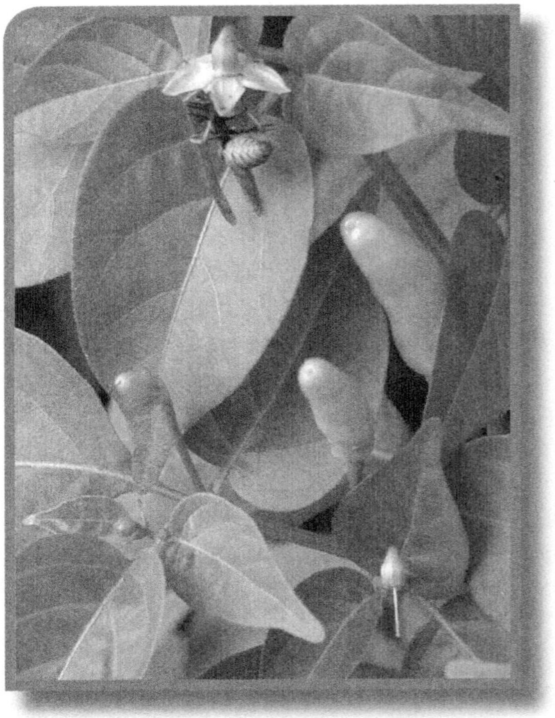

Capsicum spp. (Nīoi)

PLANT NAME: *Capsicum* spp.

SIMILARLY USED SPECIES: *Capsicum annum; C. annuum; C. baccatum; C. cerasiforme; C. chinense; C. chlorocladum; C. cordiforme; C. frutescens; C. frytescens; C. grossum; C. hispidum; C. longum; C. microcarpum.; C. minimum; C. pubescens.*

Status: Alien. Low pest factor.

Habitat: Hot, dry, and sunny.

COMMON NAMES: **Nīoi** [Hawai'i]; **cayenne**, paprika, sweet pepper, tabasco pepper, red bird pepper, africa pepper, cockspur pepper, goat's pepper [English]; aji, chile [Panama, Peru]; caja, kapur, rocoto [Cuna (Panama)]; cayennepfeffer [Germany]; hupo'o, 'upo'o [Marquesas]; ic [Ancient Mayans]; khursani [Nepal]; la jiao, zhi tian jiao [China]; locoto [Quechua]; marichi-phalam ("pepper of the sun") [Sanskrit]; mpilipili [Swahili]; oporo [Tahiti]; peberfrugt [Sweden]; pimentao, locoto, aji picante [Spanish]; pimente de cayenne, poivre de guienee [France]; polo feu [Samoa]; polo fifisi [Tonga]; polo mangiho [Niue]; uchu [Quechua]; vavalagi [Fiji]; waik'a [Aymara].

PHARMACEUTICAL NAME: Da Chili Peppa, Brah.

NOMENCLATURE: "Cayenne" is taken from the Greek word "to bite." Other sources claim that the genus name comes from the Latin "cirpsa," meaning a capsule. Only Linnaeus knows for sure.

FAMILY: Solanaceae.

CATEGORY: Herbs that Warm the Interior.

PROPERTIES: Acrid hot [China, India].

PLANT PART USED: Fruit.

TOXICITY:
- Chronic toxic doses have caused eye abnormalities in lab animals due to substance P's reduction of pain and corneal protective reflexes [Agarwal 1985]. This appears to be unrelated to blood levels of vitamin A.
- Capsaicinoids in toxic doses cause hypotension, respiratory failure, and bradycardia [Monsereenusorn 1982]. See *Cautions and Contraindications* below.

CAUTIONS AND CONTRAINDICATIONS:
- "*Bartender... I'll have what he's having.*" Overdose produces vomiting, purging, stomach pain, giddiness, and intoxication [Eclectics] and can cause chronic gastritis, hypothermia, kidney damage, and liver damage [Gruenwald 1998]. Overdose is a rare occurrence if one uses common sense, but common sense may be uncommon.
- Caution in hypoglycemia, liver disorders, kidney disorders, irritable bowel, and hemorrhoids [Kowalchik 1987]. High doses may cause gastroenteritis.
- While counter-intuitive, it is sometimes used under professional supervision for gastric or duodenal ulcers [Kang 1995; Yeoh 1995], although Michael Moore reports it as not appropriate for active inflammation. Capsaicin inhibits *H. pylori* in vitro, but not *E. coli* [Jones 1997].
- It is not known if metabolites of *Capsicum* are secreted in breast milk.
- Topical use can cause dermatitis and blistering. Don't get it in your eyes: *Trust me on this....*

Oncology

- With mounds of conflicting data [Surh 1995(b), 1996, 1998], the jury is still out regarding the relationship of *Capsicum* spp. to various forms of cancer.
- The bad news is that there are many studies linking nīoi to specific cancers [Surh 1996]. Correlations to specific cancers include liver cancer [Agrawal 1986, Jang 1998], stomach cancer [Lopez-Carrillo 1994, Kim 1985], and oral cancers [Notani 1987]. Different organs may have different responses to nīoi [Jang 1991]. There are data implicating *Capsicum* with chromosome breaks [Richeux 1999, Singh 2001], but these may only occur at high doses [Richeux 2000].
- The good news is that there is significant research demonstrating *Capsicum*'s anti-tumor activity [Han 2001; Surh 1995(b), 1996, 1998 & 2000; Park 1997, & 2004; Kim 2004].

ENERGETIC CAUTIONS:
- Not for bleeding due to heat or for dry wind conditions.
- Not in qi deficiency.
- Not in excess heat.
- Caution during pregnancy.

With mounds of conflicting data [Surh 1995(b), 1996, 1998], the jury is still out regarding the relationship of *Capsicum* spp. to various forms of cancer.

PREPARATION OF MEDICINE: Powdered, cooked, infused, decocted, tinctured, juiced, mashed, eaten, and swallowed whole ("Kahan style"). When the peppers are red, cut them off at the stem or pull up the entire plant and hang it up to dry. Powdered cayenne should always be kept in dark.
As with most other herbal remedies, it is often better to use whole plant materials rather than isolated constituents (the whole herb nīoi rather than the chemical derivative capsaicin) [Monsereenusorn 1983].
Tinctured fresh 1:2, 95% alcohol; or dried 1:3, 65% alcohol.

DOSAGE: Used in small doses to warm, in larger doses will cause a cooling effect. Cayenne is a clear example of the Chinese adage "Extreme Yang turns to Yin, Extreme Yin turns to Yang."
Internally: 1 teaspoon in 1 cup water; 400-500 milligrams in capsules; 10-15 drops of tincture.

MERIDIAN AFFINITIES: Liver, Lungs, Stomach.

WESTERN FUNCTIONS REPORTED: **Abortifacient**; **aids in assimilating foods**; **alterative**; **anthelmintic**; **anti-fatigue**; **anti-scorbutic**; **antibacterial** (topical); **antibiotic**; **anticoagulant**; **antidote to poison**; **anti-infective**; **antimicrobial**; **anti rheumatic**; **antiseptic**; **antispasmodic**; **aphrodisiac**; **benefits digestion**; **blood detoxification**; **boosts immunity**; **cardiotonic**; **carminative**; **circulatory stimulant**; **counter-irritant**; **decongestant**; **diaphoretic**; **digestive aid**; ; **expectorant**; **febrifuge**; **gargle**; **hemostatic**; **improves metabolism**;

increases appetite; invigorates blood; irritant; lowers blood pressure; lowers blood sugar; lowers cholesterol; nutritive; opens the chest; opens the nasal passages; promotes sound sleep; psychedelic; purifies blood; regulates blood pressure; relieves gas; relieves pain and inflammation; retards aging; rubefacient; shark repellent; sialagogue; stimulant; stimulates gastric secretion; stimulates endorphins; stimulates saliva; stomachic; tonic; vesicant (*whew!*)

TRADITIONAL CHINESE ENERGETIC FUNCTIONS (~ = extrapolated):

1) Warms the interior.
2) Invigorates blood.
3) Regulates qi.
4) Releases the exterior.
5) Benefits the digestion.

OTHER ENERGETIC FUNCTIONS: increases pitta, reduces kapha and vata.

Nīoi (Cayenne)
Common Medicinal Uses

- **Cold extremities**
- **Poor digestion**
- **Colds and flus**
- **Topical in a cream base for pain**
- **In formulations as an herbal harmonizer**

Nioi (Cayenne) Cross-Cultural Medicinal Uses

BITES & STINGS

- **Snakebite** [Nepal].

COSMETIC

- **Balding**.
- **Dandruff**.

CARDIOVASCULAR

- **Angina pectoris** (with a "cold" presentation) [Eclectics].
- **Arteriosclerosis** (to prevent and ongoing).
- **Stroke and heart disease**.
- **High blood pressure**.
- **Topical for bleeding** [India].
- **Poor circulation** (cream).

DERMATOLOGICAL

- **Burns** [India].
- **Frost bite** (topical) [China (roots), Eclectics].
- **Psoriasis**.
- **Skin inflammation** [Tonga (crushed leaves topical)].

DIGESTIVE

- **"Stomach problems"; abdominal pain & distension with poor absorption** [China, Eclectics, India]; **indigestion** [China, India, Nepal, Trinidad]; **gas** [Eclectics].
- **Nausea**; **low appetite** [China].
- **Enteritis**, **gastritis** [India]; **duodenal ulcers**; **gastric ulcers.**
- **Constipation** [Eclectics].
- **Diarrhea** [Ancient Mayans, Eclectics, Nepal]; **dysentery with blood & mucous** [Eclectics (especially with poor digestion)].

ENDOCRINE

- **Diabetic neuropathy**.
- **Thyroid disorders**.

HEAD & THROAT

- **Mucous membrane inflammation** [Eclectics]; **nasal sinus congestion** [India].
- **Eye pains** [Brazilian Indians (juiced)]; **chronic ophthalmia** [Eclectics]; **"chronic or indolent ulceration of the cornea"** [Eclectics]; **conjunctivitis** [Peru, Tonga]; **poor vision** [South American Indians].
- **Sore throat** (gargle but don't swallow) [Nepal, Trinidad]; **ulcerated throat** [Eclectics (infusion and tincture)]; **hoarseness**, **throat infection** [Eclectics].
- **Headaches** [Philippines]; **episodic cluster headaches and migraines**; **trigeminal neuralgia** (cream topical).
- **Earache** [ancient Mayans], **vertigo**; **relaxed uvula** [Eclectics]; **toothache** (oil topical) [Eclectics].

HEPATIC

- **Liver disorders**; **jaundice** [Tonga].

INFECTION

- **Abscesses** (mashed leaves topical) [Samoa, Tonga].
- **Boils and sores** (fruit or leaves chewed, crushed, or heated, topical) [Cook Islands, India, Panama, Philippines, Samoa, Tahiti, Tonga].
- **Fevers** [Cherokee (topical on the soles of the feet), Jethro Kloss (specific), Nepal, West Indies].

- **Low grade fevers** [Eclectics].
- **Malarial fevers**; **yellow fever**; **cholera** [Eclectic]; **typhus**.

MUSCULOSKELETAL / TRAUMA

- **Osteo or rheumatoid arthritis**, **stiff joints** (topical in a cream) [Eclectics, Physiomedicalists].
- **Inflammation** [Tonga (mashed leaves topical)].
- **Bursitis, shoulder pain.**
- **Carpal tunnel syndrome**.
- **Low back pain**.
- **Tired**, **painful muscles** [Eclectics]; **muscle aches, tension and spasm**; **cramps** [Ancient Mayans].
- **Wounds** (topical and internal use) [Samoa, Tonga].
- **Sprains and bruises.**

NEUROLOGICAL

- **Neuralgia**.
- **Post herpetic neuralgia**; **shingles** (topical in a cream).
- **Paralysis "without organic lesions"** [Eclectics].
- **Senility** (**also to prevent senility** by increasing blood flow to the brain) [USA folk medicine].

ONCOLOGY

- **Carcinoma** [Mongolia].
- **Nasal cancer** [Gabon].
- **Tumors** [Aztec, India, Native American].
- **Epithelioma**.
- **Mouth pain from chemotherapy or radiation.**

PARASITES

- **Parasites** [South America].
- **Worms** [India].

PEDIATRIC

- **Chicken pox**.
- Topical on breast **to wean a child** [Navaho].

PSYCHOSPIRITUAL

- **Depression** [Eclectics, Physiomedicalists].
- **Emotional or personal stagnation: lack of direction, procrastination, resistance to change or growth.**
- Cayenne is burned with cacao in Ailigandi to drive off **evil spirits** & used for **the "evil eye"** in Panama and India. Used in Peruvian **magickal rituals**.
- In India, cayenne is **associated with the third chakra.**

REPRODUCTIVE

- **Delayed menstruation**; [England], **unwanted pregnancy** [Indonesia].
- **Abnormal or passive uterine bleeding**, **uterine hemorrhage**.
- **Gonorrhea** [Samoa].
- **Infertility** [Japan].
- **Prostate problems**.
- **Female orgasm stimulant** (cream).

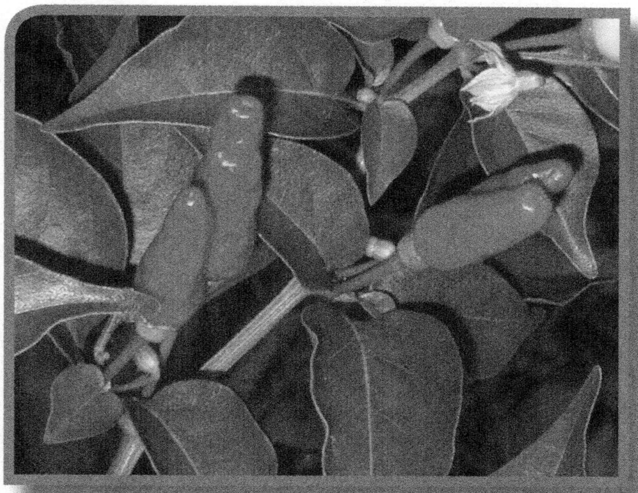

Capsicum spp.: Nīoi fruit

RESPIRATORY

- **Asthma** [Trinidad]; **hay fever**; **respiratory difficulties** [Samoa (crushed leaves or fruit infused)].
- **Common cold** [Cherokee, Eclectics, India, Trinidad]; **influenza**; **coughs** (crushed leaves or fruit infused) [Samoa, Trinidad].
- **Chest congestion** [Samoa]; **bronchitis** [India]; **chronic bronchitis**; **damp mucous conditions of the lungs and colon**; **thick white mucous**.
- **Tuberculosis** [Tonga, Trinidad]; **lungs bleeding.**
- **Emphysema**.
- **Pneumonia**.
- Internally, **protects the lungs from pollution and cigarette smoke** (irritant to mucous membranes if inhaled).

URINARY

- Seeds for **urinary tract infection**; **"yellow urine"** [ancient Mayans], **painful urination** [India].
- **Chronic renal congestion** [Eclectics]; **edema**.

VETERINARY

- **For ticks on cattle** [Ethiopia].

OTHER MEDICINAL USES

- **Alcoholism**; **"atonic dyspepsia of drunkards"** [Eclectics]; **intoxication** [Ifugao (Philippines)]; **hangover**; **delirium tremens** [Eclectics].
- **Pain internally**, **topically**, **and in aromatherapy**. Cayenne triggers endorphins when tasted. In Samoa the leaves are crushed or the fruit is infused. **Pain from breast reconstruction or mastectomy**,

post amputation pain.

- **Chills** [Eclectics, India, Physiomedicalists], **cold extremities, with blanched lips and small, weak pulse** [Eclectics]; **breathlessness** [Samoa]; **debility** [Eclectics]; **fatigue**; **sluggishness** [King's Dispensatory].
- **Misc: hemorrhoids** [Eclectics, Nepal]; **gangrene** (topical poultice) [Cherokee]; **seasickness**; **scrofula** ("the king's evil").

USE AS FOOD:

- The leaves have been used as a potherb. Please note: While *Capsicum* leaf has been used traditionally as food, I would not eat it until more research is done regarding its toxicity. The leaf and stem are reported to be uterine stimulants [Farnsworth 1975].
- The fruits or leaves are used as antidote to poisonous fish [Africa].
- Added to food to keep it from spoiling [Native American].
- Used to "cleanse" in diets high in animal products [American Hippie Medicine].
- Fire Eaters: The international consumption of *Capsicum* ranges from 2.5g/person/day in India, 5.0g/person/day in Thailand, and up to 20g/person/day in Mexico.

OTHER USES:

- Sprinkled in socks to keep the feet warm.
- Smoke from burning chillis has reportedly been used in torture.
- Indians in San Bas drag hot peppers behind their boats as shark repellents.
- Burned to drive off rats (both rodents and the human type). Also sprinkled in a garden to keep away feral pigs: One snoutful and they move on. *Quickly.*
- If you really want to remove unwanted guests from your home, just microwave a bowl of cayenne peppers. They'll leave... but then so will you....

CONSTITUENTS: Capsaicinoids usually constitute.11% in the fruit, but can be as high as 1.5%, 48% of which is capsaicin. *Capsicum* contains the steroidal alkaloidal glycosides solanidine, solanine and solasodine as well as coumarin / scopoletin.

- There are carotenoid pigments capsanthin, capsorubin, carotene, and lutein, as well as 9-17% fats and 12-15% proteins. Cayenne has 369 milligrams of vitamin C and 21,600 I.U. of vitamin A per 3.5 ounces [Kowalchik 1987]. A complete list of constituents is available on request.

POSSIBLE DRUG INTERACTIONS:

- Can enhance theophylline absorption in rabbits [Bouraoui 1988].
- Can potentiate anticoagulants (speculative) as it reduces platelet aggregation [Tsuchiya 2001].
- May cause coughing when used topically with ACE inhibitors [Brinker 2001].
- Cayenne when taken 30 minutes before aspirin can reduce mucosal damage [Holzer 1989].
- One of the possible reasons why Nīoi is used as a stimulant is its ability to release catecholemine secretions, specifically epinephrine [Watanabe 1987 & 1988(a); Kawada 1988]. This may warrant caution when used with antihypertensive medications (speculative).
- The sleeping time, plasma concentration and hypnotic effect of barbiturates was increased by capsaicin in rats [Miller 1983, Surh 1995(c)].

Nioi (Cayenne) Local Combinations

Common cold with a "cold" presentation (chills, white tongue coat, neck ache): Add *Cymbopogon refractus* (wāpine / lemongrass), *Zingiber officinale* ('awapuhi pākē / ginger).

Cold hands and feet: Add *Foeniculum vulgare* (xiao hui xiang / fennel) fruit.

Bronchitis with clear or white phelgm: Add *Curcuma longa* ('ōlena / Turmeric) and *Zingiber officinale* ('awapuhi pākē / ginger).

Salsa: Add tomato and onion.

Nioi (Cayenne) Cross-Cultural Combiations

Alcoholism: With *Hydrastis* (golden seal).

Laryngitis: As a gargle add *Commiphora myrrha* (myrrh).

Arthritis: With kelp for, and in small quantities as a catalyst to harmonize an herb formula.

High cholesterol: With *Crateaegus* spp. (hawthorne).

Cold sores, joint pain, muscle aches: Topical with olive oil.

Sprains, sore joints and muscle aches: Topical with alcohol or cider vinegar (especially good with gin... made from juniper)

Body aches and pains: With sea salt (pa'a kai) [Old Hawai'i].

Boils: Crushed leaves with coconut oil (topical) [Cook Islands, Samoa, Tahiti].

Dysentery: With sweetened Sumac leaves, bark and fruits [Samuel Thompson 1769 - 1843].

Dysentery: With poor digestion and without rectal burning add *Aloe* spp. [Eclectics].
Fever: With sugar and sour orange juice [West Indies].
Indigestion, weak digestion and loss of appetite: With cucumbers, chives or onions, shallots, lemon or lime juice, and red wine. (*Is this to relieve or create indigestion?*) [West Indies].
Malaria: With *Cinchona officinalis* (Quinine)
Post partum bleeding: With powdered *Cephaēlis ipecacuanha* (Ipacac).
Vomiting and nausea: With salt, vinegar, and water [Eclectics].
To harmonize herb formulas: [Eclectics].

Capsaicin is reported to first stimulate and then sedate the heat detecting ability of the hypothalamus gland. This could result in a lowering of body temperature, a useful characteristic hot in tropical climates.

RANGE: Tropical America. India.

HABITAT: Nīoi grows on the dry leeward coastal areas of the islands, often a welcome friend living among unfriendly Kiawe trees.

GATHERING: Don't touch your eyes, or any other sensitive parts of your anatomy, after gathering!

RESEARCH:
- There have been indications of increased gastric cancer risk at higher doses [Notani 1987] but other studies have failed to demonstrate carcinogenicity [Akagi 1998]. Chemoprotective and anti-inflammatory [Han 2001]. See *Cautions and Contraindications* above.
- Antioxidant in low doses (possibly because of carotene) [Henderson 1999; Rosa 2002; Kogure 2002].
- Weight loss has been demonstrated in female rats [Akagi 1998]. Nīoi can increase metabolism and reduce the amount of fat stored in the body [Kawada 1986; Lejeune 2003; Rhamakrishna 2003].
- Lowers triglycerides in rats [Kawada 1986].
- When used topically, Capsaicin first stimulates and then drains pain fibers of "substance P" (a transmitter of pain impulses) [Sicuteri1988, 1990]. Substance P may also play a role in the tissue inflammation of osteoarthritis and rheumatoid arthritis [Biggs 1990]. Capsaicin is anti-inflammatory [Kim 2003]. High levels of substance P have been linked to psoriasis, and capsaicin has been found to reduce the signs and symptoms of psoriasis [Bernstein 1986].
- Capsaicin has a chemical structure similar to vanilla [Kato 2003] (Hard to believe...)
- Capsaicin is hypoglycemic in animal studies [Tolan 2004].
- Increases endurance in rats [Oh 2003] and swim time in mice [Kim 1997, 1998]. See Possible Drug Interactions above.
- *Capsicum* spp. are lung protective in lab animals, offering protection against cigarette smoke and lung mucosal edema [Lundberg 1983(a)].
- Prevents the formation of gallstones in rats [Hussain 1994].

NOTES 'N QUOTES

- Cayenne has been found in ancient Peruvian burial sites, and may have been cultivated as long ago as 4000 BCE. It was brought back to Europe by Christopher Columbus on his second voyage to the West Indies, and was first described in 1494 by Diego Alvarez Chanca, a physician working with Columbus. 16th century sailors later used cayenne peppers to prevent scurvy. (Later still, a Hungarian scientist who was investigating cayenne pepper discovered Vitamin C.)
- Carolus Linnaeus named the genus *Capsicum* in the mid 1700's and identified two species. By the early 20th century the number of species had risen to more than 100. A recent reevaluation of the *Capsicum* determined that there are, in fact, only two species, and that it is a "polymorph" (a plant that takes on many shapes and varieties). The two species recognized today are *Capsicum annuum* and *Capsicum frutescens.* Linnaeus was right all along....
- The stuff that burns your mouth in cayenne pepper is called capsaicin. It will also burn your eyes. It is used in self-defense "pepper sprays." To be hit in the eyes with pepper spray is reported to be an unforgettable experience and a remarkably effective form of behavior modification. The physiological results, though, are not pretty [Reilly 2003].
- The hot qualities of peppers (determined by the capsaicinoid ingredients) are measured in "Scoville Units," which were invented by pharmacist Wilbur Scoville. The hottest peppers (the Caribbean "Scotch Bonnet" and the Mexican Habanero) rate as 300,000 Scoville Units. Cayenne and Tabasco are at 30,000 - 50,000 units. Jalapenos come in at 2500 - 5000. And bell peppers are at zero. Capasaicin is 1,600,000 units on the Scolville scale. Ap-

parently the Habanero still has a way to go [David Presti]. A simpler system uses a 0 to 10 rating.

- Cayenne from Sierra Leone is said to be the best to use for medicine.
- Tabasco sauce is made from *C. frutescens.*
- The species *C. annuum* includes chili peppers, cayenne peppers, and bell peppers.
- Fire in the Hole! To put out the fire in your mouth after a strong dose of cayenne use alcohol (like beer), fat (like milk or yogurt), salt on the tongue, or chocolate.
- The name of one of the brothers ("Ucho") of the founders of the Inca Empire means "chili pepper." The others brothers were named Cachi ("salt"), and Auca ("soldier"). Taken together, these three things were considered essential ingredients for creating such an empire.

Nīoi Pros And Cons: You Decide

Those for:

"*The all-supporting stimulating effect of Capsicum is the infallible action of internal success.*"
- - Alma R. Hutchens

"*A supreme and harmless internal disinfectant.*"
- - Juliette de Bairacli

"*The purest and most certain stimulant in Herbal Materia Medica.*"
- - R. C. Wren

"*One of the most wonderful medicines we have.*"
- - Jethro Kloss

"*The only mistake a practitioner can make with Cayenne is 'not giving enough'.*" - - W.H. Cook

And those opposed:

"*The greedy merchants, led by lucre, run*
To the parched Indies and the rising sun;
From thence hot pepper and rich drugs they bear
Barter for spices their Italian ware".
- - John Dryden (1631 - 1700)

"*It hath in it a malitious qualitie, whereby it is an enemie to the liver and other of the entrails... it killeth dogs.*"
- - John Gerard, 1597

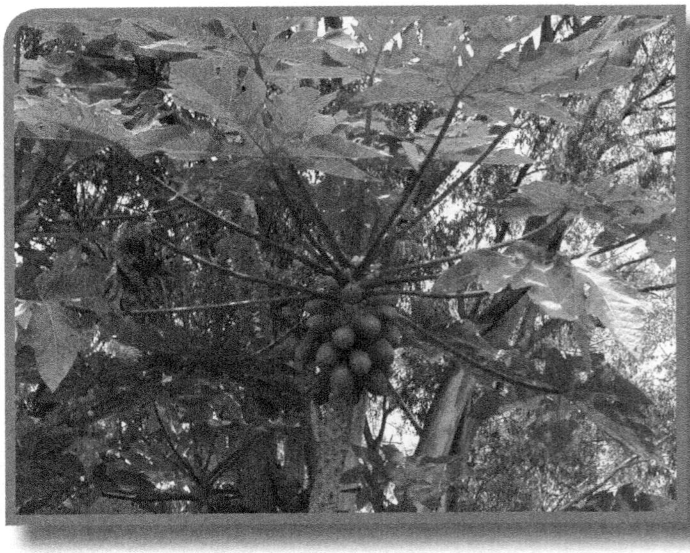

Carica papaya (Mīkana)

PLANT NAME: *Carica papaya* L.

OTHER NAMES: *Papaya vulgaris* (D.C.)

SIMILARLY USED SPECIES: *C. spinosa; Well, C. dodecaphylla; C. jaracatia; C. candamarcensis; Papaya carica; C. quercifolia.*

Status: Alien. Low pest factor.

Habitat: Full sun. Low elevation.

COMMON NAMES: **Mīkana**, **hē'ī** [Hawai'i]; **papaya** [English]; papaw [Eclectics]; mamaeiro (plant), mamao (fruit) [Brazil]; ababaī [Caribbean]; fruta de bomba [Cuba]; esi [Samoa]; lesi [Tonga]; 'I'ita [Tahiti]; weleti [Fiji]; nita [Cook Islands].

NOMENCLATURE: Carica is from the Greek "karike," a type of fig. Papaya leaves are thought to resemble fig leaves.

FAMILY: Caricaceae.

CATEGORY: Herbs that Relieve Food Stagnation~.

PLANT PART USED: All of it.

TOXICITY: Tannins are present and can be harmful in large doses.

CAUTIONS AND CONTRAINDICATIONS:

- Not during pregnancy. The raw seeds are used as birth control in some places.
- All parts can cause allergic reactions but particularly the sap. The sap can cause serious skin irritation topically and severe gastritis if taken internally.

- Papain can trigger asthma. There is a single human case report of hives and bronchial asthma from occupational airborne contact with papain [Quinones 1999]. Papaya flower pollen is also known to cause allergic responses [Blanco 1998].
- Do not use when there is the possibility of coagulation disorders, as papaine is anticoagulant [Gruenwald 1998].

Some people believe that the "mustard" seeds referred to in the Bible are Mīkana (papaya) seeds.

PREPARATION OF MEDICINE: The juice of the plant is sometimes preserved with glycerin.

DOSAGE: Sap or leaves topical as needed. For parasites, 1 tablespoon of the juiced green fruit for adults is taken with warm water and sweetener. Fruit is eaten as desired.

STATUS IN HAWAI'I: Alien. Low pest factor.

WESTERN FUNCTIONS REPORTED: **Abortifacient** (seeds); **amoebicidal** (leaves); **anodyne**; **anthelmintic** (leaf; seed; and Papain); **anti inflammatory**; **antiascariasis**; **antiasthmatic** (leaves); **antibacterial**; **antibiotic**; **anticlastogenic**; **anticoagulant**; **anticonvulsant**; **antihepatotoxic**; **anti-inflammatory**; **antioxidant**; **antiparasitic**; **antiphlogistic**; **antiyeast**; **bactericide**; **benefits digestion** (leaves and fruit); **cardiotonic**; **chologogue** (ripe fruit); **counter-irritant** (seeds); **decoagulant**; **digestive agent**; **discutient**; **diuretic**; **ecbolic** (seeds; unripe fruit); **embryocytoxic**; **emmenagogic** (leaves; seeds); **expectorant**; **febrifugal** (leaves); **fungicide**; **hypoglycemic**; **insecticidal**; **kills lice [Haiti]**; **laxative**; **livestock dewormer**; **oxytocic**; **pectoral**; **pediculicide**; **stomachic**; **suppurative**; **tenderizer**; **vermifuge.**

Mīkana (Papaya)
Common Medicinal Uses

- Indigestion (green fruit)
- Birth control (seeds, but not recommended)
- Cancer (seeds)
- Sores and skin ulcers (sap topical)

Mīkana (Papaya) Cross-Cultural Medicinal Uses

BITES & STINGS

- "**Chiggers**" [Bahamas (sap topical)].
- Topical for **scorpion stings** [Trinidad (male plant root)].
- **Bee stings** [Hawai'i (sap topical)].

COSMETIC

- Papaya juice is used **to beautify the skin** and the sap or fruit pulp is used **to lighten freckles or blemishes** [India, Tahiti]. The ripe fruit pulp is used as **a facial cosmetic and in shampoo**.

CARDIOVASCULAR

- **Heart problems** [Philippines (leaves), Turkey].
- **High blood pressure** [Honduras, South Pacific, Tahiti (flowers infused), Trinidad, (male plant root as tea)].

DERMATOLOGICAL

- **Abscesses, boils, infected sores** [Caribbean (leaf, stem, or root sap topical), France (sap topical), Hawai'i (sap topical), India (unripe fruit topical), Malaya, Marquesas, Panama (sap topical), Philippines].
- The fruit meat is applied to **a sloughing ulcer** and left for 24 hours [Bahamas].
- The unripe fruit is commonly used in hospitals in Jamaica for **chronic skin ulcers**.
- Used on swellings **to prevent pus** (raw fruit juiced) [India].
- **Ringworm** [Caribbean (leaf, stem, or root sap), India (seeds ground and poulticed), Trinidad (green fruit rubbed vigorously topically)]; **psoriasis**; **itching** [Panama].
- **Vitilago** [Haiti].
- **Corns**, **warts**, **skin growths** [India (raw fruit juiced), Indonesia, Jamaica, Malagasy, Malaya, Peru, Philippines, South Africa, Sri Lanka].
- **Epithelioma** [St Vincent].
- In Africa, papaya is **used in pediatric burn units**.

DIGESTIVE

- **Digestive problems**, **indigestion** [Caribbean (green fruit), China, Dominican Republic, India (raw fruit or seeds juiced), Mexico, Panama, Turkey]. "**Atonic and fermentative dyspepsia**" [Eclectics]; **stomach problems due to lack of gastric juices** [Fiji, Hawai'i].
- **Acid reflux** (fruit, eaten); **peptic and duodenal ul-**

cers; **intestinal irritation** [India (green fruit), Philippines]; **enteritis** [Cuba (green fruit)].
- The leaves are sometimes used for **diseases of the GI tract.**
- **Diarrhea** [Honduras, Japan, Panama, Tonga (immature seeds internal), West Africa].
- **Chronic diarrhea**, **dysentery** [France (ripe fruit decocted), India (ripe fruit), Japan, Panama].
- **Constipation**, **laxative** [Asia, Honduras, India (ripe fruit), Panama, Trinidad (male plant root as tea)].
- Ripe fruit are eaten daily **to promote regularity**.
- **Bleeding hemorroids** (ripe fruit or seeds juiced) [India].

HEAD AND THROAT
- **Headache**, **nervous headaches** (heated leaves, topical).
- **Opthalmology treatments** [Soviet Union].
- **Tonsilitis**.
- **Toothhache** [Ivory Coast, Samoa (inner bark infused as a mouth wash)].

HEPATIC
- **"Bilious" conditions** (the fruit); liver problems [Honduras, South America, Turkey].
- **Jaundice** (flowers); **cirrhosis of the liver** [India (ground seeds with lime juice)].

LYMPHATIC
- **Enlarged spleen** (dried fruit).
- **Elephantiasis** (leaves decocted, topical).

MUSCULOSKELETAL / TRAUMA
- **Arthritis**, **rheumatism** [Haiti, Java], **swelling** [Philippines].
- In Java, it is thought that eating Papaya will **prevent arthritis.**
- **Wounds**, **deep cuts** [Hawai'i (sap topical and in combination), Marquesas].
- The leaves can also be used **to dress wounds**.

ONCOLOGY
- **Cancer** [Australia, Cuba, France (sap topical), Hawai'i (seeds, half-ripened fruit), Mexico].
- **Uterine tumors** [Ghana, Nigeria, S.E. Asia].

PARASITES
- **Intestinal worms** [Caribbean (leaf, stem, or root sap), Malaysia, Tahiti (seeds grated)]; **roundworms** (unripe fruit {papain}, seeds {caricin}, or leaves {carpaine}) [India].
- Benzyl-isothiocyanate is also thought to be responsible for papaya seed's **anti-parasitic** effect [Kermanshai 2001].
- The latex reportedly is a stronger **vermifuge** than the seeds.

PEDIATRIC
- **Colic** [Malaya].
- **Diphtheria** (raw fruit juice with honey on tonsils) [India].
- In some South American tribes, **lactating mothers will not eat Papaya**, believing it will disturb their babies' digestion.
- Used **to stimulate lactation**. [Malaysia and Hawai'i]

PSYCHOSPIRITUAL
- **Depression** [Tonga (immature seeds internally).
- **Madness** [Ivory Coast].

REPRODUCTIVE
- **Venereal disease** [Africa (root infused); Trinidad (male plant root)].
- In Asia, the sap is smeared on the cervix **to stimulate uterine contractions.**
- The plant is used for **birth control** in many cultures, especially the seeds. For late menses, the flowers are infused in France, and eaten other places. The unripe fruit is used in India for young "unmarried" women who stop menstruating due to "fright" or from "exposure to the cold." These may be euphemisms for an unwanted pregnancy, possibly due to sexual assault.

RESPIRATORY
- **Upper respiratory problems** [Nigeria]; **common cold** [Caribbean (green fruit)]; **flu** [Trinidad (male plant root as tea)]; **fevers** [Java, Mexico].
- **Asthma** [Mauritius, Mexico, Philippines, Tonga (young fruit sap infused)].
- **Coughs and bronchitis** (flowers eaten).
- **Coughing blood**; **tuberculosis** [Mexico].

URINARY
- **Kidney and urological complaints** [Cameroon, Honduras, Soviet Union].
- **Painful urination**, **stones** [Java].
- **Lack of urine** [Trinidad (male plant root as tea)].

VETERINARY
- Farm animals are sometimes fed papaya seeds in order **to "tenderize" their meat before slaughter.**
- Seeds are used for **parasites in dogs** [Trinidad & Tobago].

OTHER MEDICINAL USES
- **Leprosy** [Asia].
- Thought **to increase longevity** [China].

USE AS FOOD:

- Papaya fruit is made into candies, syrup, and numerous beverages.
- There are 119 calories per papaya.
- The green fruit is boiled as a vegetable and eaten with limejuice and sugar.
- The leaves and flower buds are sometimes used as food, but this may be a dangerous practice because of digestive enzymes in the plant. Water used for boiling should be changed numerous times.

OTHER USES:

- Different parts of *Carica* spp. have a multitude of uses. The leaves can be used as a stain remover and rope or twine can be made from the bark fiber. In Haiti, soap is made from the plant. Papaya is used remove hair on hides before tanning; and to process wool, silk, and rubber.
- Papain, from the dried sap of immature papayas is used to make chewing gum and commercial meat-tenderizer. For those more inclined to "do it yourself" meat can be rubbed with leaves or green fruit. Meat can also be wrapped overnight in leaves, or a small amount of sap placed in the cooking pot.
- Many American beers are processed with papain, which eliminates precipitated proteins in the brew. Papain is also used to extract fish-oil from tuna liver.
- In Kīpahulu, Maui, a hollow papaya stem is used as "pipe" from which to smoke certain intoxicating plant materials. This is a dubious practice. (The papaya stem, that is) Papaya enzymes are known to break down protein. Lung tissue may not be the optimum "meat" that one would wish to "tenderize."

CONSTITUENTS:

- 4-terpineol, 5-hydro-caffeic acid, 6,7-epoxylinalool, alkaloids, alpha glutaric acid (fruit), alpha-linolenic acid, alpha-phellandrene, alpha-terpinene, ascorbic acid (fruit), avenasterol, benzylglucosinolate, benzyl-isothiocyanate, butanoic acid, caricin (a glucoside), carotenes, carpaine, chymopapain-a and b, cis- and trans-linalool oxide, citric acid (fruit), cotinine, cryptoxanthin, cycloartenol, dehydrocarpaines, flavonols, galacturonic acid (fruit), gamma-terpinene, glycoside carposide (leaves), linalool, long chain fatty acids (seeds), malic acid (fruit), methyl butanoate, methyl-thiocyanate, myosmine, myrosin, nicotine, papain, phenyl acetonitrile, potassium, magnesium,and calcium, pseudocarpaine, tannins, tartaric acid (fruit), terpinolene, vitamin A, vitamin C.
- Papain is used to treat arthritis.
- Six enzymes including papain, lysozyme, callose, chymopapain A & B, glutamine-cyclospherase and lipase.
- High in vitamin A (contains more beta-carotine than carrots).

POSSIBLE DRUG INTERACTIONS: Papaya enzyme may increase the INR (international normalized ratio) when used with warfarin [Gruenwald 1998].

Mīkana (Papaya) Local Combinations

Boils: Topically - add *Musa* spp. (mai'a / banana) sap to papaya sap and apply topical (clean the wound well!). Internally - take *Musa* spp. (banana) sap, *Usnea* spp ('umi koa). tincture or decoction, and *Taraxacum officinale* (laulele / dandelion) decocted.

High blood pressure: Juice from the fruit with *Cymbopogon refractus* (wāpine / lemongrass) and *Taraxacum officinale* (laulele / dandelion) tea.

Mīkana (Papaya) Cross-Cultural Combinations

Infertility in women: Half of a green fruit boiled with salt and taken internally [Trinidad].

Hypertension: Add ripe or unripe papaya fruit to sour orange juice [Trinidad].

Roundworms: Juiced with honey, hot water and followed with castor oil for roundworms [India].

Enlarged spleen due to malaria: Raw fruit with cumin seeds and pepper, or vinegar [India].

Birth control: In traditional Indian folk medicine, *Carica papaya* is used with the resin of *Ferula narthex* to cause sterility.

Boils and carbuncles: Green fruit as a poultice with coconut oil [Cook Islands].

RANGE: Native to Mexico and Central America, papaya was brought to the Philippines in the 1500s. It is now found throughout the Pacific, South America, Indonesia, Australia, and Southern Africa.

PROPAGATION & CULTIVATION:

- Certain papaya plants are male and bear no fruit. Traditional peoples will sometimes scar male plants and the resulting trauma causes them to become hermaphroditic, flower, and bear fruit. The techni-

cal term for this is "traumatic reversion."
- One papaya plant can produce fruit for more than twenty years.
- In Venezuela, varieties of papaya grow to 120 centimeters.
- Grows best below 1500 meters. Papain is harvested much similar to opium; the fruit is cut and the dried sap collected.

RESEARCH:
- Carpaine lowers blood pressure, reduces respiration, and slows the heart rate [Whistler 1992].
- May be hypoglycemic [Duke 1984].
- Papain has been shown to reduce edema [Gruenwald 1998].
- Papain is an active ingredient in the skin ointments Accuzyme and Panafil, which are used for wounds and skin ulcers. Papain is used to dissolve dead skin tissue without damaging living tissue [Hewitt 2000; Starley 1999].
- Papain, a protein-digesting enzyme in papaya aids the digestion of other foods and is used commercially as meat tenderizer [Duke 1984].
- Papaya fruit reduces urine acidity in humans [Duke, 1984].
- Recently chymopapain has been injected into ruptured disks in an attempt to avoid back surgery [FDA Drug Bulletin. 12(3): 17-18].
- Seed extracts are spermicidal in vitro [Lohiya 2000]. Chloroform extract of the seeds temporarily lower sperm counts in rabbits [Lohiya 1999]. Water extracts of the seeds temporarily lower sperm counts in rats [Lohiya 1994; Udoh 1999].
- The unripe fruit is bacteriostatic and antioxidant [Osato 1993]. Fruit extracts are stronger against gram-positive bacteria. Gram-negative bacteria require higher doses [Emeruwa 1982]. The sap inhibits *Candida albicans* growth in vitro [Giordani 1996].
- The unripe fruit extract is antihypertensive [Eno 2000] and gastroprotective in rats [Chen 1981].

NOTES 'N QUOTES
- It is said that Native Americans fed Christopher Columbus so much food that he developed digestive pains. He was then taken into the forest and fed papaya.
- *Carica papaya* was first described in the Caribbean by the Spaniard Oviedo in 1526.
- One of four "power herbs" in the Philippines.

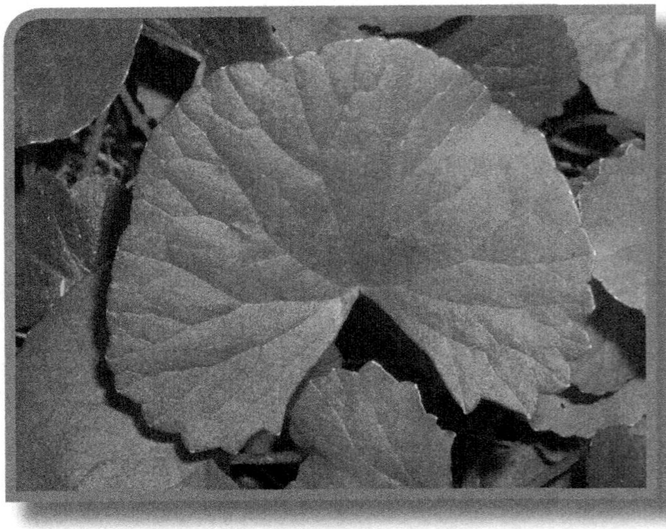

Centella asiatica (Pohe kula / Gotu kola)

PLANT NAME: *Centella asiatica* (L.) Urb.

OTHER NAMES: *Centella biflora, C. coriacea, C. erecta, Hydrocotyle asiatica, H. biflora, H. erecta.*

Status: Alien. Pest factor low to moderate.

Habitat: In your yard.

COMMON NAMES: **Pohe kula** [Hawai'i]; **gotu kola**, marsh pennywort [USA]; **ji xue cao** ("accumulated snow"), luo dei da ("drop will strike"), ma ti cao ("horse's hoof") [China]; brahmi, mandukaparni, muttil, kutannal [India]; kapukapu [Cook Islands]; tohetupou [Tahiti]; ghod tapre [Nepal]; totodro [Fiji]; tono [Samoa, Tonga].

NOMENCLATURE:
Centella is derived from the Latin "centrum," meaning prickle. The fruit of *Centella* resembles two tiny needles.
The Chinese name luo dei da ("drop will strike") is a reference to pohe kula's use for bruises, sprains and injuries.
In Hawaiian, *Hydrocotyle verticillata* is called pohe, *Tropaeolum majus* is called pohe haole, and *Centella asiatica* is called pohe kula, or sometimes pohe for short.

FAMILY: Apiaceae (carrot family).

CATEGORY: Clear heat, cool the blood.

PROPERTIES: Sweet, bland, pungent. Bitter but tasty. Cool to cold.

PLANT PART USED: Whole plant.

TOXICITY: None noted.

CAUTIONS AND CONTRAINDICATIONS: Some sources state that *Centella* may reduce fertility in animal studies, thins the blood, and may be hypoglycemic. I could not verify any of this with research studies, but I would not use it during pregnancy or with blood thinners. See *Possible Drug Interactions.*

PREPARATION OF MEDICINE: Fresh or dried. Can be used in salads.

DOSAGE: For trauma 5 - 30 grams dried, 3 times per day. Fresh 3 - 20 leaves per day.

STATUS IN HAWAI'I: Alien. Pest factor is minimal to moderate.

MERIDIAN AFFINITIES: Liver, spleen, kidney, heart, lung, large intestine.

WESTERN FUNCTIONS REPORTED: **Alterative**; **analgesic**; **antidepressant**; **antimicrobial**; **antitoxic**; **antiviral**; **anodyne**; **anti-infectious**; **antipyretic**; **aphrodisiac**; **astringent**; **diuretic**; **immunomodulatory**; **improves circulation**; **increases longevity**; **insecticide**; **narcotic**; **nervine**; **refrigerant**; **sedative**; **stimulant**; **tonic**; **veterinary lactogogue**.

TRADITIONAL CHINESE ENERGETIC FUNCTIONS (~ = extrapolated):

1) Clear heat, drain damp.
2) Cool the blood.
3) Invigorate blood.
4) Clears heat and toxins.

Pohe Kula (Gotu Kola) Common Medicinal Uses

- Low immunity
- Impotence
- Vascular problems
- Connective tissue enhancer
- Poor memory
- Heart disease

Pohe Kula (Gotu Kola) Cross-Cultural Medicinal Uses

CARDIOVASCULAR

- **Bleeding** [China]; **varicose veins** [Europe]; **hypertension**; **venous insufficiency.**

COSMETIC

- **Pregnancy-related stretch marks** (striae gravidarum).
- Used **to strengthen fingernails and speed their growth.** A common ingredient in French cosmetics.

DERMATOLOGICAL

- **Blotchy skin** [Hawai'i]; **dermatosis** [Malaya]; **eczema** [India (chronic)]; **scabies and tinea / ringworm** [China]; **skin ulcers**, **rash, and redness** [China, Fiji (leaf juice), India]; **skin irritation due to "prickly heat"**.
- **Pimples** [Fiji (leaf juice)].
- **Boils** [Samoa]; **abscesses** [India].

DIGESTIVE

- **Stomach ache** [Fiji (leaf juice)]; **abdominal pain** [China]; **peptic ulcer** [India]; **bleeding ulcer** [Fiji (leaf juice)].
- **Diarrhea** [China]; **dysentery** [China, Philippines, South Pacific]; **indigestion** [Nepal, General]; **vomiting** [China].
- **Constipation** [Fiji (leaf juice)].
- **Hemorrhoids** [Fiji (leaves)].

HEAD AND THROAT

- Juiced for eye ailments and inhaled nasally for **migraines** [Tonga]; **red eyes** [China]; **cataract** [India]; **eye problems** [Fiji (leaf juice), India, Samoa].
- **Headache** [Philippines, South Pacific]; **migraines** [Samoa].
- **Swollen throat**, **tonsilitis** [China].
- **Nosebleeds** [China].

HEPATIC

- **Jaundice**, **infectious hepatitis** [China].

INFECTION

- **Boils**, **fistulas, furuncles and carbuncles with toxic swelling** [China, Samoa].
- **Fever** [China (high fever), India, Philippines, South Pacific]; **chills and fever that come and go each season** [China].
- **Cholera** [India].

LYMPHATIC

- **Elephantiasis** [Brazil].

MUSCULOSKELETAL / TRAUMA

- Used as a connective tissue and collagen rebuilder, gotu kola is reported to stimulate the regeneration of capillary beds.
- **Trauma**, **falls**, **contusion** [China]; **wounds** [Indonesia, Philippines]; **fractures** [China, Fiji (leaves and coconut oil)].
- **Rheumatism** [Nepal]; **painful and swollen joints** [Fiji (leaf juice)]; **spasms** [Turkey].
- **Rib pain** [Fiji].

NEUROLOGICAL

- **Cold extremities**, **white fingers** [Hawai'i].
- **Convulsions** [Tonga].

ONCOLOGY

- **Cancer** [Mauritius]; **abdominal tumor** [India]; **uterine cancer** [Brazil].

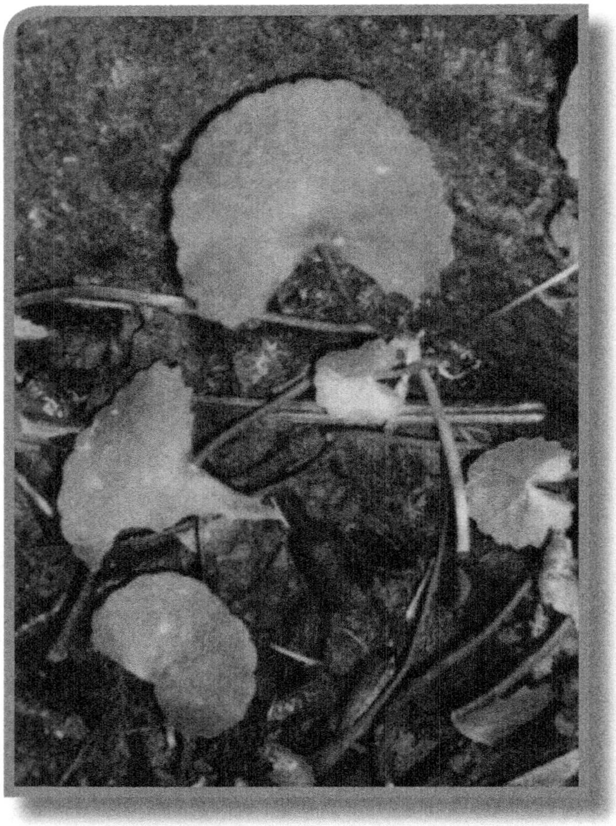

Centella asiatica: Pohe kula

PEDIATRIC

- **Delayed closure of the fontanel** [Tonga (leaves poulticed)].
- **Dysentery in children**.
- **Childhood tidal fevers** [China]; **childhood convulsions** [Fiji (leaf juice)].
- **Navel infection in babies** [Tonga (leaves poulticed)].
- **Measles** [China].

PSYCHOSPIRITUAL

- **Anxiety neurosis**; **insanity** [India].
- **Poor memory** [Hawai'i, India, Nepal].

> ***"Legend has it that gotu kola was introduced to Hawai'i as medicine by a victim of Hansen's Disease (leprosy) who had cured himself of the affliction."***

REPRODUCTIVE

- **Impotence due to vascular disease** [Hawai'i]. One of my Hawaiian teachers used to say "*Pohe makes your rooster stand up and crow!*"
- **Venereal disease** [Samoa]; **syphilis** [Nepal].
- **Post partum weakness** [Fiji (leaf juice)].
- **Unwanted pregnancy** [Fiji (leaves in combination)].

RESPIRATORY

- **Asthma**, **bronchitis**; **respiratory problems** [China].
- **Tuberculosis**; **coughing blood** [China]; **pleurisy** [China].

URINARY

- **Urinary difficulty with stones or bleeding** [China].

OTHER MEDICINAL USES

- Used for **arsenic poisoning** [China].
- **General debility** [India, Nepal].
- **Aversion / fear of cold** [China].
- **Dizziness** [China].
- **Hansen's Disease** (leprosy) [Brazil, China, India, Malagasy, Nepal, Samoa, Turkey].
- **Scrofula** [China].

USE AS FOOD: Gotu kola is juiced fresh in Thailand to make a refreshing beverage. One part of the fresh juice is mixed with two parts water, then blended with palm sugar and shreded ice. Yum!

CONSTITUENTS: 3 glucosylkaempferol, 3 glucosylquercetin, 7 glucosylkaempferol, alpha alanine, aluminum, aminobutyrate, ascorbic acid, asiatic acid, asiaticoside, aspartic acid, beta carotene, beta caryophyllene, beta elemene, beta farnesene, beta sitosterol, betulic acid, betulinic acid, bicycloelemene, brahmic acid, brahminoside, brahmoside, calcium, campesterol, camphor, carbohydrates, centellic acid, centellinic acid, centellose, centelloside, centoic acid, chromium, cineole, cobalt, elaidic acid, essential oils, fat, fiber, germacrene, germacrene-d, glucose, glutamic acid, glycine, histidine, hydrocotyline, indocentelloside, indocentoic acid, inositol, iron, isobrahmic acid, isothankunic acid, isothankuniside, kaempferol, lignoceric acid, linoleic acid, lysine, madasiatic acid, madecassic acid, madecassoside, magnesium, manganese, medicassic acid, mesoinosital, methanol, myo inositol, n-dodecane, niacin, oleic acid, oxyasiaticoside, palmitic acid, p-cymol, pectin, pyridoxin (B6), phosphorus, potassium, protein, raffinose, rhamnose, riboflavin (B2), saponin, selenium, serine, silicon, sodium, stearic acid, stigmasterol, thankunic acid, thankuniside, thiamine (B1), threonine, tin, trans beta farnesene, vellarine, zinc.

POSSIBLE DRUG INTERACTIONS: Caution with Aspirin, Coumadin, Heparin, or any blood thinner. (speculative).

Pohe Kula (Gotu Kola) Local Combinations

Skin disorders: Add *Trifolium pratense* (red clover) and *Oxalis* spp. ('ihi / sorrel).
Impotence: Add *Bacopa monnieri* ('ae'ae / brahmi).
Low immunity: Add *Trametes versicolor* (yun zhi / turkey tails) and *Morinda citrifolia* (noni).
Poor memory or heart disease: Add *Bacopa monnieri* ('ae'ae / brahmi).

Pohe Kula (Gotu Kola) Cross-Cultural Combinations

Toxic swelling: Topical with salt [China].
Bleeding: 30 grams with *Eclipta prostrata* (han lian cao) [China].
Sore throat: Mix juice with vinegar [China].
Vomiting blood or blood in urine: With *Eclipta prostrata* (han lian cao) and *Biota orientalis* leaves [China].
Food poisoning: With *Ipomoea reptans* (water spinach) [China].

RANGE: From Australia and New Zealand, to South America and South Africa. Native to Asia.

HABITAT: In Hawai'i, (if it's not too dry) somewhere in your yard. Grows from sea level to 5000'.

PROPAGATION & CULTIVATION: No need.

RESEARCH:

Antimicrobial: Constituents are antimicrobial in vitro and in vivo against *Mycobacterium leprae* and *Mycobacterium tuberculosis* [Medda 1995]. May inhibit *Herpes simplex* II Virus [Zheng 1989].

Cancer: Cytotoxic against Dalton's lymphoma ascites tumor and Erlich ascites tumor in mice [Babu & Kuttan 1995].

Cardiovascular: Demonstrates significant improvement in chronic insufficiency of the veins [Incandela & Cesarone 2001(c)], possibly through modifying mucopolysaccharide metabolism [Arpaia 1990]. It improves microcirculation in diabetics [Cesarone, Incandela, De Sanctis, & Bavera 2001(b)] and in airline passengers with varicose veins [Cesarone, Incandela, De Sanctis & Belcaro 2001(c)]. It is effective for venous hypertension [Belcaro 1990; Incandela, Belcaro, & De Sanctis 2001(a)] and secondary leg edema [Cesarone, Belcaro, & Rulo 2001(a)].
Constituents reduce atherosclerotic plaques in humans [Incandela, Belcaro & Nicolaides 2001(b)].

Cognitive: Various *Centella* extractions may increase cognition in rats [Veerendra 2003; Gupta 2003]. Certain asiatic acid derivatives are neuroprotective in rats, as well as being anti-oxidant and neuroprotective [Lee 2000(c), Veerendra 2003].

Digestion: Reduces digestive ulcer formation in rats [Cheng / Koo 2000; Cheng / Guo 2004; Sairam 2001; Chatterjee 1992].

Wounds: *Centella* is often used to speed the healing of wounds. Constituents speed wound healing in guinea pigs, [Shukla 1999] in rats, [Suguna 1996; Sunilkumar 1998] and increase human skin collagen levels in vitro [Bonte 1994, 1995; Maquart 1990]. Ingredients appear to be able to alter collagen production in such a way as to inhibit formation of hypertrophic scars, keloids, and stretch marks (striae gravidarum / striae distensae) [Bosse 1979; Widgerow 2000].

> ***"Eat one leaf per day, live an extra 25 years... two leaves per day, an extra 50 years... three leaves per day, live forever."***
> **- - Chinese saying**

NOTES 'N QUOTES

- Used by Confucius.
- Legend has it that gotu kola was introduced to Hawai'i as medicine by a victim of Hansen's Disease (leprosy) who had cured himself of the affliction.
- Called "Kūpuna medicine" ("Elders medicine") in Hawai'i because of its function of improving memory.
- Special thanks to Robert Newman for his helpful translations.

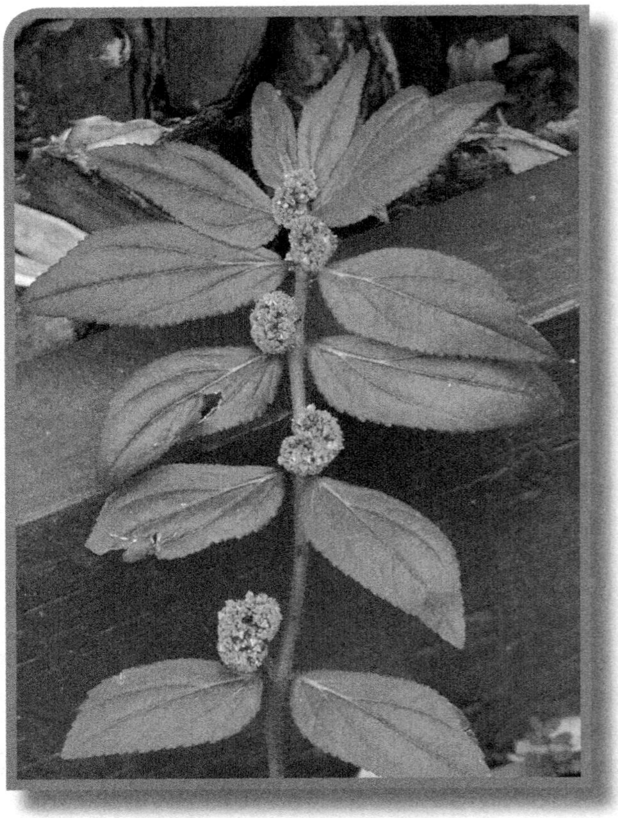

Chamaesyce hirta (Koko kahiki / Spurge)

PLANT NAME: *Chamaesyce hirta* (L.) Millsp.

OTHER NAMES: *Euphorbia hirta, Euphorbia pilulifera, Euphorbia capitata*

SIMILARLY USED SPECIES: *Euphorbia parviflora*

Status: Alien. Moderate pest factor.

Habitat: Sunny disturbed areas.

COMMON NAMES: **Koko kahiki** [Hawai'i]; pill bearing **spurge** [USA]; lal dudhi, paala, ariki thala [India]; amampatchaiarisi [Tamil]; boro-keruie [Bengali]; chara [Sanskrit]; tawatawa [Philippines]

NOMENCLATURE: *Chamaesyce* is from the Greek chamai, meaning "on the ground," and sykon, which means "fig" (an oblique reference to the shape of the capsules).
Koko is a Hawaiian word for numerous euphorbiaceae family plants, and koko kahiki means "foreign koko."

FAMILY: Euphorbiaceae.

CATEGORY: Clear damp heat.

PROPERTIES: Acrid, bitter [Great Britain]. Bitter, sour, cool, slightly toxic [China].

PLANT PART USED: All of it.

TOXICITY: Reports of toxicity have been conflicting. **Until more definitive research has been done, I do not recommend using this plant.**
Some sources list it as toxic [Huxley 1992] and possibly carcinogenic [Matthews 1994]. One animal study [Lanhers 1990] reported no toxic effects when the water extract was given either i.p. or orally.
Photosensitivity, and severe inflammation have been reported from topical use. I have used it on myself topically many times with no untoward results, but everyone's skin and system are different.

CAUTIONS AND CONTRAINDICATIONS: **Until more definitive research has been done, I do not recommend using this plant.** See *Toxicity*. Do not use during pregnancy. Can irritate the digestive system and cause vomiting. Sap can cause dermatitis and may be carcinogenic in large doses.

PREPARATION OF MEDICINE: Tincture 1:5 60%. Infused.

DOSAGE: 15-30 gm in decoction. In China up to 300 grams is used for severe digestive conditions. Tincture 10 - 60 drops.

WESTERN FUNCTIONS REPORTED: **Anodyne**; **anthelmintic for children**; **antiasthmatic**; **anti-bacterial**; **anti-cancer**; **anti-catarrhal**; **anti-emetic or emetic depending on dose**; **antipruritic**; **antiseptic**; **antispasmodic** (leaves); **anti-viral**; **aphrodisiac**; **bronchodilator**; **carminative**; **cyanogenetic**; **depurative**; **discutient**; **diuretic**; **emetic** (large doses); **expectorant**; **febrifuge**; **galactogogue**; **gastric irritant**; **heart depressant**; **lactogogue**; **laxative**; **promotes hair growth** (sap topical); **purgative**; **purifies the blood**; **reduces gas**; **relaxes the bronchioles**; **respiration depressant**; **respiratory antispasmodic**; **sedate fever** (leaves); **soothes the skin and mucous membranes**; **stop bleeding** (leaves); **stops itching**; **vermifuge**; **vesicant**.

TRADITIONAL CHINESE ENERGETIC FUNCTIONS (~ = extrapolated):
Clears heat, drains fire.

OTHER ENERGETIC FUNCTIONS: Treats disharmonies of kapha or vata.

Koko Kahiki (Spurge)
Common Medicinal Uses

- **Asthma & bronchial asthma**
- **Skin disorders**

Koko Kahiki (Spurge) Cross-Cultural Medicinal Uses

BITES & STINGS

- **Snake bite and scorpion sting**.

CARDIOVASCULAR

- **Cardiac disharmonies** [Eclectic].
- **Hypertension** [Trinidad].

DERMATOLOGICAL

- **Skin diseases** [China, Guatemala, India (sap topical) Samoa].
- **Fungus** [China]; **athlete's-foot** [China (herb decocted, **topical**)]; **ringworm** [India (poulticed), Java].
- **Dermatitis**, **dermatosis** [China (topical), Java]; **eruptions** [Samoa]; **eczema** [China (topical), India (poulticed)].
- **Skin growths** [Barbados]; **warts** [Africa, India (sap topical), Jamaica, Panama].
- **Scabies itching** [China, Guatemala].
- **Skin ulcers** [India (leaves)]; **pyodermas** [China (poulticed or wash topical)]; **sores** [Africa, Malaya, Mexico].
- **Herpes zoster** [China (poulticed or wash topical)].

DIGESTIVE

- **Indigestion** [China (decocted), India (with molasses internal)]; **nausea** [Sudan]; **vomiting**.
- **Stomach ache** [India (leaves and flower used as a "chew," once a day for four days), Mexico, Mozambique].
- **Amoebic and bacillary dysentery** [China (decocted), India (juice internal), Mozambique, New Caledonia, Upper Volta]. **Blood in the stools** [India (juiced or with milk)].
- **Diarrhea** [India (in combination), Panama].
- **Enteritis** [China (herb decocted)].

HEAD AND THROAT

- In Borneo, *Chamaesyce hirta* is a specific for eye diseases including **cancer of the cornea and conjunctivitis**.
- **Eye pain and disease** [India (sap topical)]; cornea problems [Malaya]; **eyelid problems** [Guatemala]; **conjunctivitis** [Ghana (young leaves), India (sap topical), Malaya]; **ophthalmia** [Africa].
- **Boils of mouth**; **chapped lips or tongue** [India (sap topical)]; **upper laryngeal spasm**; **toothache**.
- **Headache** [Upper Volta].

INFECTION

- **Abscess**.
- **Fever** [China, Haiti, Trinidad]. Dengue fever [Philippines

MUSCULOSKELETAL / TRAUMA

- **Wounds** [Ghana (sap topical), India (paste), Upper Volta]; **broken bones** [India (poulticed with salt)]; **bruises** [Malaya].
- **Pain in the joints**; **spasms** [Haiti].
- **Burns** [India (paste)].
- **Splinters** [Africa].

ONCOLOGY

- **Tumors** [Indonesia].

PARASITES

- **Enteric trichomoniasis** [China (decocted)]; **amoebas** [USA]; **intestinal worms** [Africa].

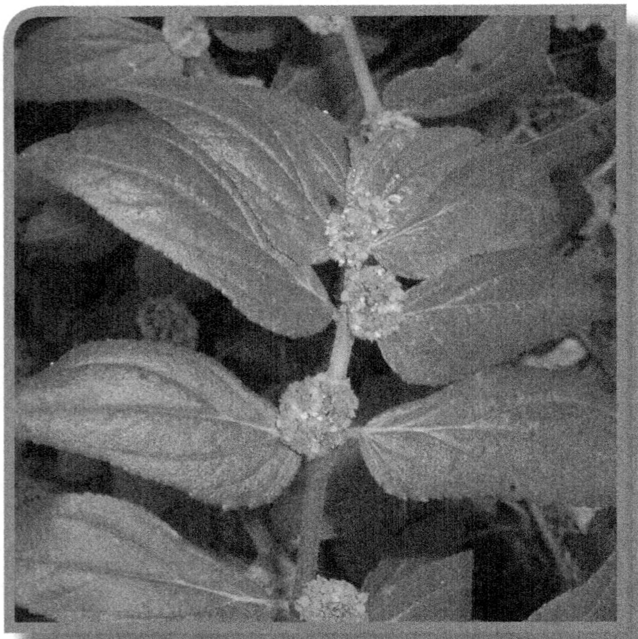

Chamaesyce hirta: Koko Kahiki

PEDIATRIC

- **Children's digestive problems** [India (seeds and leaves)].
- **Colic** [India].
- **Worms in children** [India (juice, seeds, or leaves)].
- **Measles** [Trinidad].

REPRODUCTIVE

- **Breast problems** [India]; **to increase lactation** [India (juice with molasses internal)]; **breast abscess** [China (poulticed or wash topical)]. In Jamaica, the sap is put on the nipples of young girls **to stimulate breast growth**.
- **Post-natal issues** [India].
- **Impotence** [India]; **premature ejaculatio**n [India].
- **Syphilis** (herb decocted); **gonorrhea** [Africa, India].

RESPIRATORY

- **Respiratory problems**, **spasms** [Eclectic, India]; **cough** [Africa, Australia, India (decocted), Panama].
- **Asthma** [Australian Aborigines, Eclectic, Ethiopia, Haiti, India (decocted), Samoa]; **paroxysmal asthma** [Eclectic (leaves smoked)].
- **Colds & flu** [Australia, India, Trinidad]; **hay fever**.
- **Bronchial infection** [Australia, Dominican Republic, Eclectic (in the elderly), India (decocted)]; **chronic bronchitis** [China (decocted)]; **phlegm** [Java].
- **Emphysema** [Eclectic].
- **Pain of pulmonary tuberculosis** [Eclectic].

URINARY

- **Urogenital problems** [India].
- **Kidney disease**; **nephritis** [China (decocted)]; **inflammation of the kidney and pelvis** [China (decocted)].

VETERINARY

- **Broken bones in cows** [India].

OTHER MEDICINAL USES

- **Debility** [Bahamas].
- **Rickets**.
- **Poisonous conditions** [India].

USE AS FOOD: Young shoots cooked as famine food.
CONSTITUENTS: Alkaloids, beta-sterol, flavonoids, gallic acid, glycosides, quercitrin (antidiarrheal), sterols, tannin, triterpenoids

Koko Kahiki (Spurge) Cross-Cultural Combinations

Chronic bronchitis: With *Platycodon grandiflorum* (jie geng) [China].
Urinary disorders: With *Albizia lebbeck*, *Cassia fis-*

tula, and cow's milk [Malaya].

Asthma and bronchitis: With *Grindelia camporum*, *Grindelia robusta* (gumweed) or *Lobelia inflata*.

Wounds: Leaves fried with coconut oil topical [India].

Malaria: With **Cassia occidentalis**, *Cryptolepis sanguinolenta, Garcinia kola, Morinda lucida* leaves & *Phyllanthus niruri* [Congo].

RANGE: Pantropical. Native to Australia and India.

HABITAT: It likes sun and thrives on abusive pathways and roadsides.

GATHERING: If you have sensitive skin, wear gloves while gathering to avoid dermatitis. Gather when flowering. The aerial parts can be dried for later use.

PROPAGATION & CULTIVATION: No need.

RESEARCH:

- Antibacterial against *Shigella* spp. dysentery [Vijaya 1995]. Antiamoebic [Tona 1999, 2000]. Antimalarial [Tona 1999].
- Increases urination in rats. Diuretic function is similar to acetazolamide [Johnson 1999].
- Antispasmodic [Tona 1999].
- Analgesic, anti-inflammatory, antipyretic, CNS depressant in lab animals [Lanhers 1991].
- Sedative in lab animals [Lanhers 1990].

NOTES 'N QUOTES

Introduced into Europe in 1884.

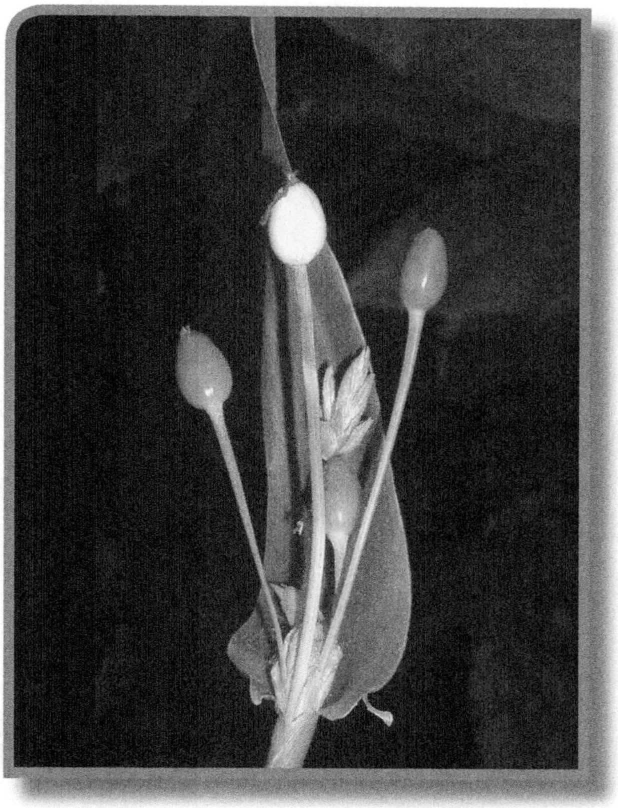

Coix lachryma-jobi (Pū'ohe'ohe / Jobs Tears)

PLANT NAME: *Coix lachryma-jobi* L.

OTHER NAMES: *Coix agrestis, C. chinensis, C. lachryma, C. lachrymajobi.*

COMMON NAMES: **Pū'ohe'ohe**, kūkaekōlea [Hawai'i]; **job's tears**, pearl barley, adlay [USA]; **yi yi ren** (kernel), yi yi gen (root) [China]; yee yee yun, yi yi yan, san yi mai (kernal), yi yi gan (root) [Canton]; bhirkoulo, jabe [Nepal]; sanasana [Samoa]; lagrimas de san pedro [Colombia, Panama], santa maria, santa juana, capin rosario, lagrimas de job, lagrimas de cristo, capin de nossa, cuenta de la virgen [Spanish]; boukon, bonkori, ewuruwura [Nigeria]; kali bugi [Sierra Leone]; mtasubihi, mtasbihi [Swahili]; gromwell, false gromwell [Shaker]; larmes de job [Martinique]; mullu [Aymara]; kuymi [Quechua].

Status: Alien beast. Moderate pest factor.

Habitat: Likes it wet.

NOMENCLATURE: The name *Coix* is from the Greek "koix," a type of palm. Job's tears seeds were thought to resemble the seed of this palm.

FAMILY: Poaceae (Grass family).

CATEGORY: Herbs that drain dampness.

PROPERTIES: Kernels and roots: Sweet, bland, cool to cold. Leaves are neutral.

PLANT PART USED: Roots, kernels, leaves.

CAUTIONS AND CONTRAINDICATIONS: Not in pregnancy.

PREPARATION OF MEDICINE: Roots can be wildcrafted. Because the seeds are processed through some method apparently known only to the Chinese, I wild craft all parts of the plant except the seeds. Decoct in formula.

DOSAGE: 5 - 30 grams.

Pū'ohe'ohe Common Medicinal Uses

- Urinary tract infections
- Poor digestion
- Joint pain
- Cancer

WESTERN FUNCTIONS REPORTED: **Anodyne**; **anthelmintic**; **antidiarrheal**; **anti-inflammatory**; **antiphlogistic**; **antipyretic**; **antirheumatic**; **antiseptic**; **antispasmodic**; **beautifies the skin**; **blood purifier**; **cathartic**; **decongestant**; **demulcent**; **depurative**; **digestive**; **discharges pus** (kernel decocted); **dissolves calculi**; **diuretic**; **hypoglycemic**; **hypotensive**; **insecticidal** (roots); **intoxicant**; **litholytic**; **nutritive**; **pectoral**; **promotes absorption**; **refrigerant**; **sedative**; **stimulant**; **stops pain** (kernel decocted); **tonic**; **vermifuge**.

TRADITIONAL CHINESE ENERGETIC FUNCTIONS (~ = extrapolated):

Kernel

1) Drains dampness.
2) Tonifies the spleen and stops diarrhea.
3) Tonifies the lungs.
4) Clears damp heat.
5) Clears heat and expels pus.
6) Expels wind dampness.
7) Benefits the skin.

Leaves

1) Warms the stomach.
2) Tonifies blood.
3) Tonifies qi.

Roots

1) Clears internal heat.
2) Drains damp.
3) Benefits the spleen.

Pū'ohe'ohe (Jobs Tears) Cross-Cultural Medicinal Uses

COSMETIC

- Internally **to beautify the skin** [China (kernels decocted and eaten)].

DERMATOLOGICAL

- **Warts**, **plantar warts** (kernels decocted or used as food up to 16 days) [China]; **eczema** (kernels decocted) [China], **puerperium** [India].
- Specific for **acne** [China].

DIGESTIVE

- **Appendicitis** (kernels decocted) [China]; **chronic enteritis** (kernels decocted) [China]; **diarrhea** (kernels decocted) [China; India]; **dysentery** [India]; **enteritis**; **gastric ulcers** (kernel decocted) [China]; **intestinal abscess** [China]; **stomach problems** [Japan]; **tenesmus** [Haiti].

ENDOCRINE

- **Diabetes** [Hawai'i].
- **Goiter** [Philippines].

HEAD AND THROAT

- **Chronic headache** (roots decocted) [Colombia]; **headache** [Panama].

HEPATIC

- **Ascites** (seeds decocted) [Caribbean, China].
- **Jaundice** (roots decocted) [China].

INFECTION

- **Abscess** [China], **anthrax** [India], **carbuncles** [China], **fever** [India], **smallpox** [India].

MUSCULOSKELETAL / TRAUMA

- **"Wind damp bi pain"**; **arthralgia and joint pain** [China Brazil], **arthritis** [China], **joint pain & stiffness** [China], **muscle twitching** (kernel decocted) [China], **rheumatism** [leaves and stems in bath in Brazil, fermented in China, Panama], **spasm** (kernel decocted) [China].

ONCOLOGY

- **Cancer** [China]; **cervical cancer** [China (kernels decocted)], **intestinal cancer** [Taiwan]; **lung cancer** [Japan]; **stomach cancer** (kernels decocted) [China, Japan].

PARASITES

- **Round worms** (ascariasis) [China (roots decocted)].

PEDIATRIC

- Seeds strung around a baby's neck for **teething** [Cherokee], as a necklace for **rheumatism**, **cavities, and to promote tooth development in children** [Cuba, Colombia].
- Newborn infants bathed in this **to prevent disease** [China].

REPRODUCTIVE

- **Menstrual disorders** [Nepal (root)]; **vaginal discharge** [China (roots, kernels decocted)].

RESPIRATORY

- **Bronchitis** [China], catarrh, chest congestion [China, Venezuela]; **cough** [China (kernel decocted)].
- **Lung abscess, lung fistula** [China (kernels decocted)].
- **Tuberculosis** [China (kernels decocted)].
- **Pleurisy** [Caribbean (seeds decocted)]; **pneumonia** [China].

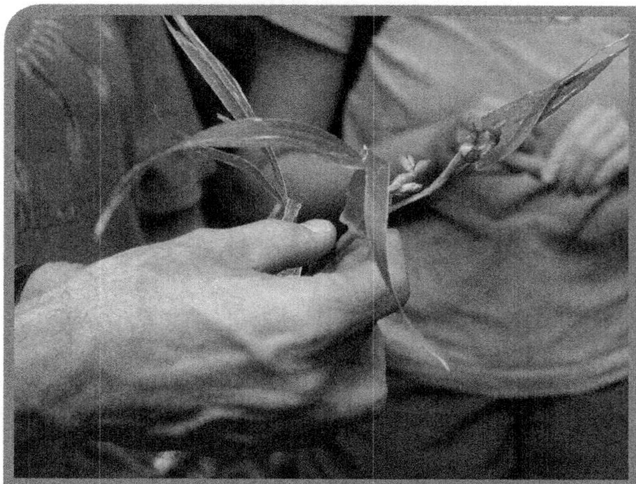

Coix lachryma-jobi: Pū'ohe'ohe tops

URINARY

- **Difficult or painful urination, urinary tract infection; kidney & bladder problems** [Brazil (leaves and stems), China (kernels or roots decocted)].
- **Edema** [Brazil (leaves and stems in bath), Caribbean, China (kernels or roots decocted), Shaker]; **hydrothorax** [China].
- **Incontinence** [Shaker].
- **Urinary stones** [China (roots decocted)]; **strangury** [India].

OTHER MEDICINAL USES

- Leaves decocted **to "benefit the breath and blood"**[China]; **"damp leg qi"** [China]; **bad breath** [China]; **beri-beri** [China (roots decocted)]; **thirst** (kernel decocted) [China, India].
- **Hernia** [China (roots)].

> ***Because Pū'ohe'ohe seeds are processed through some method apparently known only to the Chinese, I wild-craft all parts of the plant except the seeds.***

USE AS FOOD: Kernels used as food, bread and cake [Cherokee], coffee [Japan], food for convalescents [Samoa]. I buy my yi yi ren from China, rather than wild crafting them. See *Preparation of Medicine* above. You should be careful to clean the kernels very well before using as a grain, unless you wish to put your dentist in a higher tax bracket: there are often small stones mixed in with the kernels.

OTHER USES:
- Stems are used to make matting.
- The seeds are used in lei making in Hawai'i and as rosaries in China.
- Dried stalks used by the author as a straw to sip banana sap or coconut water.

ESSENTIAL OIL: Essential oil causes vasodialation. An injection of the oil causes a hypoglycemic response in rabbits, and decreases muscle spasms in frogs [Bensky 1986].

Pū'ohe'ohe (Jobs Tears) Local Combinations

Urinary infections: Roots or kernals. Add *Bidens pilosa* (kīnehi / spanish needle) and *Taraxacum officinale* (laulele / dandelion). With pain add *Hibiscus tiliaceus* (hau) and *Commelina* spp. (honohono

/ wandering Jew). With bleeding add *Capsella rubella* (shepherds purse).

Fatigue, shortness of breath: Kernals and leaves. Add *Morinda citrifolia* (noni), *Trametes versicolor* (yun zhi / turkey tails), and *Auricularia auricula* (pepeiao).

Joint pain: Kernals. Add *Siegesbeckia orientalis* (xi xian cao), *Portulaca oleracea* ('ākulikuli / purslane), *Curcuma longa* ('ōlena / Turmeric), and *Kyllinga* spp. (kili'o'opu).

Pū'ohe'ohe (Jobs Tears) Cross-Cultural Combinations

Diarrhea, dysentery, edema, or blood in the urine: With *Phragmitis communis* (lu gen), *Poria cocos* (fu ling), and/or *Atractylodes macrocephala* (bai zhu) [China].

Intestinal abscess: With *Trichosanthis kirilowii* (gua lou ren), *Prunus persica* (tao ren) *Patrinia* spp. (bai jiang cao) and/or *Paeonia suffruticosa* (mu dan pi) [China].

Lung abscess: With *Phragmitis communis* (lu gen), *Prunus persica* (tao ren) and/or *Benincasa hispida* (dong gua ren) [China].

Bladder infections: With *Akebia trifoliata* (mu tong) [China].

Diarrhea: With *Atractylodes macrocephala* (bai zhu) and / or *Poria cocos* (fu ling) [China].

Jaundice: With *Artemesia capillaris* (yin chen hao). For infantile jaundice: With *Coptis chinense* (huang lian) (just try getting children to drink this!)

Edema and to benefit digestion: As tea prepared with peanuts and brown sugar [China].

Joint pain: as a gruel (congee) add *Cinnamomum cassia* (gui zhi) as a base.

GATHERING: Gather anytime.

RESEARCH:

- The oil injected into rabbits lowers blood sugar [Hsu 1986] as does the water extract [Roman 1992].
- *Coix*ol is anti-convulsant in rats [Gomita 1981].
- Methanol extracts of yi yi ren may function as a COX-2 inhibitor and inhibit human lung cancer in vitro and in vivo. [Hung 2003, Chang 2003].
- Anti-inflammatory, possibly through the suppression of macrophage activity [Seo 2000, Otsuka 1988].
- The oil of *Coix* reduces liver and plasma cholesterol levels in rats [Park 1988].

NOTES 'N QUOTES

- Native to East Indies.
- *Coix* was introduced to China in 49 A.D. by General Ma Yuen and first appeared in Hawai'i about 1895.
- Wandering around China town in San Francisco or Honolulu one will often (literally) stumble across a large cardboard box sitting smack dab in the middle of the sidewalk. Sometimes these obstructions are filled with inscrutable little 1950s-style plastic bags, stuffed with extraterrestrial substances and used for God-only-knows-what nefarious purpose. It turns out that the peculiar white breakfast-cereal-like seeds in these bags are *Coix lachryma-jobi* (job's tears), and the little bundles of delicately wrapped grass are *Juncus* grass, (another of our Hawaiian herbs). The bags are used as a soup to benefit the digestion and to treat bladder infections.

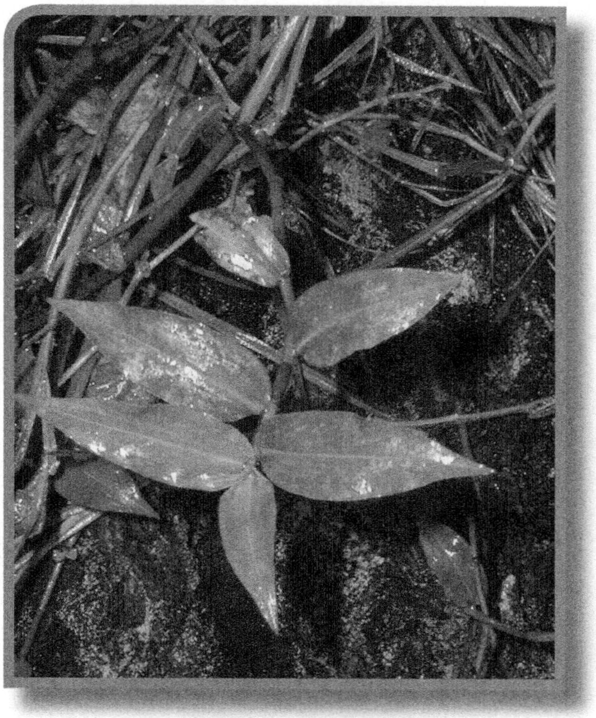

Commelina diffusa (Honohono / Wandering Jew)

PLANT NAME: *Commelina diffusa* N. L. Burm.

SIMILARLY USED SPECIES: *C. communis, C. africana, C. angustifolia, C. bengalensis, C. benghalensis, C. cayennensis, C. coelestis, C. elegans, C. erecta, C. forsskalei, C. nudiflora L., C. nudiflora, C. obliqua, C. polygama, C. rumphii, C. salicifolia, C. suffruticosa, C. virginica, Aneilema nudiflora*

Status: Alien. High pest factor.

Habitat: Wet and shady to 3600'.

COMMON NAMES: **Honohono**, mākolokolo [Hawai'i]; **wandering jew**, day flower [USA]; **ya zhi cao** [China]; ban kane [Nepal] mau'utoga [Samoa]; french weed [West Indies]; watergrass [Trinidad]; zeb gwa [Dominica]; curage [Guadaloupe]; codillo (Spanish); tsuyu kusa (dewy herb) [Japan]; kabocola [Fiji].

NOMENCLATURE: The plant is named after three Dutch botanists named Commelijn. One petal of the flower was said to be for Jan Commelijn (1629-1692), another for his nephew Caspar Commelijn (1667-1731), and the third petal was for one of their relatives who died before achieving fame. That's why we don't know his name. Honohono means "to stitch".

FAMILY: Commelinaceae.

CATEGORY: Herbs that clear heat and fire.

PROPERTIES: Sweet, bitter, cool.

PLANT PART USED: All of it.

TOXICITY: There is one reference to *Commelina forsskalei* as being toxic, [http: / / www.ars-grin.gov / cgi-bin / duke / ethnobot.pl] but other than that I could find no other evidence of toxicity within this genus. As far as I know *C. forsskalei* does not grow in Hawai'i.

CAUTIONS AND CONTRAINDICATIONS: Not during pregnancy.

PREPARATION OF MEDICINE: Infused, decocted, juiced, steamed.

DOSAGE: 1-2 oz. of fresh herb in decoction; or crushed for topical use.

MERIDIAN AFFINITIES: Bladder, liver, lung, and stomach.

WESTERN FUNCTIONS REPORTED: **Abortifacient** (*C. diffusa*; *C. coelestis*); **anti-inflammatory**; **anti-swelling**; **antibacterial**; **antibiotic**; **antipyretic**; **antitussive**; **astringent**; **bactericidal**; **demulcent** [China]; **depurative** [Hawaii, Japan, Trinidad]; **detoxifying**; **diuretic** [China, Fiji, Haiti]; **emennagogue** [India]; **emetic** (*C. nudiflora*) [Samoa]; **emmoliant**; **expectorant**; **febrifuge**; **hemostat**; **laxative** [Samoa]; **lenitive** [China]; **refrigerant**; **tonic** [Egypt].

TRADITIONAL CHINESE ENERGETIC FUNCTIONS (~ = extrapolated):

1) Cools the blood and stops bleeding (int or ext).
2) Clears heat, quells fire.
3) Expels wind dampness, reduces swelling and inflammation.
4) Clears the lungs & opens the chest (sticky phlegm)
5) Clears lower burner damp heat.

Honohono (Wandering Jew)
Common Medicinal Uses

- Urinary tract infections
- Cough with sticky phlegm
- Irritated eyes
- Fever
- Polticed for cuts
- Stop bleeding topically
- Used as a soup base (strained)

Honohono (Wandering Jew) Cross-Cultural Medicinal Uses

COSMETIC

- **Red inflamed eyes** [Hawai'i (sap topical)].

CARDIOVASCULAR

- **Bleeding** [China, Mexico]; **heart problems** [Japan, South Africa]; **hypertension** [China].

DERMATOLOGICAL

- **Irritated tissue** [Hawai'i (sap topical), Seminole]; **itching**; **rash** [Fiji]; **dermatitis** [Latin America];
- **Burns**.

DIGESTIVE

- **Abdominal obstructions** [China]; **diarrhea** (decocted) [China, Japan]; **enteritis** [China (acute), Latin America]; **hemorrhoids** (topical and internal) [China, Mexico]; **stomach problems** [Egypt]; **aid to digestion** [Fiji].

HEAD AND THROAT

- **Conjunctivitis**; **eye problems** (juice topical) [China, Egypt, Fiji, Hawai'i, Latin America, Zanzibar]; **ophthalmia** [Africa, China]; juice of stem used **to remove dirt and grit from the eyes** [Hawai'i].
- **Headache**.
- **Laryngitis** [China]; **sore throats**, **acute tonsillitis**, **pharyngitis** (gargled juice or decoction) [China].
- **Otitis media** [China, India].
- **Nosebleed**.
- In Hawai'i the stem sap is used to remove dirt from the eye, and **to soothe inflamed eyes**. I have used it numerous times for my own eye problems including a turpentine splash in the eye.

HEPATIC

- **Ascites** [China].

INFECTION

- **Abscess**, **boils** (topical & internal) [China, India, Malaya, Trinidad]; **fever** (decocted) [China, Haiti, Trinidad]; **Hansen's disease** (leprosy) [Nepal]; **malaria** [China, South America]; **to prevent infection** [China].

MUSCULOSKELETAL / TRAUMA

- **Insect and snake bites** (topical) [China, India].
- Juice dripped into cuts **to stop bleeding** [Fiji, Hawai'i, Samoa].
- **Rheumatoid arthritis** (acute) [China].
- **Swelling** [Ghana, Japan]; **spasms** [Haiti].
- **Broken bones** [Fiji].
- **Cramps**.

ONCOLOGY

- **Tumor** [Indochina, Mexico].

PARASITES

- **Malaria** [China, Latin America].

PEDIATRIC

- **Mumps** [China].

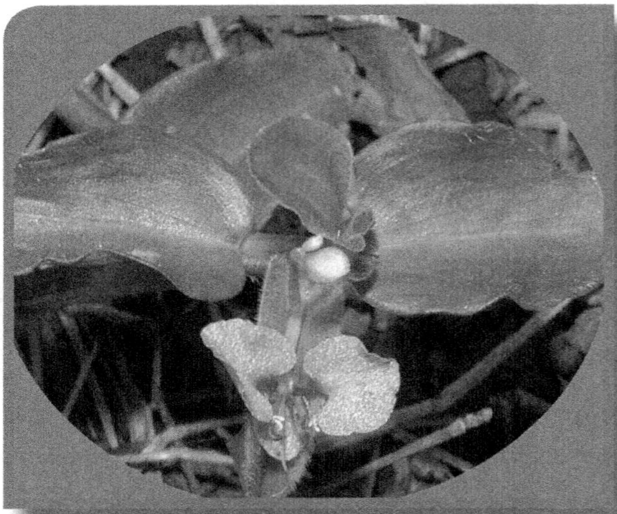

Commelina diffusa: Honohono flower

PSYCHOSPIRITUAL

- **"The evil eye"** [Bolivia].
- **Nervous conditions** [Dominican Republic, Haiti, South Africa].

REPRODUCTIVE

- **Inflammed uterus**; **painful menses** [India, Latin America]; **abnormal uterine bleeding** [Mexico].
- **Vaginal discharge** [Latin America].

- **Infertility** [Paraguay, South Africa (*C. benghalensis*)].
- **Gonorrhea** [China, Latin America]; **groin "problems"** [Egypt, Ghana].
- **Post partum discomfort** [Mexico].

RESPIRATORY

- **Common cold**, **cough**, **influenza** [Carribean, China, Trinidad].
- **Coughing up blood** [Carribean, China, Mexico]; **tuberculosis** (infused) [Acoma, Laguna, Mexico].
- Specific for **cough with sticky phlegm**.

URINARY

- **Bladder infection** [China, Trinidad], **painful or difficult urination** [China].
- **Edema** [China]; **kidney ailments** [Latin America].
- A punahele (favorite) for **cystitis with painful urination**.

> Honohono (*Commelina* spp.) is a good example of the Hawaiian herbal description of "puhi" (literally "eel"), which means "slippery." A great remedy where mucous membranes are inflamed or there is eye irritation. Works on that dry hacking cough.

VETERINARY

- **Food for livestock** [Carribean, Hawai'i, India]; infusion used as **aphrodisiac for livestock** (*C. dianthifolia*) [Navaho].

OTHER MEDICINAL USES

- **Snake bite**, **bug bite** [China].
- **Weight loss from chronic disease**.
- **Hansen's disease** (leprosy).
- **Lymph swelling**.

USE AS FOOD: Use the tips fresh in salads or as a vegetable (cooked 10 minutes) [Universal]; famine food; pot herb eaten in spring [China].
OTHER USES: Blue flower as a dye.

Honohono (Wandering Jew) Local Combinations

Painful urination or dry cough: With *Hibiscus tiliaceus* (hau) inner bark or flowers.

Honohono (Wandering Jew) Cross-Cultural Combinations

Respiratory infection: Decocted with *Taraxacum* spp. (dandelion) herb and *Morus alba* (mulberry) leaf [China].

GATHERING: Anytime.

PROPAGATION & CULTIVATION: Don't.

RESEARCH: Antitussive [Tang 1994].

NOTES 'N QUOTES

- There are 170 species of *Commelina*.
- The Japanese reportedly use *Commelina* flowers for making a kind of paper called Awobana.
- A favorite for moistening poultices. Vodka will also work.

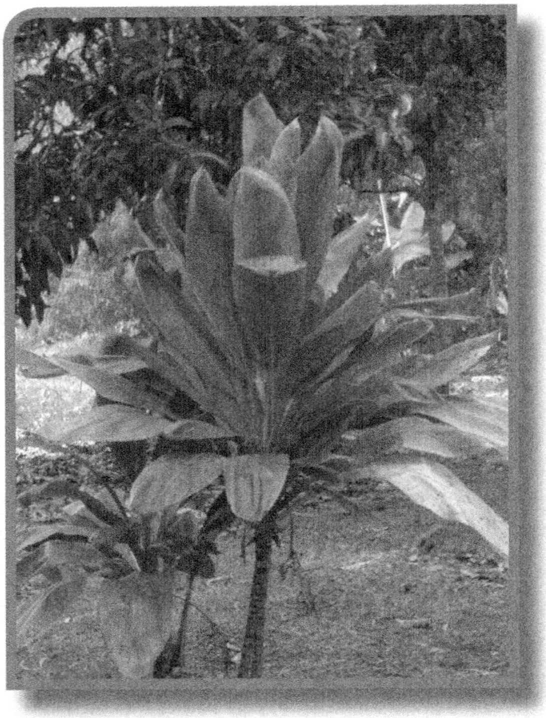

Cordyline fruticosa (Lā'ī / Ti)

PLANT NAME: *Cordyline fruticosa* (L.) *A.* Chev.

OTHER NAMES: *Cordyline terminalis*; *Dracaena terminalis*.

COMMON NAMES: **Lā'ī**, **kī** [Hawai'i]; **ti** [USA];asikuga [Solomon Islands]; cana la india [Venuzuela]; Dracena, bloddracena [Sweden]; jeluang [Sumatra]; litik, idahan [Borneo]; mak pu mak mia [Thailand]; sawang [Borneo]; si [Tonga]; ti kouka, cabbage tree (*Cordyline australis*) [New Zealand].

Status: Polynesian introduction. Low pest factor.

Habitat: Along previously inhabited streams to 2000'.

NOMENCLATURE: The name *Cordyline* comes from "kordyle," the Greek word for club. This is a reference to the root ball that is club-like. The epithet "*terminalis*" describes the flowers resting at the terminal end of the leaf cluster. The term "cabbage tree" refers to the fact that the sailors of Captain Cook ate the young shoots of *Cordyline* like cabbage.

FAMILY: Agavaceae.

CATEGORY: Clear heat, cool the blood.
PROPERTIES: Bland, sweet, cool.

PLANT PART USED: Flower, leaf, root.

TOXICITY: Some leaves are reported to contain calcium oxalate raphides, so they should be cooked. However, the young raw leaf shoots are sweet and edible.

CAUTIONS AND CONTRAINDICATIONS: Not recommended in pregnancy until more research is done.

ENERGETIC CAUTIONS: Caution with cold Spleen / Stomach~.

PREPARATION OF MEDICINE: Infused, decocted. Used fresh. Gather flowers in summer. Roots and leaves can be gathered all year. Leaves are "de-boned" by removing the midrib (kua) and the shiny side (the "alo" side) is placed against the skin.

DOSAGE: Leaves 6-10 grams, Roots 3-5 grams, Flowers 10-15 grams.

WESTERN FUNCTIONS REPORTED: **Antiseptic**; **aphrodisiac**; **depurative**; **diuretic**; **febrifuge**; **hemostatic**; **laxative**; **purgative**; and **tonic**.

TRADITIONAL CHINESE ENERGETIC FUNCTIONS (~ = extrapolated):

1) Cools the blood and stops bleeding.
2) Clears heat, quells fire.
3) Reduces swelling.
4) Clears the lungs and opens the chest.
5) Clears lower burner damp heat.

Lā'ī (Ti) Common Medicinal Uses

- **Blessings & Offerings**
- **Lung infections**
- **Bandages**
- **Topical for fevers and headaches**

Lā'ī (Ti) Cross-Cultural Medicinal Uses

CARDIOVASCULAR

- **Bleeding** [Hawai'i]; **bleeding hemorrhoids** [China].

COSMETIC

- **Baldness** [Fiji (root)].

DERMATOLOGICAL

- **Skin ailments** (juiced); **dermatosis** [Malaya].
- Topical for **boils** [Hawai'i]; **burns** [Samoa].
- **Eczema** [Fiji (leaf juice)].

DIGESTIVE

- **Indigestion** [Java]; **stomach problems** [Caroline Islands].
- **Abdominal disease and pain** [Fiji (leaf juice), Samoa, Tahiti]; **gastritis** [Fiji (leaf juice)]; **lower chest pain** [Fiji (leaf bud)].
- **Diarrhea** [Malaya, Samoa, Tahiti]; **enteritis, dysentery** [China, hawai'i, Malaya].
- **Severe constipation** [Hawai'i].
- **"Lump in the stomach"** [Hawai'i].

HEAD AND THROAT

- **Eye problems** [Samoa, Tonga]; **eye strain and inflammation** (juice; unfurled terminal leaves stirred in water and used as an eye wash) [Hawai'i]; **eye infection** [Fiji (leaf juice)].
- **Gingivitis**, **gum abscess**, **and toothache** [Fiji (root), Sumatra, Tonga (leaf with oil)]; **laryngitis** [Fiji (root)].
- **Headache** [Hawai'i (leaf topical)].
- **Nasal polyps** [Hawai'i (flowers juiced and snorted)].
- **Earache** [Fiji (leaf juice), Samoa, Tahiti].

HEPATIC

- **Liver cancer** [China]; **malarial fevers** [Malaya].

INFECTION

- **Fevers**, **dry fevers** [Hawai'i (leaves topical), Samoa (leaves infused), Tonga (leaf juice), Trinidad]; **smallpox** [Malaya, Philippines]; **abscess** [Tahiti, Tonga].

LYMPHATIC

- **Elephantiasis** [Samoa].

MUSCULOSKELETAL / TRAUMA

- **Arthritis** [Hawai'i, Malaya, Samoa]; **back pain** [Hawai'i]; **gout** [Samoa]. For **rheumatic pain**, a Hawaiian "hot pack" is made with heated leaves and sometimes heated "lomi stones" wrapped in lā'ī leaves and applied topically. Also **used for massage** in Samoa.
- **Traumatic injury**, **broken bones** [Hawai'i]; **as a bandage** [Hawai'i (terminal leaf unfurled)]; **wounds** [Hawai'i, Malaya, Samoa].
- For **blisters on the feet** a leaf can be placed into the lining of shoes. **Burns** [Cook Islands (topical, leaves infused)].
- **Swelling** [Samoa (leaves infused)].
- **Aching limbs** [Tonga (leaf juice)].

NEUROLOGICAL

- Leaves infused for **inflammations** [Samoa]; **swelling and neuritis** [Hawai'i].

ONCOLOGY

- **Lung tumors** [China], **growths** [Hawai'i].

> **In New Guinea, warriors placed their life spirits into a red lā'ī plant before going off to battle, and it was a "Wise Woman" tradition for a wife to place a red *Cordyline* flower on the outside of her house to let her husband know when she was menstruating.**

PARASITES

- Used to kill **"guinea worms"** [Fiji (young shoots)].

PEDIATRIC

- **Croup** [Samoa].

PSYCHOSPIRITUAL

- **Blessings and purifications**, **offerings** (ho'okupu) [Hawai'i].
- **For exorcisms**, **to ward off evil spirits**, **to dispel curses** with pa'akai (Hawaiian salt) [Hawai'i] and to **relieve astral possession** (occult traditions) [USA]. Some Hawaiian women have been known to wear lā'ī leaves under their bras for protection.
- **Agitated psychological states** [Hawai'i (leaves brushed down the body)]; **insanity** [Malaya]; and **the "evil eye"** [Philippines].

REPRODUCTIVE

- **Venereal disease**, **vaginal discharge**, **"groin swelling"** [Hawai'i]; **scrotal swelling** [Samoa]; **amenorrhea** [Trinidad]; **pregnancy** [China, Hawai'i]; **threatened miscarriage** [China].
- **Post partum sickness** [Fiji (stem juice)].
- **To expel afterbirth** [Fiji (stem juice)].

RESPIRATORY

- **Asthma** (flowers and leaves) [Hawai'i, Samoa].
- **Cough** [Fiji (leaf juice), India, Malaya, Trinidad]; **common cold** [Fiji (leaf juice), Samoa].

- **Chest congestion**, **bronchitis**, **sticky phlegm** ("pa'a") [Hawai'i (leaves and shoots), Samoa].
- **Shortness of breath** [Samoa].
- **Tuberculosis**, **cough with blood**.

URINARY

- **Urinary complaints** [Samoa].

OTHER MEDICINAL USES

- A body cover or a "girdle" was made with the leaves **to induce sweating** [Hawai'i].
- **Inflammation** [Samoa (leaves infused), Tonga (root)].

USE AS FOOD:

- The lā'ī roots were boiled or baked and made into food, a sweet candy, and into a fermented drink (see below).
- The leaves were used in Hawai'i to preserve breadfruit. Also used for cooking in underground ovens (called an 'imu) in Hawai'i, and as a sweetener in Fiji.
- While the leaves of various introduced and native New Zealand *Cordyline* reportedly have been eaten by the Maori [Cambie 2003], it would be hard to find an edible preparation for lā'ī leaves unless one is eating the young shoots.

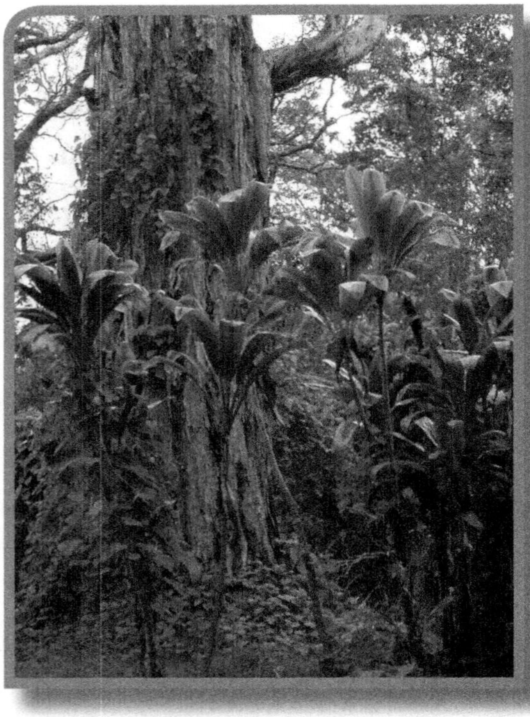

Cordyline fruticosa: Lā'ī in native forest

OTHER USES:

- The most sacred of all Hawaiian plants, lā'ī leaves have been used as wrappers, house thatching, sandals, cheerleader pom poms, plates, cooking utensils, rain coats, cordage, bandages, and almost anything else you can imagine.
- Lā'ī was used to make whistles, balls, and even used for sledding (holua) down muddy or grassy slopes.
- Used to wrap meat or yams before cooking in an underground oven (imu).
- As fringing for fishnets and to add spiritual power (mana) to fishing lures.
- Used as a lei carrier.
- In New Zealand the Maori used lā'ī to make string, rope, and even paper.
- In Hawai'i, stones wrapped in lā'ī leaves are often seen placed along hiking trails as a blessing. This is a popular activity among non-Hawaiians.

CONSTITUENTS: Imidazole alkaloids, linoleic acid, saponins, sarsapogenin, smilagenin, sterols, tyramine.

Lā'ī (Ti) Local Combinations

Bronchitis with sticky phlegm: Young leaves. Add *Commelina diffusa* (honohono / wandering Jew).
Dry cough: Young leaves. Add *Hibiscus tiliaceus* (hau).

Lā'ī (Ti) Cross-Cultural Combinations

Please note some of the ingredients in the following combinations are toxic! Do not self-administer without the supervision of a licensed practitioner or an experienced Elder.

To clear heat and reduce inflammation: With *Solanum americanum* (pōpolo) [Old Hawai'i].
Common cold, fever, earache and headache: With *Solanum americanum* (pōpolo) [Old Hawai'i].
As an emetic (causes vomiting): With *Ipomoea* spp. (morning glory) to clear the lungs [Old Hawai'i].
As a laxative: Juiced and mixed with castor oil [Cook Islands].
Boils: With heated *Morinda citrifolia* (noni) [Hawai'i].
Eye swelling (mata pupula) from supernatural causes: With *Euodia hortensis* (uhi) [Tonga].
Asthma: Flowers used as food, mixed with poi or potato [Hawai'i].
Nasal polyps and nose ailments: Juiced with *Zingiber officinale* ('awapuhi pākē / ginger), Liquid snorted with fern fiddleheads (probably *Cibotium* spp. - hāpu'u) as a "cotton ball." [Hawai'i].

RANGE: Globally, tropics and sub tropics. Native to tropical Asia, or possibly the Himalayas.

GATHERING: Kinolau of Kāne and possibly Lono. When possible, I always try to gather lā'ī before other herbs and use it as a gathering lei and medicine bundle. The lei may be offered as a gift to Wao Akua (the forest), or worn to purify the gatherer. As a medicine bundle, it is given to the patient, who removes the herbs for preparation and then replants the "wrapping" in their yard, where it will grow as a reminder of their healing process and relationship to the divine.

PROPAGATION & CULTIVATION: Place a broken stem in the ground and watch it grow.

RESEARCH: Constituents in *Cordyline terminalis* inhibit human breast cancer cells in vitro [Ooi 1993].

"... grows at the place of promising with the highest god.... as man lives or dies the Sawang (*Cordyline*) is used. People always erect it. If there is a promise between the living the wood must be planted, when there is a promise with the dead it is finally thrown into the river. The Sawang is planted for the newly married, for the dead it is thrown into the water."
- - A Ngaju, Borneo ritual practitioner

NOTES 'N QUOTES:

- A symbol of purity and spiritual power in ancient (and modern) Hawai'i, lā'ī is planted around houses, made into healer's leis, and used in ceremonial blessings. It was often grown at temples of the medicine god Lono and the hula goddess Laka. Temples to Lono were thatched with lā'ī leaves and those to Kū (the war god) were thatched with other plants.
- The first Hawaiian settlers brought lā'ī as a canoe plant. It is lovely and indispensable to Hawaiian herbalists. The green lā'ī is sacred to Hawaiians, other varieties are sacred in Malaysia, Philippines, Indonesia, New Guinea, and other places in Polynesia. Red lā'ī is sacred in many parts of Malaysia, and the Iban of Borneo plant both red and green lā'ī after certain ceremonies. In Indonesia green lā'ī is used for white magick and red lā'ī for black magick. There are almost fifty varieties of *Cordyline* grown by the Maenge of New Britain including thick and thin, striped and mottled leaves. These include a kaleidoscope of red, green, yellow, black and purple leaves.
- Legend has it that a lā'ī stalk was used to test the waters of Waipi'o stream to protect against a shark that lived there.
- A "white lightning" called "'Ōkolehao" (bearing a remarkable resemblance to an industrial solvent) was distilled in old Hawai'i. "'Ōkolehao " means "iron ass" in Hawaiian, perhaps an indication that this beverage burns upon both entry and exit.
- 'Ōkolehao may be a Hawaiian derivative of the English word alcohol.

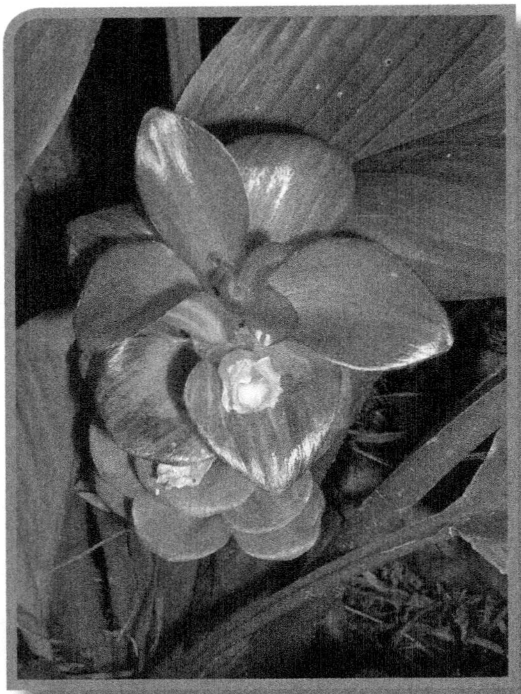

Curcuma longa ('Ōlena / Turmeric)

PLANT NAME: *Curcuma longa* L.

COMMON NAMES: **'Ōlena** ("yellow") [Hawai'i]; **turmeric** [English]; yu jin ("constrained gold" - tuber), jiang huang ("ginger yellow" - rhizome) [China]; açafrão-da-índia [Portuguese]; achirilla [Colombia]; ago, ango [Samoan, Tongan]; azafrán de la india [Spanish]; avea [Fiji]; cu nghe (fresh), bot nghe (dried) [Vietnam]; dilaw [Tagalog]; 'ena [Marquesas]; geelwortel [Holland]; gelbwurz [Germany]; gurkemeie [Norway]; gurkemeje [Denmark]; gurkmeja [Sweeden]; haldi [Hindi]; halodhi [Assami]; halud [Bengali]; haridra, gauri [India]; hsanwen [Burma]; kanghwang [Korea]; keltajuuri [Finland]; kha min [Thailand]; klacze kurkumy [Poland]; kunyit [Malaysia]; kurcum [Arabia]; manjal [Tamil]; manjano [Swahili]; re'a [Tahiti]; renga [Cook Islands]; romiet [Khmer]; safran des indes [French]; tœrmerik [Iceland]; ukon [Japan]; yuquilla [Costa Rica]; zholty imbir [Russia].

Status: Polynesian introduction. No pest factor.

Habitat: Wet, shady, rich soil to 3000'.

PHARMACEUTICAL NAMES: Tuber Curcumae / Rhizoma Curcumae Longae.

NOMENCLATURE: *Curcuma* comes from "kerkum," a yellow dye from the East Indies.

FAMILY: Zingiberaceae.

CATEGORY: Herbs that invigorate blood.

PROPERTIES: Acrid, bitter. In China the tuber (yu jin) is considered cool, and the rhizome (jiang huang) is considered warm.

PLANT PART USED: Tuber and rhizome

TOXICITY:
Curcumin antioxidants are safe and powerful anti-inflammatory agents. [Miquel 2002, Chainani-Wu 2003]
Turmeric is known to be safe in low and moderate doses. The constituent curcumin is not toxic to humans at doses ranging from 8-10 g / day [Cheng 2001, Aggarwal 2003].
In mice, 100 mg / kg / day for 90 days dose of *C. longa* ethanol extracts had no acute or chronic toxicity [Qureshi 1992].

CAUTIONS AND CONTRAINDICATIONS
- Not in pregnancy.
- Not with acute jaundice, hepatitis, bile duct obstruction, or gall stones. (Note: in China, the tuber yu jin is considered cooling and is used for damp heat jaundice... your call....)
- High doses may aggravate the GI system. Not with gastric ulcers or hyperacidity.
- In China the tuber is not used with *Eugenia caryophyllata* (cloves).
- High doses can cause dry eyes.

ENERGETIC CAUTIONS: Not in excess pitta. Not with Liver or Gall Bladder Heat. See Cautions above.

PREPARATION OF MEDICINE
Tincture [1:5, 50% alcohol]. Infused, decocted, prepared fresh, dried and powdered.
For increased absorption, some naturopaths recommend taking with Bromelain 20 minutes before meals; or, with essential fatty acids, lecithin, or fish oil during meals. Juice should be refrigerated and used within two weeks. Or just eat it.
Please Note: 'Ōlena will stain ANYTHING within reach, including your hands, blender, aura, dog, kitchen counter and children. If you don't use gloves while straining it, be prepared to have orange hands for a few days.

DOSAGE

In formula 5 - 10 grams in decoction.
I always prefer fresh, but some use 1g / day of dry, powdered curcumin in divided doses.1 teaspoon of powder in water or juice.

MERIDIAN AFFINITIES: Stomach, spleen, liver

WESTERN FUNCTIONS REPORTED: **Alexeteric** [India]; **alterative** [India]; **anodyne** [India]; **antheimintic** [India]; **anti fungal** [India]; **anti-arthritic** [India]; **antibacterial** [India]; **antibilious** [China]; **anticoagulant**; **antihelmintic** [India]; **anti-infectious**; **anti-inflammatory**; **anti-mutagenic**; **antioxidant**; **antiperiodic** [India]; **anti-pyretic** [India]; **antitumour**; **antiviral** [India]; **aromatic** [India]; **balsamic** [China]; **blood cleanser** (juiced internal) [Hawai'i, India]; **carminative** [India]; **cholagogue** [Brazil, China, India]; **depurative** [Nepal]; **digestive aid**; **diuretic** [Malaya]; **emollient** [India]; **escharotic**; **eye cleanser** [India]; **fumitory**; **hemostatic** [China, Hawai'i]; **increases intelligence**, **wisdom**, **maturity** (red on third eye) [India]; **lactagogue** [Java]; **liver protective**; **maintains balance of intestinal flora** [India]; **metabolism regulator**; **stimulant** [India]; **stimulates the secretion of pancreatic enzymes**; **stomachic** [China]; **thermogenic** [India]; **tonic** [India, Malaya]; **uterine-stimulant**; **vulnerary** [Philippines].

TRADITIONAL CHINESE ENERGETIC FUNCTIONS (~ = extrapolated):
1) Invigorates blood and removes blood stagnation (rhizome and tuber).
2) Invigorates menstrual blood (rhizome).
3) Moves qi & stops pain (rhizome and tuber).
4) Clears hot phlegm in the heart channel and cools the blood (tuber).
5) Expels wind and leads to the shoulder (rhizome).

OTHER ENERGETIC FUNCTIONS: Decreases kapha and vata, increases pitta.

'Ōlena (Turmeric)
Common Medicinal Uses

- **Inflammation**
- **Liver disorders**
- **Digestive aid**
- **Shoulder pain**
- **Sinus and ear problems**
- **Topical for infections**

'Ōlena (Turmeric) Cross-Cultural Medicinal Uses

COSMETIC

- **Beauty care treatments** [India]; **skin dye** [India]; **to remove excess hair** (topical).

CARDIOVASCULAR

- **Anemia** [India].
- **Angina pain**.
- **Capillary fragility**; **poor circulation** [India].

DERMATOLOGICAL

- **Acne pimples** [Hawai'i, India].
- **Dermatitis**, **eczema**, **fungus**, **itching**, **psoriasis**, **rash**, **& warts** [India]; **athlete's foot** (paste topical); **dermatosis** [Nepal]; **impetigo** (paste topical).
- **Diabetic wounds** (topical after debridment) [India]

DIGESTIVE

- **Abdominal pain** [China (tuber)]; **Crohn's disease** [India]; **diarrhea** [Malaya]; **dysentery** (fights protozoan parasites) [Brazil, India, Malaya, Research]; **ulcerative colitis** [India].
- **Hemorroids** [India].
- **Indigestion**, **gas**, **low appetite**, **obesity** [India].
- **Added to high-protein meal to benefit digestion and prevent gas** [India].

ENDOCRINE

- **Diabetes** [India].

HEAD AND THROAT

- **Conjunctivitis** [India, Java]; **eye infections** [Arabia]; **eye problems**, **purulent ophthalmia**, **sore eyes** [India].
- **Earaches** (juice topical) [Hawai'i].
- **Hoarse voice** [India]; **inflammation of the tonsils or throat congestion** (chewed raw) [Hawai'i]; **pharyngitis**, **tonsillitis** [India].
- **Nose growths or odors** (juiced topical) [Hawai'i]; **sinusitis**, **runny nose** [India].

HEPATIC

- **Alcohol or acetaminophin induced liver damage** (preventive) [India]; **chronic hepatitis** [India]; **hepatosis** [Malaya]; **jaundice and liver problems** [China, India, Java].
- Specific for **gall bladder infection due to suspected staphylococcus** [India].
- Michael T. Murray compares curcumin to silymarin

for its **liver protective** effects.

INFECTION

- **Abscess** [India, Java]; **chronic sores** (tuber topical and internal) [China]; **infections and non-healing wounds** [Arabia, India]; **sores** [Malaya].
- **Common cold** [China, Hawai'i, India, Java]; **fever** [India].
- **Chronic strep** [India]; tuberculosis [Hawai'i]; **HIV** [India, Research]; **smallpox** [Brazil]; **tuberculosis** [Hawai'i].

LYMPHATIC

- **Hodgkin's disease**.

MUSCULOSKELETAL / TRAUMA

- **Arthralgia**, **arthritis**, **& traumatic arthritis** [India]; **bursitis** [China, India]; **fibromyalgia**; **shoulder pain** (rhizome) [China]; **sore muscles**.
- **Bruising**, **pain & swelling from trauma** (tuber & rhizome, topical and internal) [Arabia, Brazil, China, India, Malaya]; **wounds** [Arabia, Brazil, India, Java].
- **Cat scratches** [India].

NEUROLOGICAL

- **Alzheimer's disease**; **epileptic seizures** (tuber) [China]; **multiple sclerosis.**

ONCOLOGY

- **Breast tumors**; **lung tumors**; **lymphoma** [India]; **skin tumors**; **stomach tumors.**

PARASITES

- **Scabies** [India, Java].

PEDIATRIC

- **Chickenpox**; **colic** [Brazil, China]; **infant rashes**.

PSYCHOSPIRITUAL

- In traditional Hawaiian thinking, **'ōlena is thought to have much Mana** (spiritual power) and was mixed with pa'akai (sea salt) and sprinkled with a *Cordyline* fruiticosa (lā'ī) leaf **in ceremonies to purify people and homes.**
- In India, **'ōlena is thought to bestow the energy of the Divine Mother**, **cleanse the chakras**, **and is considered a symbol of prosperity** in Ayurvedic medicine. When the juice is used as a "tikal" (orange dot) on the third eye, **it is thought to increase intelligence**, **maturity**, **and wisdom.**
- **Anxiety & agitation** (tuber) [China]; **hysteria** (from "inhaling fumes" - possibly huffing) [India].
- **Attracts money and removes evil** [India]

REPRODUCTIVE

- **Lack of menses** (rhizome) [China, India, Malaya]; **menstrual pain** (rhizome or tuber) [China].
- **Gonorrhea** [Brazil, Malaya].

RESPIRATORY

- **Asthma**, **bronchial asthma**, **bronchitis** [Arabia, Hawai'i, India]; **catarrh** [Brazil]; **chest congestion** [China]; **coughs** [Arabia, India].
- **Hay fever**.
- **Smoked with organic cotton for lung infections** [India] (not recommended!)

URINARY

- **Edema** [India]; **gravel** [Java]; **kidney failure** [India]; **urogenital disorders** [India, Malaya]; **white blood cells in the urine** [Java].

VETERINARY

- Used in Trinidad and Tobago **for ruminants having endoparasites.**
- Also for **injuries and pregnancy-related conditions in animals.**

OTHER MEDICINAL USES

- **Chest**, **flank**, **or abdominal pain** (rhizome or tuber) [China]; **colic from use of cathartics** [Michael Moore]; **insect or snake bite** [India]; **leech bite** [Brazil]; **parturition** [Java].

USE AS FOOD: A major component of curry powder, providing its color. Sometimes used as an adulterant of mustard.

OTHER USES:

- Used to make yellow-orange dyes in ancient Greece and to color kapa cloth in Hawai'i.
- Used with sandalwood paste in pre-marital bathing rituals.
- In India it is used internally to stretch the ligaments in benefit the practice of yoga.
- Planted outside of homes in Hawai'i to repel termites.
- A paste is used to plug radiator leaks in cars.

ESSENTIAL OIL: Perfume component.

CONSTITUENTS: 'Ōlena contains powerful antioxidant phytonutrients known as curcuminoids. The active constituent is curcumin, an antioxidant that reduces inflammation by reducing histimine levels and possibly by increasing natural adrenal corticoids. Although curcumin is not soluble in water, it is suspected that its metabolites may be therapeutically active and responsible for its medicinal effects. Other constituents include volatile oils 4-14% (turmerone, atlantone, zingiberone), sugars, resins, protein, vitamin C, & minerals.

Turmeric is native to India and Indonesia. India, which produces and consumes almost all of the whole world's Turmeric, has a history of use dating back almost 4000 years.

POSSIBLE DRUG INTERACTIONS: May potentiate aspirin, Coumadin (Warfarin), Persantin, or Heparin (inhibits platelet aggregation) [Srivastava 1995]. Cobalt ion neutralizes the antioxidant effects of curcumin in vitro [Sakagami 2000].

'Ōlena (Turmeric) Local Combinations

Joint pain: Add *Siegesbeckia orientalis* (xi xian cao) and *Portulaca oleracea* ('ākulikuli / purslane).
Hepatitis: Add *Zingiber officinale* ('awapuhi pākē / ginger).
Indigestion, abdominal cramps: Add *Cymbopogon refractus* (wāpine / lemongrass).
Poor memory: Add *Centella asiatica* (pohe kula / gotu kola) and *Bacopa monnieri* ('ae'ae / brahmi).

'Ōlena (Turmeric) Cross-Cultural Combinations

Please note some of the ingredients in the following combinations are toxic! Do not self-administer without the supervision of a licensed practitioner or an experienced Elder.

Scabies: With *Azadirachta indica* (neem) paste topical [India].
Fungus: With *Aloe vera* [India].
Menstrual pain: Tuber with *Paeonia lactiflora* (bai shao), *Cyperus rotundus* (xiang fu / nutgrass) rhizome, *Bupleurum chinense* (chai hu) or *Angelica sinensis* (dang gui) [China].
Torso pain: Rhizome with tuber.
Chest pain from heart disease: Tuber with *Salvia miltiorrhiza* (dan shen) [China].
Urinary stones: Tuber with *Desmodium styracifolium* (pua pilipili) [China].
Sinusitis: Juice snorted with 'alaea (iron oxide) and pa'akai (sea salt). If you've never before felt the inside of your head explode, this will create an indelible memory. Keoki Sousa tells of having a Kupuna (elder) instruct him to snort 'ōlena juice mixed with pa'akai (Hawaiian sea salt) during a bout with hayfever and sinusitis. Apparently (after he "came-to"), it had "cauterized" the inside of his skull. But, he hasn't had hayfever since. For a less-than-explosive healing experience, the "pulu" (hairs) of the hāpu'u fern (*Cibotium* spp.) were soaked in 'ōlena juice and placed in the nostrils. For growth in the nostrils or bad odor in the nose it has been juiced with *Zingiber officinale* (ginger) rhizome and flower, and *Saccharum officinarum* (white sugar cane); soaked in *Cibotium* spp. (hāpu'u) pulu, and sniffed up to ten times a day [Old Hawai'i].
Offensive nose odors: Another old recipe for offensive nose odors (probably a sinus infection) calls for 'ōlena with dried *Cocos nucifera* (coconut), *Syzygium malaccense* ('ōhi'a 'ai) bark, *Saccharum officinarum* (white sugar cane), *Morinda citrifolia* (noni) fruit, *Cordyline terminalis* (lā'ī) root, *Aleurites moluccana* (kukui) bark and flowers, and *Psilotum* spp. (moa) internally. That'd do it [Old Hawai'i].
Bruising or itching: Topical with honey [India].
Vaginal discharge: Internally with honey [India].
To tonify the skin: With milk internally [India].
Bruises or sprains: Topical (crushed rhizome) with rum, salt, *Siparuna guianensis* (leaves), *Justicia pectoralis* (leaves) [Creole]. Or with honey or *Aloe* gel [India].
Painful menses and post partum pain: Rhizome with *Cinnamomum cassia* (cinammon bark) [China].
Shoulder pain: Rhizome with *Astragalus membranaceus* (huang qi), *Cinnamomum cassia* (cinammon branch), *Ledebouriella divaricata* (fang feng) or *Notopterygium incisum* (qiang huo) [China].
Sore throat: As a gargle and internally with coconut milk, *Syzygium malaccense* (mountain apple) bark, *Aleurites moluccana* (kukui) bark and flowers, and *Psilotum* spp. (moa) [Old Hawai'i].
As a "blood cleanser": The rhizome juiced with the *Curcuma longa* ('ōlena) leaves, *Punex gigauteus* shoots and leaves, *Syzygium malaccense* (mountain apple) bark, *Acacia koa* (koa) bark, and *Saccharum officinarum* (white sugar cane) [Old Hawai'i].

RANGE: Hawai'i, India, China, Philippines, Java, Malaya, Nepal, and Brazil. Native to India.

GATHERING: Any time.

PROPAGATION & CULTIVATION: 'Ōlena dies back in winter, so remember where you've planted it if you want to partake during Makahiki (winter) season.

> ***"Roots: Curcumœ. Of Turmerick, hot in the third degree, opens obstructions, is profitable against the yellow jaundice, and cold distemper of the liver and spleen, half a dram being taken at night going to bed in the pulp of a roasted apple, and if you add a little saffron to it, it will be the better by far."***
>
> **- - Nicholas Culpepper**

RESEARCH

- Redneck rodents take note: Ethanol extracts of both *Curcuma longa* and *Alpinia galanga* when given to mice resulted in an increased weight of sexual organs and sperm motility [Qureshi 1992] plus curcumin is neuro-protective for ethanol-induced brain damage [Rajakrishnan 1999].
- Ischemia induced damage is reduced by pretreatment with curcumin in cats [Dikshit 1995].
- Antioxidant [Reddy 1994; Selvam 1995].
- Reduces death rate in mice with cystic fibrosis [Egan 2004].
- Prevents the formation of gall stones in rats [Hussain 1992, 1994].
- Creates faster closure of wounds in lab animals [Sidhu 1998].
- Curcumin lowers cholesterol and inhibits LDL oxidation in rabbits [Ramirez-Tortosa 1999].

Immunity

- Curcumin stimulates macrophage activity in mice [Antony 1999], although some constituents may reduce lymphocyte proliferation and activity [Ferreira 1992].

HIV

- Curcumin is a modest inhibitor of HIV protease [Sui 1993]. It may inhibit "LTR" (long terminal repeat) sequence in HIV, which is a part of viral functioning [Barthelemy 1998]. In Trinidad, the Indian population eats large amounts of Turmeric in curry while the African population does not. Persons of African descent in Trinidad are 10 times more likely to have HIV than persons of Indian descent [Cleghorn 1990]. This may be due to genetic, dietary, or other factors.

Alzheimers disease

- Oxidative stress, disturbed protein metabolism, and the formation of beta-amyloid fibrils appear to be key factors in Alzheimer's disease [Calabrese 2003]. In lab animals, Curcumin has been shown to be protective against amyloid beta-protein damage [Lim 2001, Ono 2004(a &b)].
- Phenolic constituents in *Curcuma longa* appear to induce an anti-oxidant and anti-degenerative "heat shock response" that reduces oxidative stress [Calabrese 2003]. Curcumin has been shown to reverse cognitive deficits in rats [Frautschy 2001]. Rosmarinic acid, another constituent in *Curcuma longa*, may also play a part [Ono 2004(b)].
- Other substances that may prevent the beta-amyloid plaque formation include red wine and Vitamin E [Ono 2004(a), Ono 2004(b)].

> **Along with *Zingiber officinale* ('awapuhi pākē / ginger), 'ōlena is our best Hawaiian food-quality anti-oxidant. It is not universally used in the way ginger is, and warrants a bit more attention to create an "energetically balanced" formula.**

Oncology

- As an anticancer agent curcumin down-regulates transcription factors, inflammatory response, cell surface adhesion molecules, and growth factor receptors [Aggarwal 2003]. Known to inhibit tumor cells [Aggarwal 2003] it is chemoprotective for various cancers in both lab animals [Kuttan 1995, Ambegaokar 2003] and in humans [Cheng 2001].
- Oral and esophageal cancer: Curcumin is inhibits human oral squamous carcinoma cell in vitro [Elattar 2000], as well as chemically induced esophageal cancer in lab animals [Ushidi 2000].
- Skin cancer: Curcumin may inhibit squamous cell carcinoma through the inhibition of arachadonic acid metabolism [Spingarn 1998].
- Lymphatic cancer: Antioxidant and cytotoxic against adenocarcinoma in vitro [Fujisawa 2004].
- Nervous system cancer: May reduce human neuroblastoma in vitro [Liontas 2004].
- Breast cancer: Of 150 medicinal herbs tested, *Curcuma longa* was among the 6 best in terms of binding to progesterone and estradiol receptors in human breast cancer [Zava 1998]. It increases cytochrome P-450 detoxification in human breast cancer cells [Ciolino 1998].
- Lung cancer: Smokers who used Turmeric daily for

one month had less urinary excretion of mutagens than did controls [Polasa 1992].

- Stomach cancer: Curcumin inhibits *H. pylori* and is chemoprotective in rats [Ikezaki 2001, Mahady 2002].
- Duodenal cancer: The ethanol extract can prevent duodenal ulcers in rats [Rafatullah 1990].
- Colon cancer: Curcumin inhibits human colon carcinoma cells in vitro and in rats [Chen 1999, Kawamori 1999].

NOTES 'N QUOTES

- 'Ōlena is listed in an Assyrian herbal written around 600 BC.
- Marco Polo compared the similarities of turmeric to saffron in 1280.
- In India, Turmeric is stored in 20' deep pits and can last as long as 3 to 4 years.
- In the 1870's, turmeric was used to test the acidity or alkalinity (pH) of substances. Alkaline substances would turn the orange Turmeric powder brown.
- Potent snakebite antivenom is made in Brazil from *Curcuma longa.*
- And just in case you were wondering... *Curcuma longa* is believed to ward off snakes, ghosts, evil spirits, and used as a paste to repel crocodiles. (It is not yet known if it repels telemarketers.)

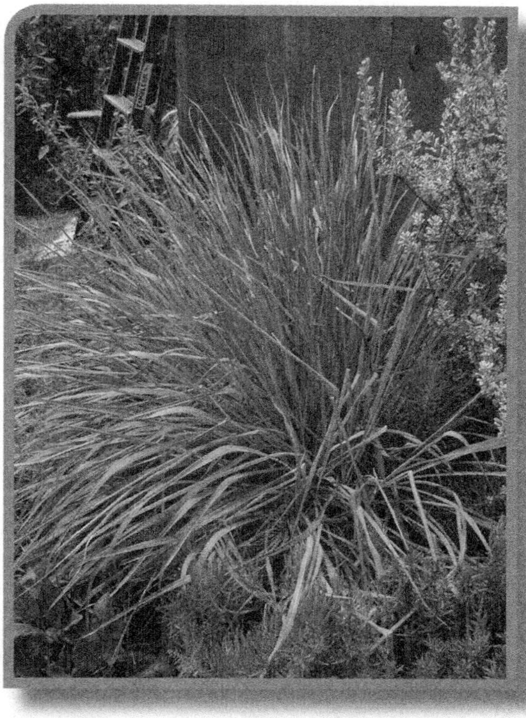

Cymbopogon citratus (Wāpine / Lemongrass)

PLANT NAME: *Cymbopogon citratus* (R. Br.) *A.* Camus.

SIMILARLY USED SPECIES: *Cymbopogon bombycinus; C. ambiguus; C. citrates; C. citrates; C. excavatus; C. flexuous; C. martini; C. nardus* (Citronella- not internally); *C. obtectus; C. procerus; C. proximus; C. winterianus.*

Status: Alien

COMMON NAMES: **Wāpine**, lāpine, lūkini [Hawai'i]; **xiang mao**, xiang ma, mao ju ma, yun xiang cao [China]; **lemongrass**, west indian lemongrass (*C. citratus*); east indian lemongrass (*C. flexuous*) [USA]; fever grass [Carribean]; moegalo [Samoa]; moengalo [Tonga]; yerba de limón, zacate de limón [Costa Rica]; calmarosa, palmarosa (*C. martini*), citronella (*C. nardus*); ilintji, kalpalpi (*C. ambiguus*) [Australian Aboriginals]; tanglad (*C. citratus*) [Phillipines]; yerba luisa [Amazonia]; suyuis, qulla waji [Aymara]; jampi ali, jich'u suqus [Quechua]; capiicati [Chiriguano]; pirhegans [Nepal].

Habitat: Dry disturbed areas to 3000'.

NOMENCLATURE: *Cymbopogon* comes from the Greek "kumbe," a cup or boat, and "pogon," beard. Parts of the flower are thought to resemble a "hairy

boat." (Doesn't make sense to me either….)
The Hawaiian name wāpine is also sometimes used for *Aloysia triphylla* (lemon vervain).

FAMILY: Poaceae (Grass family).

CATEGORY: Warm acrid release the exterior.

MERIDIAN AFFINITIES: Lung.

PROPERTIES: Acrid, bitter, warm [China]. Pungent, bitter, cooling [India].

PLANT PART USED: Whole plant.

TOXICITY: None noted for the herb.

CAUTIONS AND CONTRAINDICATIONS: NOT IN PREGNANCY. Caution with low blood pressure. Essential oil ("eo") can cause skin reaction, never put full strength essential oil directly on the skin. Always dilute well with a carrier oil for topical use.
Do not use Citronella (*C. nardus*) internally.

PREPARATION OF MEDICINE: Cut and dried. Infused or decocted.

DOSAGE: 10 - 45 grams

WESTERN FUNCTIONS REPORTED: **Analgesic**; **anodyne**; **antibacterial**; **antidepressant**; **antifungal**; **antihypertensive**; **anti-inflammatory**; **anti-oxidant**; **antiseptic**; **antispasmodic**; **astringent**; **bactericidal**; **balsamic**; **carminative**; **cyanogenetic**; **deodorant**; **depurative**; **diaphoretic**; **disinfectant** (essential oil); **diuretic**; **emmenagogue**; **expectorant**; **fungicidal**; **hypotensive**; **insect repellent**; **nervine**; **refrigerant**; **rubefacient** (essential oil); **sedative**; **strengthens the blood vessels**; **stimulant**; **sudorific**; **tonic**.

TRADITIONAL CHINESE ENERGETIC FUNCTIONS (~ = extrapolated):

1) Disperses wind damp swelling and stops pain.
2) Dispels damp cold and wind cold common cold.
3) Dredges wind and relieves the surface.
4) Removes blood stasis and opens the channels.
5) Stops watery diarrhea; relieves damp heat in the early stages.

OTHER ENERGETIC FUNCTIONS: Reduces pitta and kapha.

Wāpine' (Lemongrass) Cross-Cultural Medicinal Uses

COSMETIC

- **Cleanses dry and oily skin. Regulates oil production and astringes the skin**; **enlarged pores** [India]; **hair loss.**

CARDIOVASCULAR

- **Circulatory problems** (topical); **hypertension** [Cuba, Hawai'i].

DERMATOLOGICAL

- **Acne** (eo {essential oil} topical) [India], **athlete's foot** (eo or infused, topical) [India]; **eruptions**; **excess perspiration** (eo) [India]; **insect repellent** (eo for fleas, lice, ticks) [India, South Africa, Universal]; **ringworm** (leaf paste) [India]; **rough or loose skin** [India]; **scabies** [India]; **skin eruption** [Australian Aboriginals, China].

Wāpine (Lemongrass) Common Medicinal Uses

- **High blood pressure**
- **Common cold**
- **Use in a steam bath (pūlo'ulo'u)**

DIGESTIVE

- **Abdominal spasms** (leaves); **colitis** (leaves); **diarrhea** [Brasil, Caribbean, China]; **enteritis**; **indigestion** (leaves) [Brasil, Universal]; **gastritis**; **gastrointestinal problems** (infused) [South America]; **intestinal colic** [Amazonia, Aymara, Brasil]; **pernicious vomiting**; **stomach ache** [Caribbean, China].

ENDOCRINE

- **Diabetes** [Egypt].

HEAD AND THROAT

- **Gingivitis**; **gum and mouth diseases** (mouthwash) [Samoa, Tonga]; **sinus congestion** (eo); **thirst** (root stalk chewed); **toothache**; **sore throat** [Samoa]; **vertigo**.
- **Headache** (eo or infusion, internal or topical) [Australian Aboriginals, Caribbean, China, India, Samoa, Suriname].

INFECTION

- **Bacterial infections** (eo) [India], **boils** (eo); **cholera** (eo) [Nepal]; **fever** (infused) [Amazonia,

Australian Aboriginals, Carribean, India, South America, Trinidad]; **influenza**; **infected wounds** (infusion topical) [Australian Aboriginals]; **infections** [India]; **Hansen's disease** (leprosy); **malaria** [Amazonia].

LYMPHATIC

- **Elephantiasis** [Samoa].

MUSCULOSKELETAL / TRAUMA

- **Trauma and contusions** [China].
- **Arthritis** (eo topical) [Carribean, Cuba]; **bruises**, **cuts** [Suriname]; **gout**; **hematoma** [China]; **injuries** (oil topical) [China]; **joint pain** (infusion / soaked leaves burned and inhaled) [Aymara, Australian Aboriginals, China, Cuba]; **low back pain** (eo topical); **muscular pains** (eo or infusion topical) [Australian Aboriginals]; **neuralgia**; **neuritis**; **pain** (eo topical); **rheumatism** (eo topical) [China]; **spasm**; **sprain**; **tendonitis** (eo topical).

PEDIATRIC

- **Digestive problems**, **cramping**, **and gas in children**.

PSYCHOSPIRITUAL

- Flowers smoked for **divination** [Tanganyika (*C. densiflorus*)]; **negative thinking**, **depression**, **inertia**, **desperation**, **lack of focus or concentration** (aromatherapy); **irritability**; **mental fatigue**; **nervous exhaustion**; **nervous disorders** (infused) [South America]; **psychic awareness** (eo); **purification** (eo); **stress** (eo) [Brasil, Caribbean].
- In Western occult traditions, lemongrass is **associated with the element air, the planet Mercury, and is considered masculine**.

REPRODUCTIVE

- **Contraceptive** (infused) [Amazonia], **insufficient lactation**; **irregular menstruation** (infused) [Bolivia, China]; **post partum edema** [China].

RESPIRATORY

- **Asthma** [China, Suriname], **bronchitis** [Australian Aboriginals]; **common cold** (infusion, internal and topical) [Australian Aboriginals, China, Trinidad]; **cough** [Australian Aboriginals, China, Hawai'i, Suriname]; **pneumonia**; **tuberculosis**; **upper respiratory infections** [Australian Aboriginals].

URINARY

- **Bladder disorders** [Suriname].

VETERINARY

- **Fleas on dogs and cats** (eo topical).

OTHER MEDICINAL USES

- **Home perfume** [Amazonia]; **jet lag** [USA]; **perfume**; **steam bath** [Hawai'i].

USE AS FOOD: *C. flexous* (native to India) is sweeter than *C. citratus* and is used to make soda pop, syrup, and candy. Lemongrass (*C. citratus*) is edible; Citronella (*C. nardus*) is not.
Stalks are peeled, chopped and pounded for stir-frying or sauces. Leaf infusion is used as a curry base.

ESSENTIAL OIL (designated by "eo"):
- Topical use only. Essential oils may be toxic if taken internally.
- Lemongrass oil is sometimes referred to as "Oil of Verbena" as it smells like vervain oil.
- Citronella oil is derived from *C. nardus.*
- The plant to oil ratio is approximately 50:1.

Wāpine' (Lemongrass) Local Combinations

High blood pressure: Infused with *Pipturus albidus* (māmaki).
Common cold: Infused. Add *Zingiber officinale* ('awapuhi pākē / ginger) and *Pandanus tectorius* (hala) [Hawai'i].
As a steam bath (pūlo'ulo'u): Add *Eucalyptus* spp. (nuhōlani / palepiwa).

Wāpine' (Lemongrass) Cross-Cultural Combinations

Stretch marks: Essential oil with frankincense and lavender topical.
Bleeding: Wet leaves burned and inhaled, with *Acacia lysiphloia* [Australian Aboriginals].
Common cold and fever: With *Justicia pectoralis* (carpenter grass), *Cordia curassavica* (black sage), *Capraria biflora* (ditay payee), *Eryngium foetidum* (shado beni), *Lippia alba* (santa maria), *Ambrosia cumanensis* (tansey) [Trinidad].
Stomach ache: With chicken [China].
Trauma: With wine [China].

RANGE: It is cultivated in China, Brazil, Sri Lanka,

Indonesia, Central Africa, Madagascar and Hawai'i. Native to Australia.

GATHERING: Anytime. Slice off a handful, leaving the roots in the ground. While it is naturalized in Hawai'i, it is usually "wildcrafted" from someone's garden.

PROPAGATION & CULTIVATION: Propagated from small clumps. Does well in cultivation.

RESEARCH:
- The essential oil of *C. excavatus* provides some protection against mosquitoes [Govere 2000].
- Essential oil is antibacterial against E. coli and many other bacteria, including both gram positive and gram negative pathogens. Constituents and efficacy may differ between species of *Cymbopogon* [Pattnaik 1995; Pattnaik 1999].
- Essential oils from numerous species of *Cymbopogon* inhibit or kill many fungi including species from the genera *Aspergillus, Cladosporium, Microsporum, Mucor, Rhizopus.* and *Trichophyton* [Kishore 1993; Sarbhoy 1978].
- A 10-20% decoction (*C. citratus*) has a weak diuretic and anti-inflammatory effect in rats, and hypotensive effects when given intravenously [Carbajal 1989].
- The results of Lemongrass' use for fevers and digestive problems is inconclusive, at least in animal studies [Carlini 1986].
- *C. citratus* seems to lack sedative effects in double-blind studies [Carlini 1986].

NOTES 'N QUOTES
- Essential oil is used as an excellent alternative to those foul smelling "air fresheners" so pervasive in American automobiles.
- In some places the lemongrass rhizome is used as a toothbrush.
- One of our few Hawaiian plants that falls into the Chinese "warm acrid release the exterior" category, wāpine is a safe, useful and tasty diaphoretic and antihypertensive.

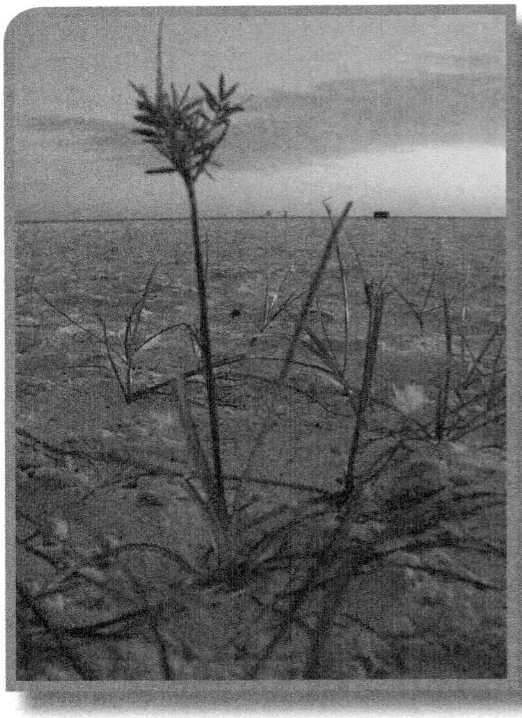

Photograph by Forest & Kim Starr (USGS)
http://www.hear.org/starr/

Cyperus rotundus (Xiang fu / Nutgrass)

PLANT NAME; *Cyperus rotundus* L.

OTHER NAMES: *Pycreus rotundus, Cyperus hexastachyos, C. hexastachys*

Status: Alien. High pest factor.

Habitat: Where ever it wants.

SIMILARLY USED SPECIES: *C. articulatus, C. esculentus, C. longus, C. laxus, C. luzulae, C. odoratus, C. prolixus, C. monocephalus, C. brevifolius, C. pilosus, C. polystachyos, C. malaccensis, C. corymbosus, C. scariosus.*

COMMON NAMES: **Xiang fu** ("fragrant appendage") [China]; **nutgrass** [English]; bathakanda, korai, musta, mustaka, mutha mutha, matasola; tiririca [Amazonia]; co cu, huong phu [Vietnam]; heung fu [Cantonese]; hyangbu [Korea]; kobushi [Japan]; mandassi [Cameroon (*C. articulatus*)], chufa [Egypt (*C. esculentus*)]; piri-piri (*C. corymbosus*) [Amazonia]; junco [Panama].

PHARMACEUTICAL NAME: Rhizoma Cyperi.

NOMENCLATURE: From "kyperos," a Greek word for sedge. "*Rotundus*" means "round."
Kili'o'opu is a Hawaiian name for *Cyperus rotundus, Kyllinga brevifolia,* and *Kyllinga nemoralis.* In order

to avoid confusion, I use the Chinese common name "xiang fu" for *Cyperus rotundus*, leaving the name "kili'o'opu" for the two species in Hawai'i of the genus *Kyllinga*.

FAMILY: Cyperaceae (sedge family).

CATEGORY: Regulate qi.

PROPERTIES: Slightly bitter, slightly sweet, pungent, neutral to warm [China]. Cooling, astringent [India].

PLANT PART USED: Rhizome.

TOXICITY: None noted.

CAUTIONS AND CONTRAINDICATIONS: Caution with constipation.

ENERGETIC CAUTIONS: Drying. Caution with Yin deficiency or Blood heat.

PREPARATION OF MEDICINE: Decoction, powder. Fried in vinegar to increase its' analgesic effects. Fried in wine to benefit assimilation.

DOSAGE: 6 - 12 grams.

STATUS IN HAWAI'I: Serious alien pain-in-the-ass (but great medicine). Pest factor is off the scale. Xiang fu is one of the world's most damaging weeds. It is an outlaw in several countries... Wanted: Dead or Decocted.

MERIDIAN AFFINITIES: Liver, san jiao.

WESTERN FUNCTIONS REPORTED: **Abortifacient** [Amazonia (*C. corymbosus*)]; **alterative** [Amazonia, Turkey]; **analgesic** [Amazonia]; **anodyne** [Amazonia, China, Japan]; **anthelmintic** [Suriname]; **antibacterial**; **antibiotic**; **antidysenteric** [Philippines, Vietnam (*C. malaccensis*)]; **anti-inflammatory** [India]; **anti-fungal**; **antimalarial**; **antimicrobial**; **antiparasitic**, **anti-pruritic**; **anti-pyretic**; **anti-rheumatic**, **antispasmodic**; **antitussive**; **aphrodisiac** [Amazonia, China]; **increases appetite** [India]; **aromatic**; **astringent** [S.E. Asia (*C. monocephalus*)]; **astringent** [Amazonia, Egypt, India, Sudan, Suriname, Turkey]; **bactericide** [Amazonia, China]; **carminative** [Amazonia, Suriname, Turkey]; **contraceptive** [Brazil (*C. corymbosus* rhizome decocted), China]; **demulcent** [Amazonia, Suriname, Turkey]; **deobstruent** [China]; **detoxifies the body through excretion** [India]; **diaphoretic** [Amazonia, Egypt, Europe (*C. longus*), S.E. Asia (*C. longus*), Sudan, Suriname]; **diuretic** [Amazonia, Egypt, Java, Philippines (*C. monocephalus*), Suriname, Turkey, Vietnam (*C. malaccensis*)]; **emmenagogue** [Amazonia, China, Egypt, Japan, Suriname, Turkey]; **emollient** [Amazonia, Egypt]; **febrifuge**; **fumigant** [Cameroon (*C. articulatus*)]; **fungistatic** [Amazonia]; **hypoglycemic**; **hypotensive**; **immunostimulant**; **improves circulation** [China]; **lactogogue** [Amazonia, China, Turkey]; **lithontripic**; **lowers blood pressure** [India]; **nervine**; **promotes memory** [India]; **purifies the blood** [India]; **reduces breast tumors**; **sedative**; **stimulant** [Amazonia, Indonesia, Suriname, Turkey]; **stomachic** [Amazonia, China, Egypt, Indonesia, Philippines (*C. malaccensis*), Turkey, Vietnam (*C. malaccensis*)]; **tonic** [Amazonia, China, S.E. Asia (*C. longus*), Suriname, Turkey]; **tranquilizer** [Amazonia]; **vasodilator** [Amazonia]; **vermifuge** [Amazonia, China (*C. brevifolius*), Egypt, India, Suriname, Turkey]; **vulnerary** [China].

TRADITIONAL CHINESE ENERGETIC FUNCTIONS (~ = extrapolated):

1) Dredges the liver, regulates qi and relieves congestion.
2) Regulates menstruation & stops pain.
3) Benefits liver spleen disharmony.
4) Strengthens the stomach and relieves distension.

Xiang Fu (Nutgrass)

Common Medicinal Uses

- **Joint pain**
- **Menstrual pain**
- **Indigestion**

Xiang Fu (Nutgrass) Cross-Cultural Medicinal Uses

BITES & STINGS

- **Scorpion bite** [Egypt, India]; **snake bite** [Peru].

COSMETIC

- **Hair tonic** [Amazonia, France]; **stimulates sebaceous glands near hair roots** [India].

CARDIOVASCULAR

- **Anemia** [Peru]; **bleeding** [Peru]; **hypertension** [Amazonia]; **palpitation** [India]; **poor circulation** [Amazonia, China].

DERMATOLOGICAL

- **Dermatosis** (*C. monocephalus* tuber with oil) [Philippines]; **scabies and skin disease** [India]; **sores** [Java]. Specific for **acne**.

DIGESTIVE

- **Abdominal pains** [China]; **bloody stool** [India]; **diarrhea** [Amazonia, China, India, Peru, Suriname]; **dysentery** [China (*C. brevifolius*), India, S.E. Asia (*C. polystachyos*), Vietnam]; **dyspepsia** [Amazonia, China, Egypt, Sudan]; **gastritis** [India]; **indigestion** [India, Pakistan]; **malabsorption** [India]; **nausea and vomiting** [China, India, Vietnam]; **stomach and bowel problems** [Amazonia, India, Zulus (*C. longus*)]; **stomach ache** [Amazonia, China, Peru, S.E. Asia (*C. polystachyos*), Vietnam]; **vomiting blood** [India].

HEAD AND THROAT

- Smoke inhaled nasally for **nose pain** [Malaysia]; **headache** [Amazonia, China, India (paste topical on forehead)]; **toothache** (*C. articulatus*) [East Africa]; **migraines** [Amazonia, China].

HEPATIC

- **"Sluggish liver"** [India]; **liver ailments** [Peru].

INFECTION

- **Cholera** [India, Pakistan].
- **Colds** [Amazonia, India]; **flu** [India]; **fever** [Amazonia, Egypt, India, Pakistan, Peru, Sudan, Suriname].

MUSCULOSKELETAL / TRAUMA

- **Trauma** [Amazonia, China]; **wounds** [Amazonia, Japan, Samoa].

NEUROLOGICAL

- **Convulsions** [India].

ONCOLOGY

- **Abdominal tumors** [Amazonia, India]; **cervical cancer** [Amazonia. China].

PARASITES

- **Parasites** [India].

PEDIATRIC

- **Colic** [Cameroon (*C. articulatus*), India, Peru].

PSYCHOSPIRITUAL

- **Depression** [Amazonia, India, China].

REPRODUCTIVE

- **Excessive menstrual bleeding**; **gynecological diseases** [Vietnam]; **irregular menstruation** [China, Vietnam]; **lack of menses** [Amazonia, China]; **PMS** [India]; **painful menses** [Amazonia, China, India]; **inflammation of the uterus** [Amazonia, China].
- **Menopause** [India].
- **Vaginal discharge** [Amazonia, Java]; **vaginal itching** [India (paste topical)].
- **Impotence** [Amazonia, China].

RESPIRATORY

- **Bronchitis** [Peru].

URINARY

- **Edema** [Amazonia, Java]; stones [Amazonia, Java]; **urinary problems** [India].

VETERINARY

- Traditionally used for: **Cracked tail**, **pneumonia**, **pox**, **scabies**, **tuberculosis & wounds in animals**.

OTHER MEDICINAL USES

- **Candida** [India]; **chest pain**, **side pains** [China]; **lesions on the fingers** [Java]; **low energy** [Amazonia, China].

Arguably one of our best local plants for the "liver qi triangle" of menstrual / musculoskeletal / digestive disharmonies.

USE AS FOOD: Reportedly edible but you wouldn't know it by me. The Native American Paiute tribe apparently ground the tubers and made them into porridge. Perhaps it was used as flavoring.

OTHER USES:

- The leaves are used for weaving.
- The dried root powder can be used like talcum powder.
- Used to make perfume [Amazonia, Cameroon (*C. articulatus*), India, Iran, Turkey].

ESSENTIAL OIL: Essential oil is antibacterial against *Staphylococcus aureus*, and stops the growth of *Micrococcus pyrogenes*.

CONSTITUENTS: A-cyperone, a-rotundol, b-cyperone, b-pinene, b-rotundol, b-selinene, camphene, cymene, cyperene, cyperenone, cyperol, cyperolone, cyperotundone, isocyperole, isokobusone, kobusone, limonene, patchoulenone, pcymene, sugenolacetate, sugetriol, sugeonol.

Xiang Fu (Nutgrass) Local Combinations

PMS: Add *Portulaca oleracea* ('ākulikuli / purslane).
Joint pain: Add *Siegesbeckia orientalis* (xi xian cao) and *Kyllinga brevifolia* or *Kyllinga nemoralis* (kili'o'opu).
Poor digestion, gas: Add *Foeniculum vulgare* (xiao hui xiang / fennel).
Menstrual cramps: Add *Piper methysticum* ('awa / kava).

Xiang Fu (Nutgrass) Cross-Cultural Combinations

Diarrhea: With *Aegle marmalos* (bilwa), *Corriandum sativum* (dhaanyaka) and *Cuminum cinimum* (jeeraka) [India].
Breast distention during menses: With *Bupleurum chinense* (chai hu) and *Trichosanthes kirilowii* (gua lou) [China].
Indigestion, nausea, vomiting, and heartburn: With *Atractylodes lancea* (cang zhu) [China].
Abdominal distention: With *Perilla frutescens* (zi su geng) [China].
Irregular menstruation and menstrual pain: With *Angelica sinensis* (dang gui) and *Ligusticum chuanxiong* (chuan xiong) [China].
Asthma: With *Piper nigrum* (bi ba), *Zingiber officinale* ('awapuhi pākē / ginger), *Syzygium aromaticum* (clove), and *Cuminum cinimum* (jeeraka) boiled in ghee. Cool and take internally [India].
Sores on the head: With *Terminalia bellirica* [India (young leaves ground and used topically)].

HABITAT: Where ever it wants, but often in moist soil with full sun.

GATHERING: Quite a bit of work, difficult to dig up. The Chinese gather summer or winter. Of course, one can always buy from Chinatown.

PROPAGATION & CULTIVATION: By rhizome. Flowers are hermaphroditic. Does not seem to set seed in Hawai'i. Don't plant it in your yard... you'll be sorry....

RESEARCH:
- Methanol extract stimulates interferon production [Seo 2001].
- Anti-inflammatory and anti-pyretic in rats. Antipyretic activity in rats is said to be six times stronger than aspirin, apparently due to triterpens [Gupta 1980].
- There are estrogen-like substances in the volatile oils [Chang 1987].
- Improves hemorrheological indexes in rats (plasma specific viscosity, whole blood specific viscosity, erythrocyte electrophoresis) [Xue 1993].
- Contains antimalarial compounds [Weenen 1990].

NOTES 'N QUOTES

- Jeffrey C. Yuen calls *Cyperus rotundus* a "Hun" herb: One that is used for dealing with the past or future. It can be used when we are frustrated that things are not turning out the way we'd planned.
- Xiang fu is rated 8th amongst 250 possible antifertility plants in China [Duke 1985].
- There is speculation as to the mechanisms of *Cyperus* ' menstrual effects, as it is sometimes reported to enhance, and sometimes reported to inhibit, fertility. Current research is centered on the relationship between the genus and a fungus *Balansia cyperi* with which it is a symbiot. There are reports of specifc beds of *Cyperus* having different functional effects due to different fungal relationships in each group.
- Special thanks to Henriette, Robyn, and the Herbal Hall crew for information on *Cyperus.*

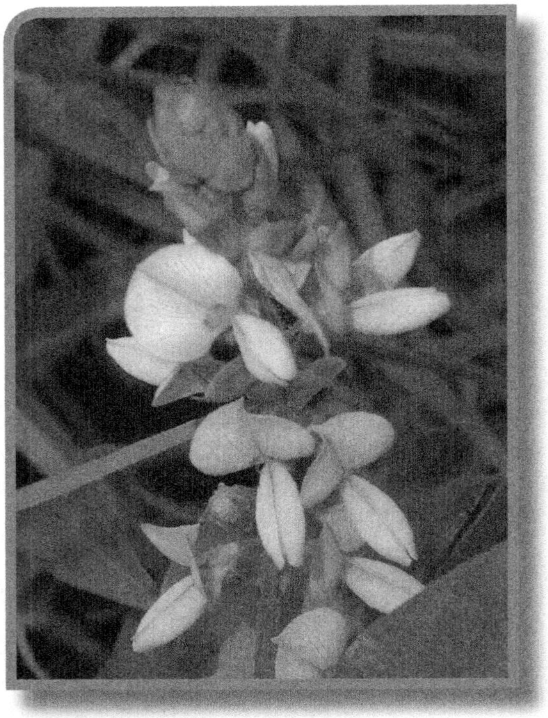

Desmodium spp. (Pua Pilipili)

PLANT NAME: *Desmodium* spp.

SIMILARLY USED SPECIES: *Bidens pilosa, Bidens bipinnata, D. adscendens, D. caespitosum, D. caudatum, D. glaucescens, D. heterophyllum, D. laxiflorum, D. mollicum, D. multiflorum, D. pseudotriquetrum, D. sambuense, D. sandwicense, D. styracifolium, D. sequax, D. sinnatum, D. triquetrum, D. uncinatum, Hedysarum triflorum.*

Status: Alien. Very high pest factor.

Habitat: Mostly on your clothes.

COMMON NAMES: **Pua pilipili** [Hawai'i]; shi lin tong (*D. styracifolium*), hu lu cha (*D. triquetrum*), jin qian cao (*D. styracifolium*) [China], long she huang (*D. triquetrum, D. pseudotriquetrum*) [China, Taiwan], nian ren hua [Taiwan (*D. sinnatum*)]; serious pain in the #%@$$%# hitchhiker! [USA]; amor do campo [Portugese (*D. adscendens*)]; amor seco [Amazonia]; amorosoes [Peru (*D. adscendens*)]; bosuku [Congo (*D. adscendens*)]; burbur [Creole (*D. adscendens*)]; carraficho beiço de boi [Brazil (*D. adscendens*)]; chuchu maiharina [Quechua (*D. adscendens*)]; cousin trois sous [France (*D. adscendens*)]; dusenesh [Peru (*D. adscendens*)]; hamsapādī ("swan feet") [India (*D. triflorum*)]; loaka [Congo (*D. adscendens*)]; lokanga [Congo (*D. adscendens*)]; manayupa [Guatemala (*D. mollicum*)]; margarita [Peru (*D. adscendens*)]; pash pam [Belize (*D. adscendens*)]; pega-pega [Brazil (*D. adscendens*)]; prishnaparni [India (*D. gingaticum*)]; salaparni (*D. giganteum*) [India, Nepal]; salia kuiva [Quechua (*D. adscendens*)]; strong back, beggar-lice, tick trefoil [English]; trèfle savane [France (*D. adscendens*)].

NOMENCLATURE: The genus name comes from the Greek "desmos," a chain. This is a reference to the chain-like seedpods that are attached to your pant legs. In Hawaiian, pua means "flower," and pilipili means to stick close to something.
Note: In China, *Desmodium* species are sometimes used as a substitute for *Bidens* spp. because they are therapeutically similar. Indeed, in China, both *Bidens bipinnata* and *Desmodium caudatum* are called nian shen cao. And in South America, *Desmodium* spp. and *Bidens pilosa* also share a same common name: amor seco. Go figure....

FAMILY: Papillionaceae (fabaceae).

CATEGORY: Varied. Clear heat and toxins. Sometimes drain damp.

PROPERTIES: Varied tastes. Often bitter, sometimes astringent. Neutral to cold.

PLANT PART USED: Leaves and stems. See Toxicity.

TOXICITY: Of 450 *Desmodium* species, none appear to be toxic with the exception of *Desmodium oojeinense* and *D. gyrans*. To my knowledge *D. oojeinense* does not grow in Hawai'i.

CAUTIONS AND CONTRAINDICATIONS: Not in pregnancy.

PREPARATION OF MEDICINE: Infused, decocted.

DOSAGE: 15 - 60 grams as a single herb. Less in forumla.

WESTERN FUNCTIONS REPORTED:
Abortifacient (*D. ascendens*); **alterative** (*D. gangeticum*) [India]; **analgesic** (*D. ascendens, D. caudatum*); **anodyne** (*D. canum, D. caudatum*) [Bahamas, China]; **anthelmintic** (*D. adscendens*) [Guinea]; **antiallergic** (*D. ascendens*); **anti-anaphylactic** (*D. adscendens*); **antiarachidonic** (*D. ascendens*); **antiasthmatic** (*D. adscendens, D. mollicum*) [Amazonia]; **anticonvulsant** (*D. ascendens*); **antihistamine** (*D. adscendens, D. mollicum*) [Amazonia]; **anti-inflammatory** (*D. adscendens, D. mollicum*) [Amazonia];

antispasmodic (*D. adscendens, D. mollicum*) [Amazonia]; **anti-toxic** (*D. mollicum*); **aphrodisiac** (*D. adscendens, D. giganteum, D. mollicum*) [India, Ivory Coast]; **blood cleanser** (*D. adscendens, D. mollicum*) [Peru]; **bronchiodilator** (*D. adscendens*) [Amazonia]; **calcium antagonist** (*D. ascendens*); **cardiotonic** (*D.* gingaticum); **carminative** (*D. heterophyllum* roots, *D. tiliaefolium, D. triflorum*); **contraceptive** (*D. adscendens*) [Amazonia]; **depurative** (*D. adscendens, D. canum, D. mollicum*) [Amazonia, Trinidad]; **detoxifying** (*D. caudatum*) [China]; **digestive aid** (*D. adscendens*, leaf decocted) [Nicaragua]; **diuretic** (*D. adscendens, D. gangeticum, D. heterophyllum, D. mollicum, D. retroflexum, D. styracifolium*) [Amazonia, China, Nepal]; **emmenagogue** (*D. retroflexum*); **excitant** (*D. ramosissimum*) [Africa]; **expectorant** (*D. gangeticum*) [India]; **febrifuge** (*D. caudatum, D. gangeticum, D. ramosissimum, D. styracifolium*) [Africa, China, India]; **galactagogue** (*D. adscendens, D. heterophyllum*) [Amazonia, Ivory Coast]; **hypothermic** (*D. ascendens*); **lactafuge** (*D. polycarpum*) [Akar entimor]; lactogogue (*D. triflorum*) [India]; **laxative** (*D. adscendens, D. mollicum*) [Amazonia, Ghana]; **liver protective** (*D. ascendens*); **magickal potion** (*D. heterocarpum*) [Panama, Philippines]; **oxytoxcic** (*D. adscendens*) [Guinea]; **potassium-channel-opener** (*D. adscendens*); **promotes lactation** (*D. adscendens*, topical) [Amazonia]; **prostaglandigenic** (*D. ascendens*); **purgative** (*D. retroflexum*); **reduces swelling** (*D. heterocarpum*) [China]; **refrigerant** (*D. styracifolium*) [China]; **sedative** (*D. gangeticum*) [Malaya]; **sterilant** (*D. ascendens*); **stomachic** (*D. retroflexum*); **tonic** (*D. gangeticum, D. heterophyllum* roots, *D. triflorum*) [India, Nepal]; **tracheorelaxant** (*D. ascendens*); **vulnerary** (*D. adscendens*) [Amazonia].

TRADITIONAL CHINESE ENERGETIC FUNCTIONS (~ = extrapolated):

1) Relieves water retention & promotes urination.
2) Clears heat.
3) Clears heat and poison.
4) Resolves dampness.
5) Disperses swelling.
6) Eliminates phlegm.
7) Resolves accumulation.
8) Kills intestinal parasites.

Pua Pilipili
Common Medicinal Uses

- Hepatitis
- Asthma
- Back pain
- Infections

Pua Pilipili
Cross-Cultural Medicinal Uses

BITES & STINGS

- **Snake bite** [China (*D. heterocarpum*), Nepal (*D. giganteum*)].
- **Scorpion sting** (*D. giganteum*) [Nepal].

CARDIOVASCULAR

- **Bleeding** (*D. mollicum, D. pulchellum*).
- **Heart disease.**
- **Circulation problems** (*D. giganteum*) [India].

DERMATOLOGICAL

- **Acne** (*D. canadense*).
- **Dermatosis** (*D. heterophyllum, D. triflorum*) [Malaya, Singapore], **itching** (*D. triflorum*) [India], **skin problems** (*D. caudatum*) [China]; **rash.**
- **Psoriasis** (*D. umbellatum*) [Fiji]; **eczema.**
- **Ringworm** (*D. adscendens*) [Africa].
- ***Treponema pertenue* infection,** also called "yaws".
- **Boils, carbuncles, and furuncles** (*D. caudatum, D. triquetrum, D. pseudotriquetrum*) [China] ; **skin sores** (*D. pulchellum*) [Java].
- **Burns** (*D. triflorum, D. heterophyllum*, topical) [India].

DIGESTIVE

- **Constipation** (*D. adscendens, D. mollicum, D. umbellatum*) [Ghana, Java].
- **Blood in the stools** (*D. triflorum*); **diarrhea** (*D. adscendens, D. cephalotes, D. gangeticum, D. pulchellum, D. triflorum*) [Brazil, Java, Malaya, Nepal, Nicaragua, Suriname]; **dysentery** (*D. adscendens, D. canadense, D. caudatum, D. giganteum, D. mollicum, D. ramosissimum, D. triflorum, D. triquetrum, D. pseudotriquetrum*) [China, Ghana, India, Java, Suriname, Upper Volta]; **enteritis** (*D. caudatum, D. triquetrum, D. pseudotriquetrum*) [China]; **enterosis** (*D. heterophyllum*) [Java, Ma-

laya].

- **Gastritis**, **gastroenteritis** (*D. caudatum*) [China]; **stomach pain** (*D. cephalotes, D. heterophyllum, D. triflorum*) [India, Malaya]; **gastric and duodenal ulcers** (*D. caudatum*) [China].
- **Indigestion**; **digestive problems** (*D. adscendens*) [Nicaragua].
- **Loss of appetite or nausea** (*D. ascendens*); **malnutrition**.
- **Hemorrhoids** (*D. triquetrum*) [Java, India].

HEAD AND THROAT

- **Cataracts** (*D. cephalotes, D. triflorum*) [India]; **eye problems** (*D. canadense, D. ramosissimum*); **ophthalmia** (*D. triflorum*) [India].
- **Earache** (*D. heterophyllum*) [Malaya].
- **Headache** (*D. gangeticum*) [Malaya].
- **Sore throat** (*D. heterocarpum, D. triquetrum, D. pseudotriquetrum*) [China]; **mouth inflammation**, **bleeding gums** [Cherokee *D. nudiflorum, D. perplexum* root chewed].

HEPATIC

- **Acute & chronic hepatitis** (*D. adscendens, D. styracifolium*) [China, Suriname]; **jaundice & hepatic lesions** (*D. ascendens. D. triquetrum, D. pseudotriquetrum*) [China]; **liver problems** (*D. cajanifolia*) [Panama]; "**biliousness**" (*D. canadense* root decocted, *D. giganteum, D. heterophyllum* root, *D. triflorum*, root) [India, Iroquois, Nepal].
- **Gall stones** (*D. styracifolium*) [China].

INFECTION

- **Abscess** (*D. caudatum, D. canadense, D. triflorum*) [China, India, Java]; **sores** (*D. adscendens, D. heterophyllum, D. triflorum*) [India, Liberia, Malaya]; **infections**.
- **Fever** (*D. canum*, D.*caudatum, D. giganteum, D. styracifolium*) [China, India, Trinidad]; **chronic fever** (*D. giganteum*) [Nepal]; **flu with fever** (*D. caudatum*) [China].
- **Consumption** (*D. adscendens*) [Amazonia (leaf decocted)]; **tuberculosis**.
- **Malaria** (*D. adscendens*) [Amazonia (root decocted), Brazil, Suriname].
- **Epidemic encephalitis** (*D. heterocarpum*) [China].

LYMPHATIC

- **Lymph enlargement**; **spleen inflammation** (*D. triflorum*) [India].

MUSCULOSKELETAL / TRAUMA

- **Aches and pains** (*D. adscendens*) [Brazil]; **back pain** (*D. adscendens* decocted, or in rum, *D. gyroides*) [Belize, Java]; **rheumatism** (*D. gyroides, D. triflorum*) [Haiti, Perak]; **rheumatic arthralgia** (*D. triquetrum, D. pseudotriquetrum*) [China].
- **Fractures** (*D. adscendens*); **wounds** (*D. adscendens*) [Africa, Amazonia, Ghana]; **trauma** [China (poulticed)].
- **Cramps** [Cherokee (*D. nudiflorum, D. perplexum* root infused, topical), Houma (*D. paniculatum* root infused in whiskey)].

NEUROLOGICAL

- **Convulsions** (*D. adscendens, D. mollicum*) [Amazonia (leaf infused), Liberia]; **epilepsy**.
- **Nerve pain**.
- **Vertigo**.

ONCOLOGY

- **Hepato-digestive side effects from chemotherapy** (*D. ascendens*).

PEDIATRIC

- **Colic** (*D. adscendens, D. capitatum*) [Africa, Ghana (leaf decocted), Perak]; **infant malnutrition** [China *D. triquetrum, D. pseudotriquetrum*]; **diarrhea in children** (*D. triflorum* or *D. heterophyllum)* leaves ground in cow's milk [India].
- **Parotitis** (*D. heterocarpum*) [China]; **measles, childhood eruptive diseases** ("tou gin") (*D. caudatum*) [China].

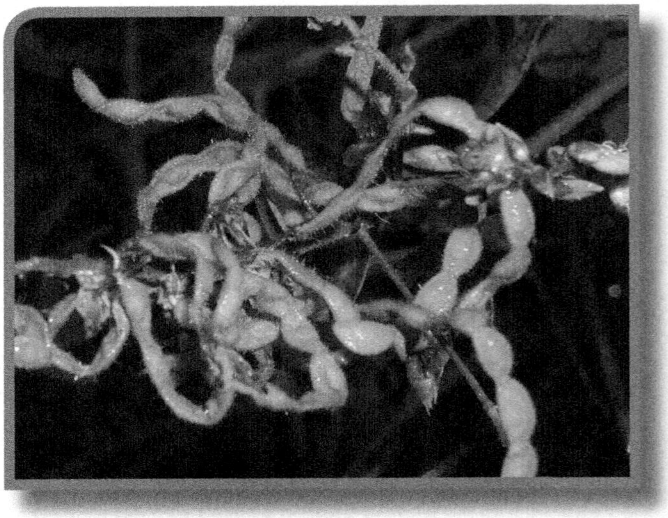

Desmodium spp.: Puapilipili seeds

PSYCHOSPIRITUAL

- **Nervousness** (*D. adscendens*) [Amazonia (infused)].
- **A "sedative for the brain"** (*D. giganteum*) [India].

REPRODUCTIVE

- **Gonorrhea** (*D. styracifolium*) [China]; **venereal disease** (*D. adscendens*) [Amazonia, Liberia, Nicaragua, Trinidad].
- **Childbirth** (*D. canum, D. pulchellum*) [Bahamas, Malaya]; **post partum** (*D. laxiflorum*) [Philippines]; **mastitis** (*D. caudatum, D. heterocarpum*) [China, Malaya]; **to increase lactation** [Rio Pastaza Indians (topical as a wash)].
- **Abnormal menstruation** (*D. canum*) [Bahamas]; **menstrual cramps** (*D. ascendens, D. caudatum*) [China]; **ovarian irritation** (*D. adscendens*) [Peru]; **uterine bleeding** (*D. adscendens*) [Peru].
- **Vaginal discharge** (*D. adscendens*) [Brazil, Peru]; **vaginal infections** (*D. adscendens* as a bath) [Amazonia]; **vaginitis** (*D. mollicum*).
- **Impotence**.
- **Emesis gravidarum** (*D. triquetrum, D. pseudotriquetrum*) [China].

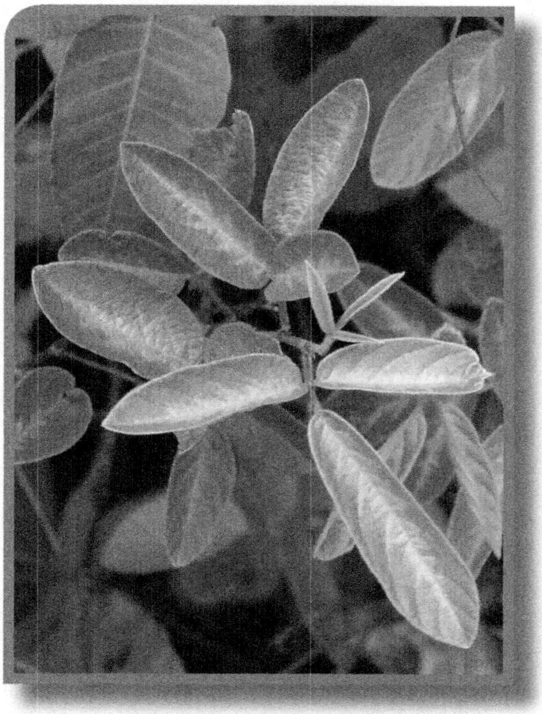

Desmodium spp.: Puapilipili leaves

RESPIRATORY

- **Allergies** (*D. adscendens*); **asthma** (*D. adscendens, D. giganteum*) [Africa, Ghana, Hawai'i (smoked), Nepal, Suriname]; **bronchitis** (*D. adscendens*) [Africa]; **congested lungs and nasal passages** (*D. ascendens*); **cough** (*D. adscendens, D. giganteum, D. heterocarpum, D. polycarpum*) [Cameroon, Malaya, Nepal, Tanganyika (leaves smoked)]; **coughing blood** (*D. triquetrum, D. pseudotriquetrum*) [China]; **phlegm** (*D. gangeticum*) [India]; **pneumonosis** (*D. triquetrum, D. pseudotriquetrum*) [China].
- **Common cold** (*D. triquetrum, D. pseudotriquetrum*) [China]; **head cold** [Tanganyika (leaves smoked)]; **common cold and lung problems** [Alabama tribe (as an emetic)].

> ***D. gyrans* is used with *Banisteriopsis caapi* in Ayahuasca mixtures**

URINARY

- **Kidney problems** (*D. adscendens, D. cajanifolia*) [Amazonia, Panama]; **kidney stones** (*D. gangeticum, D. styracifolium*) [China, Java, Malaya]; **kidney degeneration**.
- **Urinary problems** (*D. adscendens*) [Peru, Suriname]; **urinary tract infection** (*D. canum*) [Trinidad]; **urinary abscess** (*D. adscendens*) [Brazil]; **decreased urination** (*D. adscendens, D. canum, D. heterocarpum, D. heterophyllum* roots, *D. triflorum*) [China, India, Trinidad].

OTHER MEDICINAL USES

- **Environmental toxins** (*D. adscendens*) [Peru]; **fatigue** (*D. ascendens*); **wasting of the flesh** (*D. adscendens*) [Trinidad].
- **Mucous discharge**.
- **Inflammation**.
- **Hookworms** (*D. triquetrum, D. pseudotriquetrum*) [China].

USE AS FOOD: Indians in Central America eat *D. parvifolium* as a green vegetable.

OTHER USES: Given to a lover who has lost interest in his partner to make him return [Amazonia].

CONSTITUENTS: From various species: Astragalin, beta-phenylethylamines, beta-sitosterol, cosmosiin, cyanidin-3-o-sophoroside, dehydrosoyasaponin I (DHS-I), desmodimine, eicosanoic acid eicosyl ester, hordenine, isoflavones, lupenone, lupeol, pelargonidin-3-o-rhamnoside, phenethylamines, salsoline, soyasaponin I, soyasaponin II, soyasaponin III, stearic acid, tectorigenin, tetrahydroisoquinolines, triterpenoid saponins, tritriacontane, tryptamines (*D. pulchellum*), tyramine.
Some species of *Desmodium* (*D. uncinatum* & *D. canum*) contain isoflavones [Tsanuo 2003; Botta 2003]. Isoflavones may have evolved among some legumes to cause a kind of "birth control" against over-foraging animals, preventing them from reproducing.
Desmodium pulchellum contains tryptamines.

Pua Pilipili Local Combinations

Hepatitis: Add *Bidens pilosa* (kīnehi / spanish needle), *Eclipta alba* (han lian cao), and *Boerhavia* spp. (alena).
Asthma: Add *Waltheria indica* ('uhaloa) root bark, *Curcuma longa* ('ōlena / Turmeric), and *Musa* spp. (mai'a / banana) sap.
Back pain: Add *Siegesbeckia orientalis* (xi xian cao) and *Piper methysticum* ('awa).

Pua Pilipili Cross-Cultural Combinations

Wounds: *D. adscendens* leaf poulticed with lime juice (ouch!) [Amazonia].
To increase lactation: Ground leaves with "long green pepper" [Ghana].
Decreased urination: Decocted with *Plantago major* (laukahi / plantain) [China].

RANGE: Tropics and subtropics.

GATHERING: No need... da sticky li'l buggah gon' gaddah you....

PROPAGATION & CULTIVATION: No.

RESEARCH:

- Water and ethanol extracts of *D. ascendens* administered orally prevent anaphylaxis and block histimine contractions in guinea pigs [Addy 1984]. *D. ascendens* inhibits arachadonic acid metabolism and may relieve asthma through various mechanisms; including the inhibition of allergic airway muscle contractions and the blockage of histamine response in the lungs [Addy 1986; 1988; 1990; 1992].
- The ethanol extract of *D. adscendens* causes analgesia and hypothermia in mice [N'gouemo 1996].
- *D. adscendens* may function as a calcium channel blocker or potassium channel opener (DHS-I) [Barreto 2002; McManus 1993].
- *D. styracifolium* may reduce the formation of calcium oxalate renal stones [Hirayama 2003].
- Various extracts of *D. barbatum* are antibacterial in vitro [Jimenez Misas 1979].
- Ethanol extracts of *D. triflorum* are anthelmintic in vitro against roundworms [Raj 1975].

NOTES 'N QUOTES

- There are 450 listed species of *Desmodium* with 7 growing in Hawaii. For expediency I have lumped them together here. While there are many overlapping features in the genus, there are also traditional differences in usage. Some species are used more in South America for liver disease, asthma, and back pain, while others are used more in China for kidney stones and gall stones.

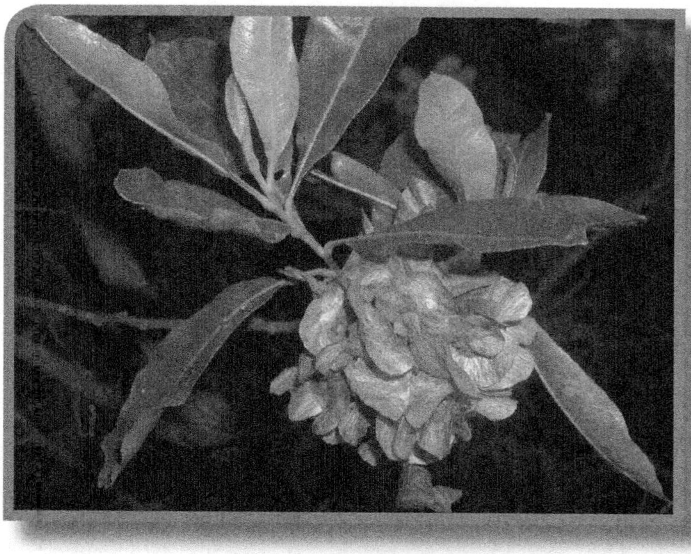

Dodonaea viscosa ('A'ali'i)

PLANT NAME: *Dodonaea viscosa* Jacq.

OTHER NAMES: 'A'ali'i was once considered many different species including *D. sandwicensis*, *D. eriocarpa*, and *D. spathulata*. These are now all considered *D. viscosa*. 'A'ali'i is a polymorph; it tends to mutate into many varieties. In Hawai'i it is a taxonomist's nightmare, with no seemingly reasonable way to organize the gene pool.

Status: Indigenous.

Habitat: Sunny, hot, dry.

COMMON NAMES: **'A'ali'i**, 'a'ali'i kū makani ("'a'ali'i upright in the wind") [Hawai'i]; ake, akeake, akerantangi [New Zealand]; alipata [Philipines (Tagalog)]; 'apiri [Tahiti]; bandari [India]; calapinai [Philipines (Tagalog)]; candlewood, dogwood [Bahamas]; chacataya [Bolivia]; chamana [Ecuador, Peru]; chamiso [Argentina]; chanamo, hayuelo [Colombia]; chapuliztle, cuerco de calva, granadina [Mexico]; chulita [Guatemala]; florida hopbush, hopshrub [England]; gansies [Afrikan]; gelampaya, serengan laut [Malaya]; gitaran [Puerto Rico]; granadillo, hayo [Venezuela]; hopbush, native hop [Australia]; hopwood [England]; kabunda [Congo]; kankerbos [Afrikan]; kayu berthi. letup letup [Malaya]; kayu mesen, kisig, mesen [Java]; kharata [India]; mai pek [Thailand]; manglier petites feuilles [Haiti]; mukusao, umusasa [Congo]; native birch, native lignum vitae [Tasmania]; sanatha [Pakistan]; sanatta [Sanskrit]; switch sorrel [Jamaica]; vassoura vermelha [Brazil]; vrali [Spain]; walaytinahndi [Hindi]; yxichapulin [Aztec].

NOMENCLATURE: The family name Sapindaceae comes from "sapo" or soap, a reference to the abundance of saponins in the family. Phillip Miller named the genus in 1754 after the 16th century Flemish botanist Rembert Dodoens (1517-1585). The epithet viscosa means "sticky" or "thick".

FAMILY: Sapindaceae.

CATEGORY: Expel wind damp~.

PROPERTIES: Astringent, cool to cold~, toxic.

PLANT PART USED: Usually leaves, but sometimes bark or roots.

TOXICITY: Mildly Toxic. *Dodonaea* contains small amounts of cyanogenic toxins: plant materials that can cause cyanide poisoning.

CAUTIONS AND CONTRAINDICATIONS: Topical use only.

PREPARATION OF MEDICINE: Poulticed or decocted for topical use only.

DOSAGE: As needed.

WESTERN FUNCTIONS REPORTED: **Analgesic**; **anodyne** (leaves); **anthelmintic** (extract); **antibiotic** (extract); **antiHIV**; **antimicrobial**; **antiseptic**; **antispasmodic**; **antitumor** (extract); **antiviral**; **astringent** (leaves); **bactericide**; **candidicide**; **carminative**; **dentifrice**; **diaphoretic** (leaves); **febrifuge** [Tahiti]; **fungicidal**; **hemostatic** (leaves infused); **hypotensive** (extract); **lactagogue**; **myorelaxant**; **odontalgic** (leaves); **panacea**; **poultice**; **sedative** (?); **purgative** [Tahiti]; **spasmolytic** (extract); **stimulant** (leaves chewed); **styptic**; **sudorific** [Reunion Island (leaves infused)]; **tonic**; **vulnerary** (leaves).

TRADITIONAL CHINESE ENERGETIC FUNCTIONS (~ = extrapolated):

1) Expels wind dampness~.
2) Clears damp heat~.
3) Calms internal wind~.

'A'ali'i Common Medicinal Uses

- Dermatological conditions

'A'ali'i Cross-Cultural Medicinal Uses

BITES & STINGS
- **Stingray wounds or just plain stings** [Australia (leaves poulticed or root decoction topical)].
- **Snake bite** [India, Pakistan].

CARDIOVASCULAR
- **Bleeding** [Colombia].
- **High blood pressure**.

COSMETIC
- **To prevent scarring** (leaf powder topical).

DERMATOLOGICAL
- In Australian aboriginal medicine, *Dodonaea* is burned and used topically **for any wound from the ocean**.
- **Abscesses, boils** [Hawai'i (leaves poulticed), Latin America (boiled leaves poulticed)].
- **Rash, itching and skin diseases** [Hawai'i (young leaf tips poulticed)]. In old Hawai'i 'A'ali'i was used as a wash for **rashes and contagious diseases**.
- **Burns & scalds** [Indonesia (topical)].
- **Eczema**.
- **Fungus**.

DIGESTIVE
- **Stomach problems** [South Africa].
- **Gas**.
- **Hemorrhoids**.

HEAD AND THROAT
- **Sore ears** [Australia (root decoction topical)].
- **Tooth ache** [Australia (leaves chewed), Panama (leaves chewed)].
- **Sore throat** [Madagascar (leaf)].

INFECTION
- **Fever** [New Caledonia, Madagascar (leaves), Mexico (leaves decocted), Pakistan, Reunion Island (wood decocted)].
- **Streptococcus**.
- **Influenza**.
- **Candida**.

MUSCULOSKELETAL / TRAUMA
- **Rheumatism and gout** [Hawai'i, Mexico (leaves decocted)].
- **Sprains & wounds, bruising**; **fractures** [Oaxacan Chinantecs (leaves)]; **swelling**.
- **Shoulder problems**.
- **Cramps**.

PEDIATRIC
- **Colic** [Mexico (leaves decocted)].

PSYCHOSPIRITUAL
- **Insomnia**.
- **'A'ali'i is sacred to Laka, the goddess of hula**.
- Used as a wash for **protection against supernatural forces** [Hawai'i].
- In Peru 'a'ali'i is sometimes chewed with, and used as an alternative to, coca leaves (not recommended!).

REPRODUCTIVE
- **Infertility** [Oaxacan Chinantecs (leaves)].
- **Painful menses** [Oaxacan Chinantecs (leaves)].
- **Post partum** [Oaxacan Chinantecs (leaves)].
- **Threatened miscarriage** [Oaxacan Chinantecs (leaves)].
- **Venereal disease** [Mexico (leaf decocted)]; **HIV**.

VETERINARY
- 'A'ali'i is **said to have harmed camels and killed calves**.

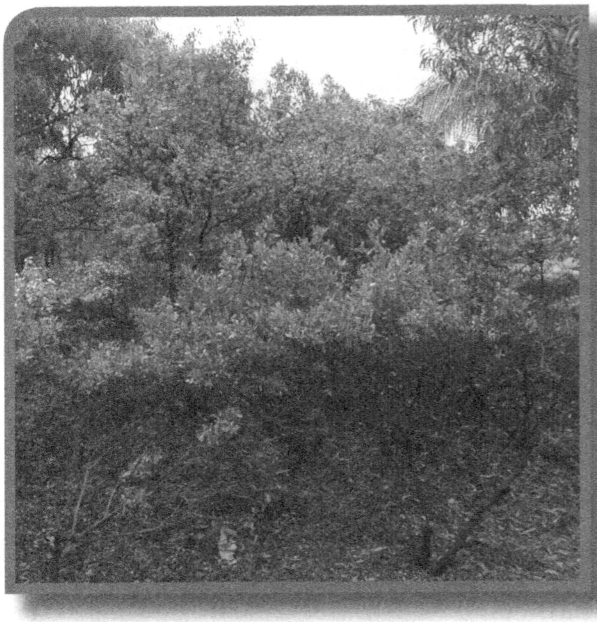

Dodonaea viscosa ('A'ali'i) tree

USE AS FOOD: Australians reportedly use the fruit instead of hops to make beer, though considering it's reported toxicity this warrants more research. The seeds are reportedly edible.

OTHER USES:
- The wood is hard and has been used in Hawai'i for woodworking, house construction, agricultural implements, and fishing equipment. 'Ō'ō (digging sticks), squid spears, and squid lures were among some of its uses.

- The fruit was used to make a red dye for kapa; and in making haku leis.
- In Bolivia, *Dodonaea viscosa* is used as a control for "ulu" (*Eloria noyesii*), a pest of the coca plant.
- The seed oil has been used to make soap.
- The Masai use the stems as a toothbrush.
- Materials in the fruit are used to stun fish.

CONSTITUENTS: 21,22-diangeloyl-barringtogenol-c (stem); 21,22-diangeloyl-r1-barringenol (stem); 21-angeloyl-r1-barringenol (stem); 3,6,4'trimethoxy-5,7-dioxyflavone; 4h-1-benzopyran-4-one; 5,7-dihydroxy-3,6-dimethoxy-2-(4-methoxyphenyl) -flavone; arachidic-acid (seed); behenic-acid (seed); beta-sitosterol (seed); cleomiscosin (stem); dodogenin (seed); dodonin (seed); erucic-acid (seed); fat (seed); hautriwaic-acid (leaf); hentriacontane (leaf); hyperin (fruit); hyperin (leaf); isorhamnetin-3-o-rutinoside (fruit & leaf); linoleic-acid (seed); oleic-acid (seed); palmitic-acid (seed); phytosterols (leaf); protein (seed); quebrachitol; resin (leaf); rutin (fruit & leaf); saponin (seed); stearic-acid (seed); stigmast-5-en-3-ol; stigmasterol (stem); tannin (bark & leaf).

- The leaves are reportedly slightly cyanogenic and are said to contain as much as 18% tannins. They also contain saponins. Saponins are glycosides that are toxic but so difficult to absorb that they often pass through the body undigested. The Saponins of some plants are used to stun fish.

'A'ali'i Local Combinations

Ringworm (*Tinea corporis, T. capitis*) or "**Haole rot**" (*Tinea versicolor*): Topical as a wash. Add *Ageratum conyzoides* (maile hohono).

Staff infections: Topical. Add *Musa* spp. (mai'a / banana) sap.

'A'ali'i Cross-Cultural Combinations

Topical for rashes - Use 'a'ali'i (*Dodonaea viscosa*).

Internal for rashes - Has been usedwith one or more of the following (see *toxicity*):

Plantago major (laukahi / plantain).
Bidens pilosa (kīnehi / spanish needle).
Stellaria media (chickweed).

RANGE: Tropics and subtropical areas world-wide.

HABITAT:

- Sandy and rocky soil from coastal regions up to 8200'. Likes it sunny, hot and dry. Wind, pruning, and drought tolerant. By Hawaiian standards, 'a'ali'i is "one tough buggah."
- 'A'ali'i is one of the few native Hawaiian plants that responds well to fire. It will reintroduce itself to an area quickly after a fire, and, along with 'ōhi'a (*Metrosideros polymorpha*) and kupukupu (*Nephrolepis multiflora*), is a frequent volunteer on recent lava flows.

GATHERING: Sacred to Kapo and Laka the hula goddesses.

PROPAGATION & CULTIVATION:

- By seed or cuttings. 'a'ali'i is dioecious (each plant is only one gender), so you'd best gather in the wild from a co-ed cluster. Scarify the seeds with boiling water and soak overnight. In Australia there has been success from long soaking, nicking, and even microwave boiling for a few seconds.
- *Dodonaea* apparently has no animal or insect pollinators, relying solely on the wind for reproduction.

RESEARCH:

- Antiseptic [Rojas 2003].
- Crude extracts are antibacterial against *Streptococcus pyogenes* and *Staphylococcus aureus* [Getie 2003].
- Antiviral against Coxsackie virus B3 and influenza A [Getie 2003].
- Chloroform-methanol extracts relax smooth muscle in lab animals, possibly through interference with calcium metabolism [Rojas 1992].

"He 'a'ali'i ku makani mai au; 'a'ohe makani nana e kulā'ī."
I stand as strong in the wind as an 'a'ali'i that no gale can knock down.
- - Traditional Hawaiian boast

NOTES 'N QUOTES

- The first written record of use in Hawai'i was 1922.
- There are 65 species in the genus *Dodonaea*, 59 of which are endemic to Australia.
- While 'a'al'i wood is reportedly termite resistant, the plant is host to the native koa bugs and the Blackburn Butterfly.

- Will reportedly sink in fresh water.
- Thanks to Jim Duke for his information on *Dodonaea.*

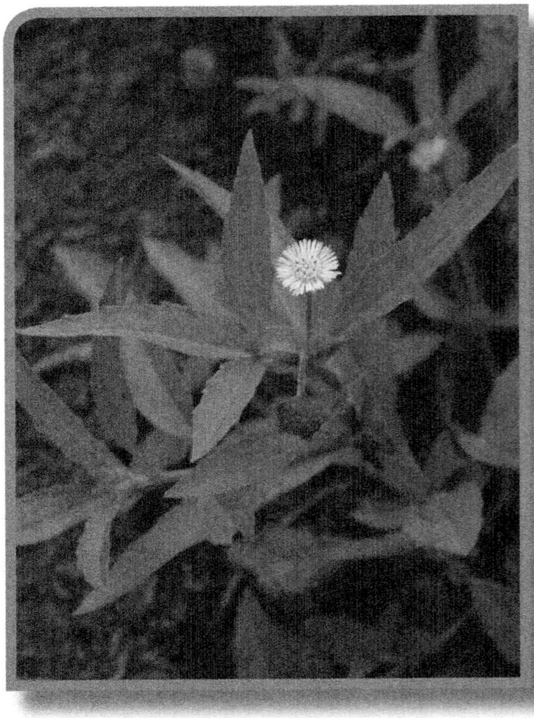

Eclipta prostrata (Han Lian Cao)

PLANT NAME: *Eclipta prostrata* (L.) L.

OTHER NAMES: *E. alba, Verbesina alba,* V. *prostrata.*

Status: Cute but alien. Low pest factor.

Habitat: Warm, wet, salty.

SIMILARLY USED SPECIES: *Alternantha sessilis.*

COMMON NAMES: **Han lian cao** [China]; false daisy, trailing eclipta [USA]; bhringaraj ("king of the tresses"), kayyunni, kannunni [India]; hong ling cho [Canton]; takasaburo [Japan].

NOMENCLATURE: From the Greek ekleipein, meaning "deficiency," a reference to *Eclipta*'s lack of a plant part called a pappus.

FAMILY: Asteraceae (Daisy family).

CATEGORY: Tonify Yin.

PROPERTIES: Sweet, sour, cool to cold. (In India: sweet, sour, and cool or… acrid bitter hot and dry… depending on the source.)

PLANT PART USED: Traditionally all of it is used. I gather flowering tops.

TOXICITY: None noted.

CAUTIONS AND CONTRAINDICATIONS: Strong doses of fresh decoction may disturb digestion.

ENERGETIC CAUTIONS: Not with diarrhea from cold Spleen / Kidneys. Can cause chills.

PREPARATION OF MEDICINE: Infused, decocted, medicated oil, medicated ghee.

DOSAGE: 10 grams dried. 30 grams fresh.

STATUS IN HAWAI'I: Cute but alien. Low pest factor... can be difficult to find, but worth it. Look near salt spray. I've also seen it in gardens at 1100' elevation.

MERIDIAN AFFINITIES: Liver, Kidney.

WESTERN FUNCTIONS REPORTED: **Alterative** [India (root)]; **antifungal**; **antipyretic** [China, India]; **antiseptic** [India (roots)]; **antitoxic** [China]; **antiviral** [India]; **astringent** [China]; **benefits hair and skin** [India]; **calms the mind** [India]; **cholagogue** [India (leaf and root)]; **cools and purifies the blood** [India]; **darkens the hair** [China (internal)]; **deobstruent** [India (leaf juice)]; **depurative**; **draws out poison** [India]; **emetic** [India (root)]; **expels intestinal worms** [India]; **febrifuge**; **hair-dye** [China]; **hair-oil** [India]; **heals ulcers** [India]; **hemostatic** [China, India]; **hepatic tonic** [India (leaf juice)]; **improves post-operative healing** [India]; **insecticide**; **laxative** [India]; **nervine** [India]; **nourishes the organism** [India]; **nourishing to liver and kidneys**; **ophthalmic**; **prevents aging** [India]; **prevents cellulite** [India]; **prevents hair loss** [India]; **promotes deep sleep** [India (oil)]; **promotes hair growth** [China (topical)]; **purgative** [India (root)]; **reduces inflammation** [India]; **reduces stomach acid** [India]; **rejuvenates bones, hair, memory, sight, and teeth** [India]; **speeds healing of cuts** [India]; **speeds internal healing** [India]; **stimulates the digestion** [India (leaf juice internal)]; **stops bleeding** [India]; **stop uterine bleeding** [India, China]; **strengthens the hair** [China]; **strengthens the spleen** [India]; **strengthens the body** [India]; **styptic**; **tonic** [China, India (root)]; **vulnerary** [India].

TRADITIONAL CHINESE ENERGETIC FUNCTIONS (~ = extrapolated):
Tonify yin, stop bleeding.

OTHER ENERGETIC FUNCTIONS: Reduces kapha and vata, rejuvenates pitta [India].

Han Lian Cao Cross-Cultural Medicinal Uses

COSMETIC

- **Premature gray hair** [China]; **topical to color the hair** [India].
- **Balding** [China, Singapore].
- **Ink for tattooing** [India].
- **Poor complexion** [India].

CARDIOVASCULAR

- **Vomiting or coughing up blood, nose bleed, blood in the stool, uterine bleeding, bleeding wounds, and especially bloody urine** [China].
- **Thrombocytopenic purpura** [China, Research].
- **Anemia** [China, Suriname].
- **Bleeding due to "yin deficiency"** [China].

Han Lian Cao
Common Medicinal Uses

- Gray hair or balding
- Bleeding
- Hepatitis
- General "tonic"

DERMATOLOGICAL

- **Skin conditions** [Caribbean (topical), India (poultice); Philippines]; **eczema** [China]; **dermatitis** (topical); **"rice-field" dermatitis** [China].
- **Ringworm** [Java].
- **Tinea pedia** (athlete's foot) [China].

DIGESTIVE

- **Constipation** [India].
- **Gastric ulcer** [India]; **duodenal ulcer**, **peptic ulcer** [India]; **melena** (tarry stools) [China].
- **Vomiting blood** [China].
- **Copremia** (blood poisoning from fecal contamination) [China].
- **Gastritis** [China]; **gastrosis** [Malaya]; **enteritis** [China]; **enterorrhagia** [China]; **dysentery** [China, Suriname].
- **Indigestion** [China].
- **Low appetite** [India (leaf juice internal)].

HEAD AND THROAT

- **Blurred vision** [Caribbean, China]; **conjunctivitis** [China]; **eye diseases** [India, Suriname]; **night blindness** (specific) [India].
- **Ear ache** [India (juice topical)].
- **Mouth ulcers** [India]; **tooth loss** [China]; **toothache** [India, Java].
- With oil topical for **headache** [India].

HEPATIC

- **Acute and chronic hepatitis**, **jaundice**, **& cirrhosis** [China, India, Suriname].

INFECTION

- **Abscess**, **boils** [China].
- **Fevers** [China, India (leaf juice internal)].

LYMPHATIC

- **Enlarged spleen** [India].
- **Swollen glands** [Caribbean, India (poulticed for respiratory infection)].
- **Elephantiasis** [India].

MUSCULOSKELETAL / TRAUMA

- **Lumbago** [China]; **rheumatic joint pains** [India (leaf juice internal)].
- **Scorpion sting** [India]; **snake bite** [China].
- **Trauma** [China]; **wounds** [Caribbean].

NEUROLOGICAL

- **Vertigo**, **dizziness** [Caribbean, China, Malaya].
- **Memory disorders** [India].
- **Tinnitus** [China].

ONCOLOGY

- **Cancer** [India].

PARASITES

- **For worms** with castor oil [India].

PEDIATRIC

- **For infants with respiratory infections**, eight drops of honey with two drops of plant juice [India].
- **Diphtheria** [China (fresh)].
- **Infantile malnutrition** [China].
- **Pertussis** [Trinidad].

PSYCHOSPIRITUAL

- **Giddiness** [Malaya].
- **Neurasthenia**, **neurosis** [China].
- **Calms the emotional body** (oil topical), insomnia (oil on the feet), for excess pitta [Ayurveda].

REPRODUCTIVE

- **Excessive menstrual bleeding** [China]; **uterine hemorrhaging** [India (30 – 60 grams leaf decocted per day)].
- **Parturition** (after giving birth) [Malaya].

RESPIRATORY

- **Asthma** [Caribbean, India, Suriname].
- **Bronchitis** [Caribbean]; **catarrh** [India].
- **Cough** [India, Trinidad].
- **Coughing blood** [China]; **tuberculosis** [China].

URINARY

- **Bladder infection** [China]; **painful urination** [India]; **urogenital problems** [China].
- **Edema** [India (leaf juice internal)].

VETERINARY

- **Skin diseases in dogs** [Trinidad, Tobago].
- **Ulcers and wounds in cattle** (roots topical)

OTHER MEDICINAL USES

- **Athlete's foot** (topical).
- **Fevers caused by imbalance of the doshas**: pitta, vata, and kapha [India].
- **Marasmus** (wasting of the flesh)[Trinidad].

USE AS FOOD: Cooked leaves are edible. Leaves eaten as a vegetable [India].

OTHER USES: Black dye used for hair. Also tattoos.

ESSENTIAL OIL: Promotes deep sleep [India].

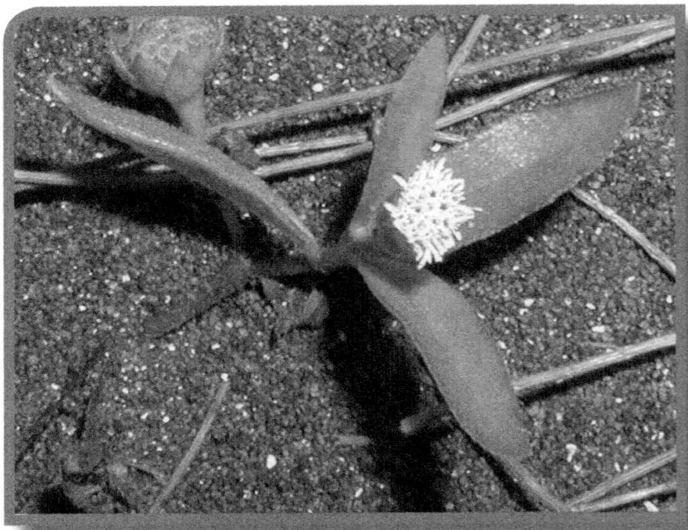

Eclipta prostrata: Han Lian Cao

CONSTITUENTS:3,4-dihydoxy benzoic acid; a-formyl-a-terthienyl; alpha-formylterthienyl; alpha-terthienyl; a-terthienylmethanol; beta-sitosterol;

c-terthienylmethanol,; demethyl wedelolactone; demethylwedelolactone; ecliptine; ediptne; isodemethylwedelolactone; lacceroic acid; nicotine; nonacosanol; saponins; stearic acid; stigmasterol; strychnolactone; thiophene derivates; wedelolactone.

- The most useful constituents seem to be various wedelolactones which research shows to be remarkably liver protective and reputed to be an "extremely aggressive" free radical scavenger. Other ingredients (stigmasterol and alpha-terthienyl) are also liver protective... at least if you're a rat [Singh 2001; Zhang 2001].

POSSIBLE DRUG INTERACTIONS: Contains coumarins. Speculative caution with anti-coagulants.

Han Lian Cao Local Combinations

Gastric bleeding: Add *Erigeron canadensis* (fleabane).
Hepatitis: Add *Bidens pilosa* (kīnehi / spanish needle).
Blood in the urine: Add *Plantago major* (plantain).
Night sweats: Add *Ophiopogon* spp. (mai men dong / mondo grass) tubers.

Han Lian Cao Cross-Cultural Combinations

Coughing blood or vomiting blood: With *Nelumbo nucifera* (he ye / lotus) leaves and *Biota orientalis* (ce bai ye) leaves [China].
Lung congestion in children: Juiced with honey.
Blood in the urine: With *Imperatae cylindrica* (bai mao gen) and *Plantago asiatica* (che qian zi / plantain); or *Rehmannia glutinosa* (sheng di huang) [China].
Premature balding: With *Ligustrum lucidum* (nu zhen zi), *Polygonum multiflorum* (he shou wu), *Rehmannia glutinosa* (shu di huang), *Angelica sinensis*, (dang gui), *Ligusticum wallichi* (chuan xiong), and *Paeonia alba* (bai shao) [China].
Skin diseases: 16 parts of *Eclipta prostrata* (bhringaraj), 1 part of Triphala formula {*Emblica officinalis* (amalaki), *Terminalia chebula*, (haritaki), *Terminalia belerica* (bibhitaki)}, 1 part of *Caltropis gigantea* (arka) and 1 part of *Smilax officinalis* (sariva) mixed with 80 parts of sesame oil and boiled to make a medicated oil [India].
Jaundice: With *Wedelia calendulacea* [India].
Hair tonic: Topical with mineral oil, or leaf juice boiled with coconut oil [India].
To boost immunity: With *Astragalus membranaceus* (huang qi) and *Ligustrum lucidum* (nu zhen zi).
Burning urination: With salt [India].
Blood in the stool: With *Sanguisorba officinalis* (di yu) [China].
Weak lungs, dizziness, and gray hair: With *Ligustrum lucidum* (nu zhen zi) [China].
Bleeding peptic ulcer: With *Juncus effusus* (deng xin cao) [China].
Sedative: With *Bacopa monnieri* (brahmi) [India].

RANGE: China, Japan, Malaysia, Philippines, Australia & Hawai'i; but native to the Americas.

HABITAT: Likes it warm and wet. Grows best near the ocean. Partial shade.

GATHERING: At the start of flowering. Because of its' affinity to the kahakai (seashore), I use Kanaloa as kinolau when gathering. It appears to be an annual.

PROPAGATION & CULTIVATION: Start seeds in a green house. Transplant to pots. It looks like it might clone well, but I've never tried.

RESEARCH:

- The Chinese patent remedy Er Zhi Wan (*Ligustrum lucidum & Eclipta prostrata*) has been clinically proven effective for yin deficiency in rats [Cao 2000]. I swear I am not making this up. Do rats get night sweats and red cheeks? How do they check the tongue & pulse?
- Extracts are liver protective [Saxena 1993]. An alcohol-extracted consituent of *Eclipta prostrata* is liver protective in rats [Han 1998; Singh 2001].
- Alkaloid extracts of E. *prostrata* are analgesic [Sawant 2004].
- Methanol extracts are antifungal and antibacterial [Wiart 2004].
- Extracts have been shown to be effective against snakebite [Martz 1992; Mors 1989 & 1991]. Alas, there are no snakes in Hawai'i.

One of the ten auspicious flowers (Dasapuspam) in Ayurveda and said to be the best herb in Ayurveda for liver cirrhosis and infectious hepatitis.

NOTES 'N QUOTES

- The first recorded use of *Eclipta prostrata* was in the Tang Materia Medica AD 659.
- *Eclipta* is used in the Chinese patent medicine Qiang sheng bu gan pian.
- *Eclipta prostrata* flowers are hermaphroditic (contain both sexes).
- *Eclipta* is one of the few "yin tonics" among Hawaiian medicinals. Although sometimes difficult to find, *Eclipta*, when needed, can be worth the hunt. In Taiwan, the Hawaiian weed *Alternanthera sessilis* (joyweed) is called (and used as) han lian cao.

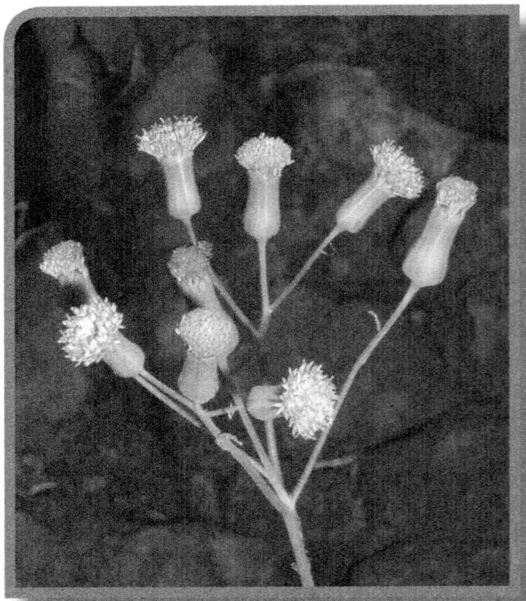

Emilia spp. (Red Pualele)

PLANT NAME: *Emilia* spp.

OTHER NAMES OR **SIMILARLY USED SPECIES**: *Cacalia sonchifolia, E. coccinea, E. sonchifolia, E. fosbergii, Hieracium javanicum.*

COMMON NAMES: **Red pualele** [Hawai'i]; yang ti cao (goatsfoot grass), yi dian hong, yang ti gen [China]; **floras paintbrush**, cupid's shaving brush, lilac tasselflower [English]; banasurya [India]; emilienkraut [German].

Status: Alien. Low pest factor.

NOMENCLATURE: Pualele means "jumping flower," a reference to the seeds of many of the asteraceae (dandelion) family that scatter in the wind.

Habitat: Dry, sunny, disturbed areas. Low elevations.

FAMILY: Asteraceae.

CATEGORY: Clear heat and toxins ~.

PROPERTIES: Bitter cool.

PLANT PART USED: Whole plant.

TOXICITY: Possibly some long term chronic toxicity. **Until more definitive research has been done, I do not recommend using this plant.**

CAUTIONS AND CONTRAINDICATIONS: May contain pyrrolizidine alkaloids. Not in pregnancy. Not in liver disease.

ENERGETIC CAUTIONS: Caution in deficient spleen stomach ~.

PREPARATION OF MEDICINE: Decocted, mashed for topical use.

DOSAGE: 10 grams in combination.

WESTERN FUNCTIONS REPORTED: **Analgesic** [China]; **antipyretic** [China]; **anti-swelling** [China]; **antitoxic** [China]; **depurative**; **diaphoretic**; **diuretic** [China]; **febrifuge** (leaves) [Africa]; **ophthalmic**; **refrigerant** [China]; **sudorific** [India].

TRADITIONAL CHINESE ENERGETIC FUNCTIONS (~ = extrapolated):

1) Clear heat and poison.
2) Lowers fever.
3) Drains dampness.
4) Reduces swelling.

Red Pualele Common Medicinal Uses

- **Colds and flu**
- **Infections**

Red Pualele Cross-Cultural Medicinal Uses

DERMATOLOGICAL

- **Eczema** [China]; **sores** [Malaya].

DIGESTIVE

- **Diarrhea** (root) [India, Java], **enteritis**, **dysentery**, **painful dysentery** [China].

HEAD AND THROAT

- **Conjunctivitis** [Africa (leaves juiced)]; **eye inflammations** (leaves juiced); **eye problems** [India]; **night blindness** (leaves juiced) [India]; **ophthalmia** [Java].
- **Ear problems** [India]; **ear ache** [Java]; **otitis** [India]; **sore ears** (leaves juiced); **tympanitis** [India].
- **Laryngitis**, **oral ulcer**, **pharyngitis** [China]; **sore throat** [China, Ghana].

INFECTION

- **Boils and abscesses** [China]; **furunculosis** [China]; **infected wounds** [China, India].
- **Colds and flu** [China]; **influenza** [China, Europe]; **upper respiratory tract infection** [China].
- **Fever** [China, Europe, India, Java].

LYMPHATIC

- **Lymphoma** [China].

MUSCULOSKELETAL / TRAUMA

- **Swelling** [Java]; **traumatic injury** [China].
- **Wounds** [China, India].

NEUROLOGICAL

- "**Fits**" [India (roots ground internal)].

ONCOLOGY

- **Leukemia** [China].
- **Tumor**.

PEDIATRIC

- **Infantile bowel complaints, abdominal distention with gas** (root).

REPRODUCTIVE

- **Mastitis** [China].
- **Orchitis** [China].

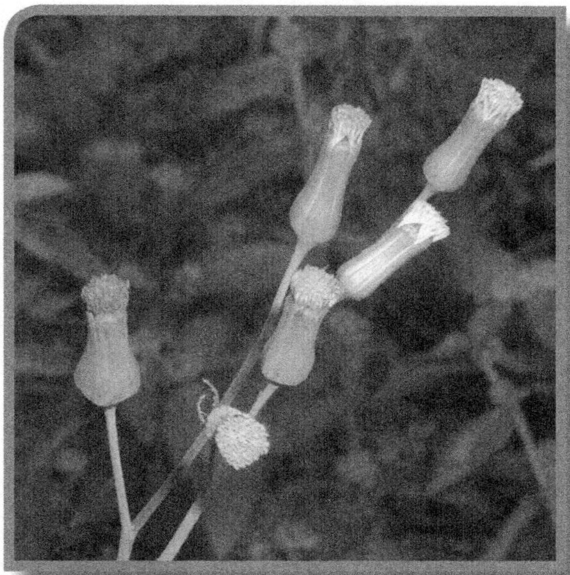

Emilia spp.: Red Pualele flowers

RESPIRATORY

- **Bronchitis** [Europe].
- **Cough** [Europe, Malaya].
- **Lung inflammation** [China].

URINARY

- **Urinary tract infection** [China].

OTHER MEDICINAL USES

- **Snake bite** [China].

USE AS FOOD: While the plant has been used as a potherb, **eating it is not recommended** because of the possibility that some species of *Emilia* may contain pyrrolizidine alkaloids. See *Cautions and Contraindications.*

CONSTITUENTS: Beta-sitosterol, doronine, stigmasterol, palmitic acid, pyrrolizidine alkaloids, senkirkine, simiral, honey acid.

Red Pualele Local Combinations

Infections: Add *Bidens pilosa* (kīnehi / spanish needle), *Youngia japonica* (hawksbeard).
Common cold: Add *Pandanus tectorius* (hala), *Cymbopogon refractus* (wāpine / lemongrass), *Zingiber officinale* ('awapuhi pākē / ginger).

Red Pualele Cross-Cultural Combinations

Enteritis or dysentery: With *Polygonum chinense* (bian xu), *Acalypha australis*, and *Pteris multifida* [China].
Lobar pneumonia: With *Ilex* asprella roots, *Mahonia japonica* [China].
Urinary tract infection: With *Phyllanthus urinaria*, *Plantago asiatica* (che qian cao / plantain), *Lygodium japonicum* (jin sha teng) [China].

RANGE: Native to southern and eastern Asia and the western Pacific.

PROPAGATION & CULTIVATION: By seed.

RESEARCH:
- Water and alcohol extracts of *Emilia sonchifolia* leaf are anti-inflammatory in rats [Muko 2000].
- Alcohol extract of *Emilia sonchifolia* is cytotoxic in vitro to Daltons lymphoma, Ehrlich ascites carcinoma and mouse lung fibroblast cells, but not in vitro to human lymphocytes [Shylesh 2000].

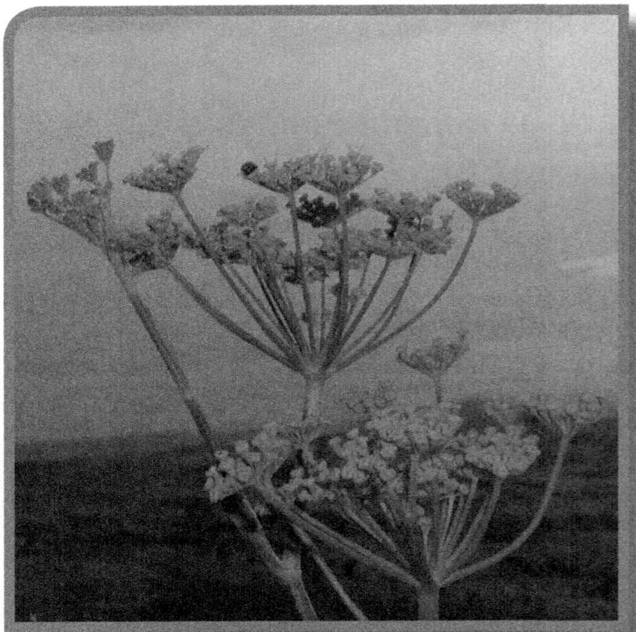

Foeniculum vulgare (Xiao Hui Xiang / Fennel)

PLANT NAME: *Foeniculum vulgare* Mill.

OTHER NAMES: *Anethum foeniculum, F. capillaceum, F. officinale.*

Status: Alien. Moderate pest factor, but fragrant.

Habitat: Upcountry, sunny.

COMMON NAMES: **Fennel** [English]; **xiao hui xiang** [China]; adas [Java, Indonesia]; almindelig [Denmark]; fenchel, fenchle [Germany]; fenikkel [Norway]; fenoll, fonoll [Catalan]; fenouille [France]; finocchio [Italian]; foeniculum, maratrum [Latin]; hinojo [Spain]; inuju [Aymara, Kechua]; jinuchchu [Kallawaya]; koper wloski [Poland]; marathron ("to grow thin") [Ancient Greek]; mieloi [Basque]; shouikyo [Japan]: sohoehyang [Korea]; sanuf, bari-sanuf [Hindi]; shatapuspha [Sanskrit].

PHARMACEUTICAL NAME: (Fructus) Foeniculi Vulgaris.

NOMENCLATURE: Linnaeus included this plant in the genus Anethum, but the botanist De Candolle later placed it in a new genus called *Foeniculum. Foeniculum* was the name used by the ancient Romans for fennel. It was derived from the Latin word "foenum" which means "hay." The specific epithet "*vulgare*" means "common."

FAMILY: Apiaceae (carrot family).

CATEGORY: Warm the interior, expel cold.

PROPERTIES: Sweet, acrid, neutral to warm [China]. Sweet, bitter, cool to cold [India]. Warm and humid [Mexico].

PLANT PART USED: Mostly the fruit (sometimes called the "seed").

TOXICITY: There is no acute toxicity of the ethanol extraction in mice at 0.5 - 3 g / kg or chronic toxicity at 100 mg / kg per day. Interestingly, male mice gained significant weight while undergoing the chronic treatment, but not female mice [Shah 1991]. The oil is toxic to the liver and irritating to the kidneys. An overdose of the volatile oil can cause nausea, vomiting, pulmonary edema, and seizures. 5-20 drops of the oil can trigger convulsions and hallucinations.

CAUTIONS AND CONTRAINDICATIONS:
- Not in pregnancy.
- Allergic reactions, while rare, can occur with *Foeniculum vulgare*. 62% of plant coumarins come from the apiaceae family of plants; of which *Foeniculum* is one genus [Nielsen 1971]. Certain coumarins are known to cause photodermatitis. Fennel is known to cause photodermatitis or contact dermatitis. Those who are allergic to one apiaceae family member are often allergic to others.
- Not with estrogen sensitive cancer.
- Caution with diverticulitis, diverticulosis, duodenal ulcer, GERD (chronic heartburn), stomach ulcer, ulcerative colitis.

ENERGETIC CAUTIONS: Caution with yin deficient heat.

PREPARATION OF MEDICINE: Infused or decocted. Seeds may be ground, chewed or steeped in tea. Does well in tincture 1:5, 60% alcohol.

DOSAGE: 5–10 grams in formula.

MERIDIAN AFFINITIES: Spleen, stomach, liver, kidney.

WESTERN FUNCTIONS REPORTED: **Abortifacient**; **alleviates the symptoms of "male menopause"**; **analgesic**; **anodyne** [China]; **anthelmintic** [India (seeds)]; **anti-fungal** (essential oil); **anti-inflammatory**; **anti-microbial**; **antipyretic**; **antiseptic**; **antispasmodic** [India, Mexico]; **antitussive**; **aphrodisiac** [China, India (seeds)]; **appetizer** [India (seeds)]; **appetite stimulant**; **aromatic**; **astringent**; **bactericidal** (essential oil); **balsamic** [Japan]; **calms the nerves** [India]; **cardiotonic** [Dominican Republic]; **carminative** [Cherokee, China, Haiti, India, Iraq, Mexico,Turkey]; **choleretic**; **calming for overactive digestive systems**; **cold remedy** [Cherokee]; **diaphoretic**; **digestive**; **diuretic** [Dominican Republic, France, Haiti, Hippocrates, India, Mexico, Turkey]; **emmenagogue** [Haiti, Hippocrates, Turkey]; **estrogenic**; **expectorant** [China, Japan, Mexico, Research, Turkey]; **facilitates birth**; **febrifuge**; **hallucinogenic**; **hepatic**; **hypotensive**; **increases libido**; **increases milk secretion**; **increases peristalsis**; **increases the digestive flora**; **lactogogue** [China, Haiti, Mexico, Turkey]; **laxative** [India (seeds)]; **mild stimulant**; **orexigenic**; **parasiticide** [Turkey]; **prevents influenza**; **promotes menstruation**; **promotes gastrointestinal motility**; **promotes mental alertness** [India]; **purgative** [India (roots)]; **reduces arterial blood pressure** (water extraction); **regulates the menses** [India (seeds)]; **respiratory stimulant**; **restorative** [Turkey]; **secretagogue**; **secretolytic**; **spasmolytic** (essential oil); **stimulant** [Dominican Republic, India, Iraq, Mexico, Turkey]; **stomachic** [China, Dominican Republic, India (seeds), Japan, Turkey, Venezuela]; **stops bleeding** [Bermuda]; **tonic** [Cherokee, China, Kurdistan, Venezuela]; **vermicide** (essential oil) [Nepal]; **weak diuretic** (leaves) [India].

TRADITIONAL CHINESE ENERGETIC FUNCTIONS (~ = extrapolated):

1) Regulates the liver qi.
2) Harmonizes the stomach.
3) Warms the kidneys.
4) Removes cold and stops pain.
5) Soothes the urinary bladder~.
6) Benefits the eyes~.
7) Opens the lungs & clears cold phlegm~.
8) Dispels wind.

OTHER ENERGETIC FUNCTIONS:
Decreases: vata, pitta, & kapha [India].

Fennel Common Medicinal Uses

- **Poor digestion, gas, abdominal pain**
- **Diminished lactation**
- **Irregular or painful menstruation**

Fennel
Cross-Cultural Medicinal Uses

CARDIOVASCULAR

- **Hypertension.**

DERMATOLOGICAL

- **Dermatosis** [Malaya]; **sores** [Haiti].

DIGESTIVE

"*Fennel seede drunke assuageth the paine of the stomache, and the wambling of the same, or desire to vomite, and breaketh winde*" - - John Gerard, 1597

- **Indigestion**, **gas**, **bloating**, **abdominal pain & distention**, **poor appetite** [China, Haiti, Iraq, Malaya Mexico, Spain Turkey]; **to prevent gas after eating** [Universal (seeds chewed)]; **dull abdominal pain with food.**
- Because Ayurveda considers fennel energetically cool, it is used for **digestive problems where hot spicy herbs might aggravate the patient** [India].
- **Nausea and vomiting** [China].
- **Acid stomach**, **heartburn** [China, Haiti, Iraq, Kashaya (seeds chewed), Mexico, Pomo (seeds chewed), Turkey].
- **Diarrhea**; **irritable bowel syndrome**; **rectal inflammation** [China].
- **Enteritis** [China]; **food poisoning** [China]; **hiatus hernia**; **weight loss** [Medieval Herbalists].

HEAD AND THROAT

"The distilled water of the whole herb, or the condensate juice dissolved, but especially the natural juice,that in some counties issues out hereof of its own accord, dropped into the eyes, cleanses them from mists and films that hinder the sight." - - Nicholas Culpepper

- **Conjunctivitis and blepharitis** (infusion topical); **eye wash** (seeds decocted) [Pomo, Kashaya]; **poor vision** [China, Hippocrates, Medieval Herbalists, Peter Holmes, Pliny].
- **Gargle for pharyngitis**; **thirst** [India (seeds)]; **sore throat** (gargle); **toothache** [China].
- **Headaches**.

HEPATIC

"The seed and the roots much more, help to open obstructions of the liver, spleen, and gall, and thereby help the painful and windy swellings of the spleen, and the yellow jaundice; as also the gout and cramps."

- - Nicholas Culpepper

- **Cirrhosis**, **gall bladder disorders**; **liver problems** [Malaya].

INFECTION

- **Dysentery**, **fever** [India (seeds)].

MUSCULOSKELETAL / TRAUMA

- **Arthritis**, **joint inflammation & muscular pain** (essential oil topical); **rheumatism** [Malaya]; gout.
- **Back pain** [China], **spasm** [Haiti].
- **Wounds** [India (seeds)]; **contusions**, **bruises**, **sprains**.

ONCOLOGY

- **Cancer** [Europe, UK]; **uterine cancer** [China]; **tumor** [Italy].
- **Side effects of chemotherapy and radiation**.

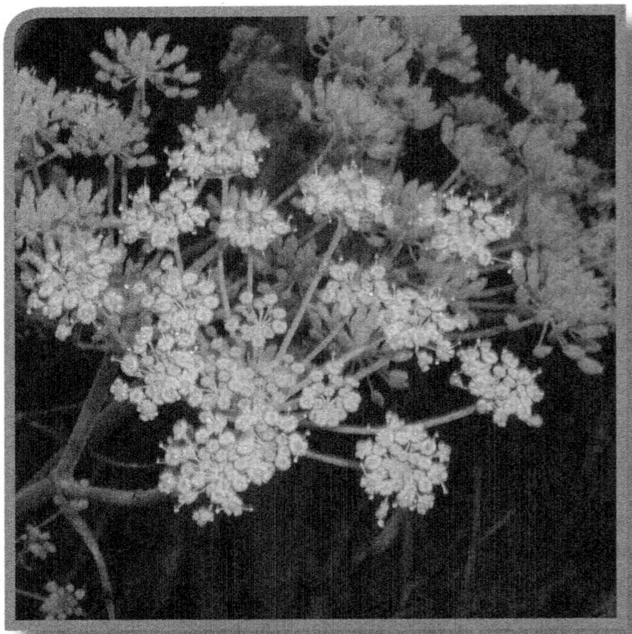

Foeniculum vulgare: Fennel flowers

PEDIATRIC

- While nursing, an infant may also absorb the fennel that is used to stimulate lactation. This can help to treat **colic** [Cherokee, China, Haiti, Mexico].
- **Summer diarrhea with fever in children** ("summer heat") [China]; **digestive tonic for children**; **gas in children** [Cherokee].
- **Bedwetting**.
- **Cough in infants**.

PSYCHOSPIRITUAL

"I suppose the reason of its benefit this way is because it is an herb of Mercury, and under Virgo, and therefore bears antipathy to Pisces."

- - Nicholas Culpepper

- **Believed to repel witches** (along with St. Johns Wort) during the Middle Ages, **fennel was one of the nine sacred herbs.**

• **Said to give strength and courage**.

REPRODUCTIVE

"The leaves or seed, boiled in barley water and drank are good for nurses, to increase their milk, and make it more wholesome for the child."

- - Nicholas Culpepper

• **Insufficient lactation** [China, Haiti, Latin America, Turkey]; **mastitis**.
• **Lack of menses.**
• **Painful menses**; **irregular or delayed menstruation with clots** [China].
• **Gonorrhea** [Ethiopia]; **venereal disease** [India (seeds)].
• **Given to women in labor** [Cherokee]; **post partum** [Iraq].
• **Virility** [China].

RESPIRATORY

"The seed is of good use in medicines to help shortness of breath and wheezing by stopping of the lungs."

- - Nicholas Culpepper

• **Respiratory problems** [China]; **bronchitis**, **chest congestion**, **cough with thick white phlegm**, **wheezing**, **hoarseness**, **voice loss** [China, Turkey]; **to loosen phlegm**; **chronic cough** (fennel syrup).
• **Cold remedy** [Cherokee].

URINARY

"Fennel is good to break wind, to provoke urine, and ease the pains of the stone, and helps to break it."

- - Nicholas Culpepper

• **Sandy deposits in urine**; **urinary stones**; **strangury** [China]; **bladder pain**; **kidney problems**.
• **Enuresis** [China].
• **Night time urination**.
• **Testicle pain** (roasted).

VETERINARY

• Small branches are placed in horses' harnesses **to keep flies away**. Crushed leaves are used as **flea repellant** on dogs.
• Used for "**cattle condiments**."

OTHER MEDICINAL USES

"The seed boiled in wine and drank, is good for those that are bitten with serpents, or have eaten poisonous herbs, or mushrooms."

- - Nicholas Culpepper

• **Used to improve the taste of other medicines**.
• **Cholera** [China].
• **Low energy** [China].
• **Longevity**.
• **Hernia** [China].
• **Leprosy** [India (seeds)].
• **Parasites**.
• **Swallowing air** [Haiti].
• **Fluid discharge** [China].
• **Snake bite** [China].

USE AS FOOD:

"*Both the seeds, leaves and root of our Garden Fennel are much used in drinks and broths for those that are grown fat, to abate their unwieldiness and cause them to grow more gaunt and lank.*"

- - William Coles, Nature's Paradise, 1650

• The Romans ate young fennel stalks, and some varieties of fennel are used today as a vegetable. The leaves are used in salads and to flavor fish. The young stems can be used in soups. The cultivated bulbs are often better to eat than the wild crafted ones.
• Young leaves can be used as a garnish, added to cooked food and salads, or to flavor fish. This can be useful to help digest greasy meals. Leaves can be harvested year round.
• Seeds can flavor bread stuffing or cakes.
• Eaten during Lent to allay hunger.
• Fennel seeds have been used as a juniper substitute for flavoring gin, and are often used for flavoring "licorice" products. In fact, some of my Hawaiian teachers called this plant "licorice".
• Fennel has more isoflavones than soy.
• The smell and taste of fennel is dependent on the proportions of two chemicals, "fenchone," which is bitter, and "anethole" is sweet.

OTHER USES:

• Flowers used as perfume [Mexico].
• Insect repellant (dried herb).
• Flowers and leaves are mixed to make yellow and brown dyes. Seeds used as a dye for wool.
• Smoked as a tobacco substitute [Hopi].

ESSENTIAL OIL:

• The oil increases smooth muscle contractions in guinea pigs [Reiter 1985].
• Anethole is mainly found in the volatile oil.
• The essential oil is used in perfumes, cosmetics, and liqueurs.
• The essential oil prevents liver damage in rats caused by carbon tetrachloride [Ozbek 2003]. It is also antioxidant and antibacterial [Ruberto 2000].
• Antioxidant effects are comparable to alpha-tocopherol and butylated hydroxytoluene (BHT) [Ruberto 2000].

CONSTITUENTS:

- Volatile oils (80% anethole, dianethole, 5% estgole, fenchone, photoanethole).
- Flavonoids (kaempferol glycosides, quercetin, rutin). Coumarins (bergapten, imperatorin, marmesin, xanthotoxin). Sterols.
- Fruits contain pentosan, pectin, trigonelline, fenchone, seselin, anethole and choline.
- The plant also contains sesquiterpene, germacrene-D, b caryophyllene, d-pinene, phellandrine, anisic acid and anisic aldehyde. (There are many more constituents, too many to list. A list of constituents will be sent on request.)

POSSIBLE DRUG INTERACTIONS: Anethole potentiates streptomycin against tuberculosis in lab animals [Bensky 1986].

Fennel Local Combinations

Menstrual cramps: Add *Piper methysticum* ('awa / kava).

Poor digestion, nausea, vomiting: Add *Zingiber officinale* ('awapuhi pākē / ginger), *Curcuma longa* ('ōlena / Turmeric).

Chronic, copious, clear or white lung phlegm: Add *Cymbopogon refractus* (wāpine), *Citrus reticulata* (tangerine) peel.

Fennel Cross-Cultural Combinations

Bacterial cystitis: With *Barosma betulina* (buchu) and *Arctostaphylos uva-ursi* (kinnikinick).

Inflammation of the mouth and throat: With *Rosmarinus officinale* (rosemary), *Salvia officinalis* (sage) and *Hamamelis virginiana* (witch hazel) as a gargle.

Colic: With *Verbena officinale* (vervain), *Glycyrrhiza glabra* (licorice) and *Melissa officinalis* (lemon balm).

Lower abdominal pain that is aggravated by cold: With *Lindera strychnofilia* (wu yao) and *Cinnamomum cassia* (rou gui) [China].

Cough: Fennel oil with warm water and honey.

Colic: With *Chamaemelum nobile* (roman chamomile), *Acorus calamus* (shi chang pu / sweet flag rhizome), *Alpinia officinale* (gao liang jiang / galangal).

Gas, indigestion and diverticulitis: With *Mentha piperita* (peppermint) or *Anthemis nobilis* (chamomile).

Common cold or flu with fever: With *Anthemis nobilis* (chamomile) and *Achillea millefolium* (yarrow).

One of the "three cooling spices" along with *Cuminum cyminum* (cumin) and *Coriandrum sativum* (coriander) [India].

Bladder infection: With *Arctostaphylos uva-ursi* (bearberry).

Facial steam: With *Achillea millefolium* (yarrow), *Lavandula officinalis* (lavender), and *Mentha piperita* (peppermint).

Poor digestion: As a "cordial" with fresh *Taraxacum officinale* (dandelion) root and leaf; *Gentiana leutea.* (gentian) root; *Mentha piperita* (peppermint) leaf; *Glycyrrhiza glabra* (licorice) root; and *Zingiber officinale* (sheng jiang / ginger) rhizome [Naturopathic].

After a greasy meal: With *Dioscorea villosa* (wild yam); *Podophyllum peltatum* (mayapple) root; *Taraxacum officinale* (dandelion) fresh root and leaf; *Chelidonium major* (celandine) fresh root and tops; *Eschscholzia californica* (california poppy) fresh herb; and *Mentha piperita* (peppermint) oil [Naturopathic].

Swollen or tired eyes: With *Monotropa uniflora* (bird's nest). Infusion topical [Native American].

To prevent griping: From the use of *Cassia marilandica* (senna) [Native American].

To raise or lower the Qi: One source states that use with salt will lower the Qi, and use with wine will raise the Qi.

RANGE: Global. Native to the Mediterranean.

HABITAT: Upcountry areas, lots of sun. I don't think I've ever seen it below 2000'.

GATHERING: Seeds ripen in autumn.
On the mainland, fennel can easily be confused for poison hemlock.

PROPAGATION & CULTIVATION: In Hawai'i it shouldn't be propagated, as there is plenty to wild craft.

RESEARCH:

- Fennel lowers blood pressure in laboratory animals. This may be due to its diuretic effects [El Bardai 2001]. Arterial blood pressure in rats is lowered without changing heart or respiratory rate in intravenous boiled fennel leaf tea. Cold infusion was inactive. A histamine antagonist blocked this action [Abdul-Ghani 1988].
- In studies of frogs, fennel seeds aid in expectoration

by stimulating the cilia of frog esophagus [Muller-Limmroth 1980].

- The seed extract is estrogenic [Albert-Puleo 1980; Malini 1985].

NOTES 'N QUOTES

"*Both leaves, seeds, and roots thereof are much used in drink or broth, to make people more lean that are too fat.*"

- - Nicholas Culpepper

"*The roots are of most use in physic drinks, and broth that are taken to cleanse the blood, to open obstructions of the liver, to provoke urine, and amend the ill color in the face after sickness, and to cause a good habit through the body.*"

- - Nicholas Culpepper

- Fennel may have been responsible for the immortality of Prometheus in Greek legends.
- Throughout history, fennel has been used as medicine in China, Egypt, Greece, & India. Hippocrates and Dioscorides both used fennel to stimulate lactation in nursing mothers. When Pliny (Caius Plinius Secundus, A.D. 23-79) noted that snakes shedding their skins would frequent patches of fennel, he commented " *...when they cast their old skins, and they sharpen their sight with the juice by rubbing against the plant.*" Thus he recommended it for visual problems, and even blindness. Pliny had no less than twenty-two formulas that included fennel.
- Fennel water and seed are mentioned in a Spanish farm document from 961 A.D.
- Charlemagne spread the use of fennel throughout Central Europe and grew it on imperial farms. And the household of King Edward I once bought 8 1/2 lb. of fennel as one month's supply.
- The common giant fennel (*Ferula communis*) is actually not fennel, but is a large cousin in the same family.
- One of the most energetically "warm" plants in the Hawaiian pharmacopea, fennel is only found at altitude. The seeds and leaves are useful for indigestion, to warm up a "cold" constitution, or for copious clear or white lung phlegm. The (cultivated) bulb as food is also good for this.

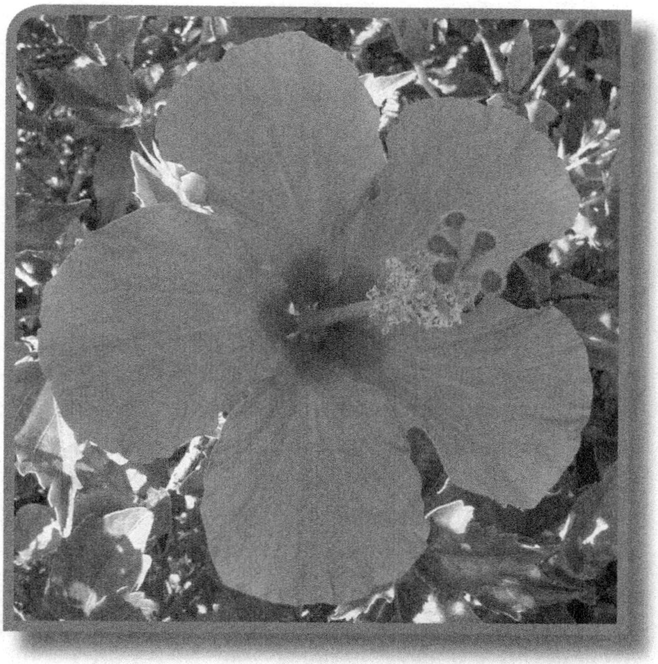

Hibiscus rosa-sinensis (Aloalo / Red Hibiscus)

PLANT NAME: *Hibiscus rosa-sinensis* L.

SIMILARLY USED SPECIES: Most of the genus.

COMMON NAMES: **Aloalo** [Hawai'i]; **red hibiscus**; china rose [English]; da hong hua ("big red flower") [China];'aute samoa [Samoa]; fu sang; gumamela [Philippines]; Hawaiian hibiscus [Australia]; japā [India]; japa puspi [Nepal]; japapushpam [India]; papo [Panama]; pejo [Colombia]; shoeflower [Jamaica].

Status: Alien. No pest factor.

Habitat: Sunny, rich well drained soil.

NOMENCLATURE: *Hibiscus* is taken from the Greek "hibiscos," a name for mallow.

FAMILY: Malvaceae.

CATEGORY: Clear heat and toxins.

PROPERTIES: Sweet, astringent, neutral to cool.

PLANT PART USED: Mostly flowers, but occasionally leaves or roots. Hawaiians often prefer using the unopened flowers.

TOXICITY: The flowers are not teratologic (do not cause birth defects) in rats at clinical doses [Nath 1992].

CAUTIONS AND CONTRAINDICATIONS: Oc-

cupational skin symptoms are suspected for *Hibiscus rosa-sinensis*.
Not in pregnancy [Brinker 2001].

PREPARATION OF MEDICINE: Infused, decocted, poulticed. I use fresh closed-flower poultices for injuries and boils, and infusions of the flowers internally.

DOSAGE: 15 – 30 grams for internal use of the flowers.

WESTERN FUNCTIONS REPORTED: **Abortifacient; analgesic; anodyne; antidiarrheic; antidote for poison; antiestrogenic; antifungal; anti-implantation; anti-infectious; anti-inflammatory; antipyretic; antispasmodic; antispermatogenic; aperient; aphrodisiac; astringent; CNS depressant; constipating; contraceptive; demulcent; dentifrice; diuretic; embryotoxic; emmenagogue; emollient; expectorant; hemostat; hypoglycemic; hypotensive; hypothermic; insect attractant; laxative; menorrhagia; mildly laxative; pectoral; promotes hair growth and color; puerperium; purgative; refrigerant; relaxes spasm; soothes irritated tissue; stops bleeding; sudorific; swelling; urogenital; venereal.**

TRADITIONAL CHINESE ENERGETIC FUNCTIONS (~ = extrapolated):
1) Clears toxins.
2) Benefits urination.
3) Regulates the menses.

Aloalo (Red Hibiscus)
Common Medicinal Uses

- **Poulticed for boils**
- **Urinary tract infections**
- **Bronchitis with sticky phlegm**

Aloalo (Red Hibiscus) Cross-Cultural Medicinal Uses

BITES & STINGS
- **Insect bites** (flower poulticed).

COSMETIC
- The flowers are used **to make mascara and eye liner** [China, India].
- In India, the flowers and leaves are mashed together to make **a "cream rinse" to blacken the hair**. It is a major ingredient in the hair oil called Cemparuttyādi.
- Sometimes the flowers are boiled in coconut oil and applied topically to stimulate hair growth and to treat **dandruff**. Use about 12 flowers per cup of oil.

CARDIOVASCULAR
- **Angina** (flower infused).

DERMATOLOGICAL
- **Abscesses and boils** [Hawai'i (flower buds topical), China (flowers internal), India (flowers & leaves), Philippines (poultice), Samoa (leaves poulticed)].
- **External swellings** [Philippines (flowers poulticed)].
- **Fissures** (flower poulticed).

DIGESTIVE
- **Anal and rectal problems** (flowers decocted for a sitz bath); **hemorrhoids** [India (flowers)].
- **Stomatitis** (flower infused); **digestive abscess** (flower); **vomiting blood**.

ENDOCRINE
- **Diabetes** [India (flowers)].

HEAD AND THROAT
- **Acute conjunctivitis** [China (root)]; **ophthalmia**.
- **Headaches** [Philippines (leaves infused or poulticed); South Pacific].
- **Adenopathy**.

INFECTION
- **Fever** (*Hibiscus* spp.) [China (flowers internal), India (flowers), Nepal (petals infused), Pakistan, Philippines (leaves decocted)].

LYMPHATIC
- **Lymphadinitis** (leaves and flowers topical).

MUSCULOSKELETAL / TRAUMA
- **Topical for bruises and sprains** [Hawai'i]; **swelling**.

ONCOLOGY
- **Cancer** [China (leaves and flowers poulticed), Philippines (poultice)].

PEDIATRIC
- **Children's fevers** (*Hibiscus* spp.).
- **Mumps** (leaves and flowers poulticed or internal) [China, Philippines].
- **Parotitis** [China (root)].

PSYCHOSPIRITUAL

- **Infections from the bite of a ghost** [Samoa (leaves poulticed)].
- **Sacred to the Hindu God, Ganesh**.
- In occult circles *Hibiscus rosa-sinensis* is **associated with the fire element** and is used **to connect to one's deepest passions**.

REPRODUCTIVE

- **Menstrual disorders** [India (flowers)]; **irregular menses** [China (root or flowers), India (flower or leaf extract)]; **excessive and painful menstruation** [India (flowers), South Pacific].
- **Used as lubricant during labor** [Philippines]; **to aid in delivery** [South Pacific]; **"post partum relapse sickness"** [Samoa].
- **Late menses** [China (root), India (leaves)], **to induce abortion** [India (flower extract), South Pacific].
- **Inflamed cervix** [China (root)].
- **Vaginal discharge** [China (root)].
- **Mastitis** (leaves and flowers topical).
- **Venereal disease** (flowers internal) [India (root)].

RESPIRATORY

- **Respiratory illnesses** [Cuba (*Hibiscus* spp.)]; **colds & flu**.
- **Asthma. bronchitis** (flowers internal) [China (root), Philippines (leaves infused)].
- **Tuberculosis**.
- The flowers are used for **coughs** in India and Nepal and are sometimes made into a cough syrup. They are also used in baths or a steam inhalation, and the root is used as a substitute for *Althaea officinalis* (marshmallow root).

URINARY

- **Urinary tract infection** [China (root), India (flowers), Philippines (decocted)].
- **Urinary stones** [India (flowers)].

OTHER MEDICINAL USES

- **Burning sensation in the body** [India (flowers)].
- **Hernia**.
- **Inflammation** (leaves poulticed) [Philippines, Samoa].
- **"Tooala"** [Samoa (pounded and decocted)].

USE AS FOOD: In China the Flower petals are added to baked goods, with sugar and lemon. Flower petals are used as a condiment with salads. The flowers are pickled. The leaves are sometimes used as a potherb. The flowers can be boiled, sweetened, and chilled for a summer drink [India].

OTHER USES:

- The flowers are used to shine shoes in China.
- Flowers are made into purple dye used as food coloring.
- Shampoo and hair conditioner.
- The stem fiber can be used for cordage, nets, even paper.

CONSTITUENTS: Alkanes, anthocyanosides (responsible for the red of the flowers), beta-sitosterol, campesterol, cholesterol, citric acid, cyanidin, cyanin glucosides, ergosterol, flavonoid glycosides, flavonoids, fructose, glucose, hibiscetin, lipids, oxalic acid, stigmasterol, sucrose, taraxeryl acetate, tartaric acid. Flowers: b-carotene, flavanoids, and vitamin c. calcium, iron, niacin, phosphorus, riboflavin, thiamine, mucilage, ramified polysaccharides, pectic polysaccharides.

POSSIBLE DRUG INTERACTIONS: Possible hypokalemia due to diuretic action of some *Hibiscus* spp. (speculative). Following this line of thought, possible interactions include: NSAIDS (toxicity), muscle relaxants (potentiation), antidiabetic medications (antagonism), lithium therapy (potentiation), corticosteroids (hypokalemia), diuretics (potentiation), antihypertensives (potentiation), sympathomimetics (antagonism). All of this is speculative.

Aloalo (Red Hibiscus) Local Combinations

Boils: Add *Plantago major* (laukahi / plantain) as a poultice.

Bronchitis with sticky phlegm: Add *Commelina* spp. (honohono / wandering jew) and *Sonchus oleraceus* (pualele / sow thistle).

Urinary tract infections: Add *Bidens pilosa* (kīnehi / spanish needle) and *Taraxacum officinale* (dandelion).

Aloalo (Red Hibiscus) Cross-Cultural Combinations

Vomiting blood: Root with *Achyranthes* spp. [Samoa].

Gonorrhea: With *Zingiber* spp., water, and sand [Samoa].

To cool the head: Leaves and flowers ground with soaked fenugreek seeds [India].

Parotitis: With *Hibiscus mutabilis.* [China]

To stimulate hair growth: Fresh flowers with olive oil [India, Philippines].

To cause miscarriage: Flowers with papaya seeds [Philippines].

Temporary and permanent birth control: Traditionally used for both temporary and permanent birth control in India, depending on the plants with which it is combined. (Note: Herbal birth control is *not* a good idea for a multitude of reasons.) For temporary birth control, *Hibiscus rosa-sinensis* is traditionally combined with *Mimosa pudica* (hilahila), *Piper nigrum* (black pepper / bi ba), and *Cissampelos pareira.* For sterilization, *Hibiscus rosa-sinensis* is traditionally used with *Heliotropum indicum*, *Plumbago zeylanica* ('ilie'e), *Salmalia malabrica*, and *Plumeria rubra* (toxic) [India].

RANGE: Native to China / India, but globally pandemic in temperate and tropical areas. The Polynesians carried *Hibiscus rosa-sinensis* across the Pacific, as far east as the Marqueses Islands. Some say that it is not native to anywhere and is a man-made hybrid. In Hawai'i some of the flowers may have crossed with our native species.

GATHERING: The closed flowers can be gathered any time. When tested as a means of birth control in rats, the flower extracts were the most effective. Flowers used in this way were most potent when gathered in winter or spring [Kholkute 1977].

PROPAGATION & CULTIVATION: Will grow by grafting, cutting, or layering.

RESEARCH:

- Water and ethanol extract of the leaves significantly improved glucose tolerance in rats, the water extract was comparable to tolbutamide [Sachdewa 2001].
- Water extract inhibits *Herpes simplex* virus (presumably in vitro) [Zheng 1989].
- There are anti-fertility effects in lab animals [Pal 1985]. The benzene extract of the flowers at 1 gm / kg body weight / day resulted in termination of pregnancy in 92% of mice studied [Pakrashi 1986]. The flower appears to block implantation of a fertilized egg. The hormonal effects of the genus are in question. One species, *H. macranthus* is reported to be estrogenic [Telefo 1998], but *H. rosa-sinensis* appears to be anti-estrogenic [Prakash 1979]. There is some evidence that for contraception, benzene extract of the flower is stronger than the rest of the plant and that it's efficacy may depend on the season in which it is gathered [Kholkute 1977].

NOTES 'N QUOTES

- The flowers are hermaphroditic (are both male and female).
- Aloalo is one of our best local plants used topically for boils. It also is useful to break up sticky lung phlegm. It should be used fresh.

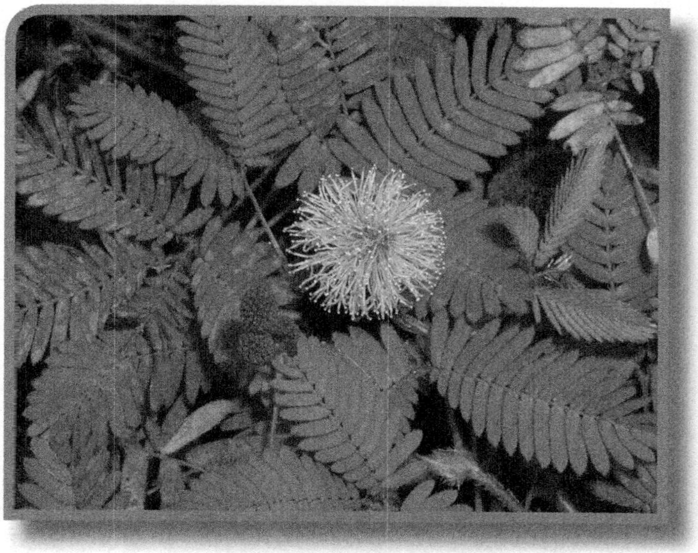

Mimosa pudica (Hilahila / Sensitive Plant)

PLANT NAME: *Mimosa pudica* L.

COMMON NAMES: **Hilahila** ("shy") [Hawai'i]; **sensitive plant**, sleeping grass [English]; han xiu cao [China]; betguen sosa [Guam]; chami [Peru]; cogadrogadro [Fiji]; lajjalu [India]; lajwania [Indo-Fijiian]; mechiuaiu [Palau]; ra kau pikikaa [Cook Islands]; sulinit [Borneo]; tchua tchu zaw [Hmong - Laos].

Status: Alien. High pest factor.

NOMENCLATURE: From "mimos" to mimic. Because the leaves close up when touched they were thought to mimic a wilting leaf. Both "*pudica*" and "hilahila" mean "ashamed" or "bashful."

Habitat: Sunny, well drained soil. Disturbed areas.

FAMILY: Fabaceae.

CATEGORY: Herbs that calm the spirit.

PROPERTIES: Sweet astringent, slightly cold.

PLANT PART USED: Whole plant.

TOXICITY: **There is some chronic toxicity**. The dried plant is reportedly toxic to cattle. **Do not use this plant without heating, including tincturing!** Mimosine, a constituent, can cause hair loss if not exposed to heat.

CAUTIONS AND CONTRAINDICATIONS: **Use only under professional supervision and not for extended periods of time**. Not in pregnancy. Not for children.

Mimosa pudica thorns can harbor the fungus *Fonsecaea pedrosoi*, a cause of chromoblastomycosis. Not that you would, but don't walk barefoot on hilahila.

PREPARATION OF MEDICINE: Infused, decocted, mashed topical.

DOSAGE: 10 - 15 grams in formula, up to 25 grams if used alone

STATUS IN HAWAI'I: Alien. High pest factor. Get rid of it! The sharp thorns make short work of unprotected feet. Wear gloves when gathering.

WESTERN FUNCTIONS REPORTED: **Anthelminthic**; **antibacterial**; **antibiotic**; **antihyperglycemic**; **anti-implantation**; **anti-inflammatory** [China]; **antimicrobial**; **anti-pyretic** [China]; **anti-spasmodic**; **antitussive** [China]; **antiviral**; **bactericide** [Trinidad]; **calmative** [Panama]; **contraceptive** [India]; **depilatory**; **diuretic** [China]; **emetic** [Haiti, Panama, Southeast Asia, Venezuela]; **expectorant** [China]; **poison**; **sedative** [China, Guatemala, Java]; **tonic** [Costa Rica, Dominican Republic, Venezuela]; **tranquilizing** [China].

TRADITIONAL CHINESE ENERGETIC FUNCTIONS (~ = extrapolated):
Dispel pain and remove swelling [Taiwan]

Hilahila (Sensitive Plant)
Common Medicinal Uses

- **Insomnia**
- **Irritability**
- **PMS**

Hilahila (Sensitive Plant) Cross-Cultural Medicinal Uses

BITES & STINGS

- **Insect bites** [Indo-Fijiian]

COSMETIC

- **Balding** [Panama].

DIGESTIVE

- **Dysentery**, **bloody dysentery** (leaves ground, internal) [Haiti, India, Indo-Fijiian]; **diarrhea** [India]; **enteritis**, **gastritis** [China].
- **Hemorrhoids** [Fiji (leaves in combination), India,

Indo-Fijiian].

ENDOCRINE

- **Diabetes** (whole plant) [India].

HEAD AND THROAT

- **Acute conjunctivitis** [China].
- **Headache** [Borneo (root), Panama].
- **Hoarseness** [Haiti]; **throat diseases** (seeds) [Southeast Asia]; **sore throat** [Brazil (decoction gargled)].
- **Sinus problems**.
- **Toothache** [India (root fried in ghee, topical)].

INFECTION

- **Fever** [Borneo (root), Cuba (root decocted), India, Indo-Fijiian].
- **Sores**.

LYMPHATIC

- **Enlarged lymph glands**; **scrofula** [Brazil (leaves)]

MUSCULOSKELETAL / TRAUMA

- **Rheumatism** [Brazil (root decocted)]; **rheumatoid arthritis** [India (root decocted)].
- **Skin wounds** [India]; **swelling** [Brazil (root decocted), Java]; **trauma** (mashed topical).
- **Gout** [Nepal (poultice)]

NEUROLOGICAL

- **Convulsions** [Madagascar]

ONCOLOGY

- **Tumors**; **glandular tumors** [South America]

PARASITES

- **Stomach worms** [Indo-Fijiian].

PEDIATRIC (NOT RECOMMENDED)

- **High fever in children** [China].
- **Whooping cough** (leaves fried, internal with honey) [India].

PSYCHOSPIRITUAL

- In the Afro-Brazillian religion Candomblé, *Mimosa pudica* is **associated with the god Exu**.
- **Hysteria** (root tied around the neck to remove evil spirits) [India]; **insomnia** [China, Indo-Fijiian, Java (placed under pillow), Panama, Peru, Trinidad]; **irritability**, **"neurasthenia"** [China]; **nervousness** [Indo-Fijiian]; **depression** [Mexico (dried leaves infused)].

REPRODUCTIVE

- **To facilitate childbirth** [Carribean]; **labour pain** [India].
- **Excess menstrual bleeding** [India]; **menstrual difficulties** [South East Asia].
- **Venereal disease**, **syphilis** [Indo-Fijian].
- **Aphrodisiac** [Bolivia (seeds), Hawai'i (root infused in oil, topical).
- **Unwanted pregnancy** [Cuba (root decocted)].

RESPIRATORY

- **Asthma** [Costa Rica, Southeast Asia]; **bronchitis**, **lung infections with fever** [China]; **cough** [Borneo (root)]; **pulmonary hemorrhage** [Bolivia].

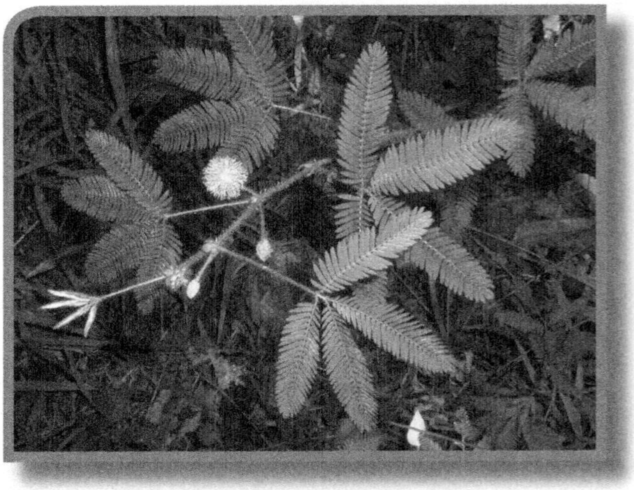

Mimosa pudica: Hilahila

URINARY

- **Urinary inflammation** [Nepal]; **kidney inflammation** [West Indies]; **reduced or burning urination** [Trinidad]; **bladder infections** [Fiji (leaves / roots in combination)].
- **Urinary stones** [Cambodia, China].

VETERINARY

- **Eaten by elephants in the wild, apparently for digestive problems and possibly for gastrointestinal parasites**.

OTHER MEDICINAL USES

- **Leprosy** [Indo-Fijian].

CONSTITUENTS: Ascorbic-acid, crocetin, crocetin-dimethyl-ether, d-glucuronic-acid, d-panitol d-xylose, gentisic acid, jasmonic acid, linoleic-acid, linolenic-acid, mimosine, mucilage, norepinephrine, oleic-acid, palmitic-acid, sitosterol, stearic-acid.

Hilahila (Sensitive Plant) Local Combinations

Urinary stones: Add *Kyllinga* spp. (kili'o'opu) and

Commelina spp. (honohono / wndering jew).

Agitation: Add *Vernonia cinerea* (yi chi xiang / ironweed), *Oxalis* spp. ('ih / sorreli), *Verbena littoralis* (ha'uoi / vervain), and *Pipturus albidus* (māmaki).

Insomnia: Add *Piper methysticum* ('awa).

Hilahila (Sensitive Plant) Cross-Cultural Combinations

Snakebite: Root internal with three leaves of *Azadirachta indica* (neem).

Diabetes: Whole plant with rice [India].

Temporary birth control: Roots with *Piper nigrum* (bi ba / black pepper), *Cissampelos pareira*, and *Hibiscus rosa-sinensis* (aloalo / red hibiscus) [India]. DO NOT COUNT ON THIS WORKING. HERBAL BIRTH CONTROL MAY NOT BE RELIABLE.

Permanent sterilization: With *Bambusa rundinacea, Heliotropium indicum, Hibiscus rosa-sinensis, Plumbago zeylanica, Plumeria rubra,* and *Salmalia malabrica.*

Wheezing: Leaf shoots with *Panicum maximum.* [Dominica].

Poisons, curses, and to facilitate childbirth: With *Cassia bicapsularis* and *Petiveria* spp. [Dominica].

RANGE: Throughout the Pacific, India, Indonesia, Southeast Asia, China, North and South America. Probably native to South America.

HABITAT: Full sun, well-drained soil, disturbed areas, and lawns. Anywhere people walk barefoot.

GATHERING: Gloves, summer and autumn.

PROPAGATION & CULTIVATION: From seed or cuttings. (Don't propagate in Hawai'i!) Does not like over watering or root disturbance.

RESEARCH

- Water extract reduces myotoxicity of *Naja kaouthia* (cobra) venom [Mahanta 2001].
- Anticonvulsant in lab animals [Ngo Bum 2004].
- May stimulate nerve regeneration in lab animals [Prasad 1975].
- Ethanol extract lowers blood sugar in mice. [Amalraj 2002]
- Showed no significant reduction of urinary stones in rats [Joyamma 1990].
- *M. scabrella* and *M. tenuiflora* contain tryptamines in the roots. It is unclear if *M. pudica* does.

NOTES 'N QUOTES

"*The proprietor of a bar in our town keeps a sensitive plant (Mimosa pudica) on his premises. When this plant is touched, the leaves fold and the stems droop. Recovery is prompt, and the action can be repeated endlessly without harm to the plant. When the bartender feels a customer has had too much to drink, he gives him an "alcohol-sensitive test" by having him touch the plant. He warns that if the plant wilts when it is touched, the drinker should not drive. The inebriated patron is usually so startled by the plant's action that he willingly calls a cab.*"

- - Mary Shier, President,
Anchorage Chapter Alaska Master Gardener.

- Nitrogen fixer.
- This beautiful and aggravating garden pest seems to find its way into most Hawaiian yards at one time or another. Its most interesting characteristic is the way the leaves fold shut when touched.

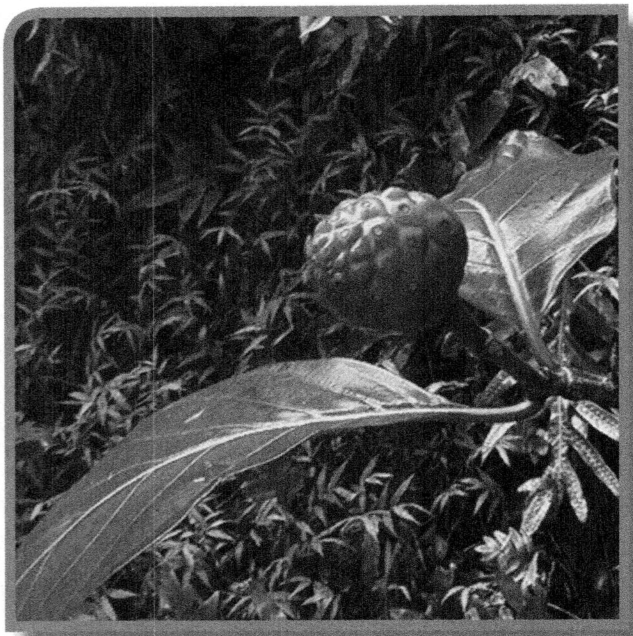

Morinda citrifolia (Noni)

PLANT NAME; *Morinda citrifolia* L.

COMMON NAMES: **Noni** [Hawai'i, Marquesas]; **hai ba ji** ("ocean ba ji") (plant), ju ye ba ji (leaf) [China]; Indian mulberry [USA]; dog dumpling [Barbados]; nonu [Samoa, Tonga]; nono [Tahiti, Cook Islands]; cheesefruit [Australia]; dilo-k [Solomon Islands]; Kura [Fiji]; nen [Marshall Islands].

Status: Polynesian introduction. No pest factor.

NOMENCLATURE: *Morinda* comes from "morus" (mulberry) and "indicus" (Indian), thus the common name "Indian mulberry."

Habitat: Low elevations.

FAMILY: Rubiaceae (coffee family).

CATEGORY: Herbs that tonify qi (fruit) ~, clear heat and toxins (root), invigorate blood (leaf) ~.

PROPERTIES: Sweet, stinky, neutral ~.

PLANT PART USED: Fruit, leaf, bark, root

TOXICITY: None noted.

CAUTIONS AND CONTRAINDICATIONS: Hold your nose. Due to high levels of potassium in the fruit, do not use with impaired kidney function [Mueller 2000]. Like other tonics, noni can cause gas if used to excess or in the wrong presentation.

ENERGETIC CAUTIONS: Not with Exterior Wind Cold / Wind Heat ~.

PREPARATION OF MEDICINE: The fruit has numerous preparations:

- "Pake" (Chinese / Armitage) style: Take a gallon jar, fill it with fruits and let it sit in the sun for 3-4 weeks, then in the shade for 1 week. Strain and bottle the juice. Refrigerate [Hawai'i - Landish Armitage].
- "Saffrey" style: Juice ripe noni fruit in a blender. Strain and refrigerate the juice. Take 2-3 "zips" by straw, 3 times per day for diabetes [Hawai'i - Rev. Nani Saffrey].

DOSAGE: Fruit: 2 oz of the juice twice a day. Root: 10 grams.

STATUS IN HAWAI'I: Most of the noni in Hawai'i is Polynesian introduction. But there is an endemic species of dry-land noni called "noni kuahiwi" (*M. trimera*).

MERIDIAN AFFINITIES: Lung spleen liver kidney ~.

WESTERN FUNCTIONS REPORTED: **Analgesic** [Haiti]; **antiascariasis**; **antibacterial**; **anodyne** [St. Thomas]; **cathartic**; **diuretic** [Samoa]; **emmenagogue** [Malaya, Philippines]; **energy tonic** [Hawai'i]; **hypotensive**; **laxative** [Java, Samoa]; **purgative** [Sierra Leone]; **sedative** [Haiti]; **tonic** [Tonga]; **uterine muscle relaxant**.

Noni Common Medicinal Uses

- **Low energy (fruit)**
- **Diabetes (fruit)**
- **High blood pressure (fruit)**
- **Sprains, injuries, (heated leaf topical)**
- **Insect stings (ripe stinky fruit topical)**

TRADITIONAL CHINESE ENERGETIC FUNCTIONS (~ = extrapolated)

Fruit

1) Tonify lung and kidney qi ~.
2) Nourishes lung and kidney yin ~.
3) Clears middle burner dampness, and calms rebellious qi ~.
4) Calms ascendant yang and sedates wind ~.
5) Clears heat and toxins and detoxifies fire poison ~.

Leaf

1) Invigorates blood, speeds the healing of wounds and strengthens bones ~.
2) Expels parasites and fungus ~.

Root bark

1) Removes / eliminates dampness.
2) Strengthens bones

Noni
Cross-Cultural Medicinal Uses

BITES & STINGS

- **Centipede stings** [New Guinea (root topical)]; **fire ant stings** [Hawai'i (ripe fruit topical)]; **fish poisoning, stings from reef fish** ("Nohu") [Polynesia]; **ciguatera fish poisoning** (wood extract) [Tahiti]; **stonefish and stingray wounds** (root topical) [Micronesia, Tahiti]; **bug bites** [Samoa].

COSMETIC

- **Bad breath and a "rustle voice"** [Tahiti (young fruit juiced, in nostril)]; **eye shadow** [Samoa]; **shampoo** [Malaya]; **skin tags** (topical) [Hawai'i].

CARDIOVASCULAR

- **Heart "troubles"** (fruit juiced, diluted with water) [Hawai'i].
- **High blood pressure** [Fiji (young fruit), Hawai'i (fruit), Polynesia].

DERMATOLOGICAL

- **Skin diseases** [New Guinea (root bark infused)]; **eruptions** [Hawai'i (roots juiced and fruit in salves)]; **eczema** (root bark) [China], **rashes** [Hawai'i]; **ringworm**
- **Abscess & ulcers** [Hawai'i (flower sap topical); Polynesia (leaf topical)]; **sores on the feet** [Micronesia, New Guinea].
- **Burns** [Tahiti].

DIGESTIVE

- **Poor digestion** [Hawai'i]; **loss of appetite** [Polynesia]; **blood poisoning from bad food** [Malaya]; **nausea** [Malaya, Samoa]; **motion sickness** [Hawai'i].
- **Constipation** (Flowers and fruit) [Hawai'i].
- **Gastric ulcer** [Hawai'i]; **stomach pain** [Marshall Islands (flower, leaves), Tonga (infused leaf or bark), New Guinea (leaves)].
- **Dysentery** (leaves) [New Guinea]; **bloody dysentery** [China (root bark), Hawai'i (charred leaf)]; **diarrhea** [Hawai'i (mashed seeds with water), Philippines, Tonga].
- **Hemorrhoids** (young fruit topical) [Tahiti].
- **Hiatal hernia** [Polynesia].

ENDOCRINE

- **Diabetes** [Hawai'i (fruit), Java, Micronesia (fruit), Polynesia, Tahiti (wood extract)].

HEAD AND THROAT

- **Toothache** (crushed fruit) [Samoa, Tonga]; **mouth and gum infection** (Ripe fruit chewed: Yum!) [Hawai'i, Polynesia;]; **gingivitis** [Tonga]; **mouth ulcers** (young fruit topical) [Tahiti].
- **Sore throat** [Samoa (crushed fruit), Tahiti, Tonga]; **tonsillitis** [Tahiti]; **"ranula"** (tongue swelling) [Tahiti].
- **Conjunctivitis** [Samoa]; **eye problems** [Samoa]; **injured eyes** (leaf juice topical) [Micronesia]; **sty** [Polynesia (flower sap), Tonga (leaves)]; **cataracts** [Hawai'i (juice in eyes)].
- **Headache** [Dominican Republic, New Guinea (heated leaves topical)].

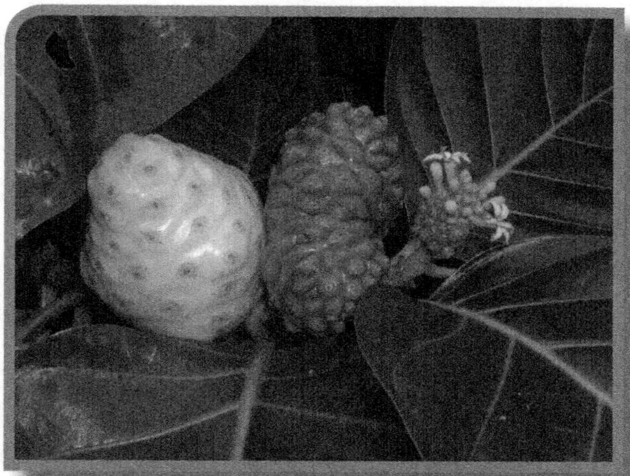

Morinda citrifolia: Noni fruit

HEPATIC

- **Fever with jaundice** [Samoa]; hepatosis [Java].

INFECTION

- **Fever** [Hawai'i (Leaf topically, root bark), Malaya, New Guinea (root juice internal), Samoa].
- **Open sores, boils, abscesses, staph infection** [Hawai'i (ripe & unripe fruit internal and topical. Leaves topical), Micronesia (root juiced topical), Philippines, Samoa, Tahiti (wood extract), Tonga]; **brings boils to a head** [Hawai'i].
- **Tuberculosis** [China (root), Hawai'i (fruit), Micronesia (unripe fruit), Samoa]; **smallpox** [Malaya, Micronesia (root salve with oil)]; **tetanus** [Samoa].

LYMPHATIC

- **Elephantiasis** [Samoa]; **enlarged spleen** [Sumatra].

MUSCULOSKELETAL / TRAUMA

- **Deep bruises, falls, contusions, fractures, sprains** [China (root), Hawai'i (leaf), Polynesia]; **broken bones** (leaf used topically) [Fiji, Hawai'i]; **concussion** (green fruit topically) [Hawai'i]; **swelling** [Java, Samoa]; **wounds** [Haiti, Hawai'i, Samoa, Polynesia (leaf topical)].
- **Arthritis** [Dominica, Fiji (leaves), Hawai'i (leaf and fruit, topically and internally), Samoa (leaves), Tonga, Trinidad (leaf topically)]; **inflammation of the fingers and toes** [Polynesia]; **joint swelling** (leaves) [Samoa]; **gout**; **muscle pain** [Tonga].
- **Burns** (leaves) [Tahiti].
- **Pain from fish barbs** (leaf stem topical) [Tahiti].

NEUROLOGICAL

- **Parkinson's disease** (fruit) [Hawai'i].
- **Convulsion** [Malaya].
- **Inflammation** [Hawai'i, Samoa].

ONCOLOGY

- **Breast cancer** (fruit) [Hawai'i]; **cancer** [Tahiti].

PARASITES

- **Worms and parasites** [Hawai'i]; **filariasis** (tropical parasite) (leaves) [Samoa].

PEDIATRIC

- **Head lice** (fruit juiced and applied topically, then shampooed with coconut) [Hawai'i].
- **Colic** [Malaya].
- **Thrush** [Hawai'i (flower sap topical)].

PSYCHOSPIRITUAL

- "**Ghost medicine**" [Polynesia].
- **Mental illness** (Root bark) [Hawai'i].

REPRODUCTIVE

- **Menstrual cramps** [Hawai'i].
- **Menopause** (fruit) [Hawai'i].
- **Childbirth** [New Guinea (bark)]; **breast hardness after childbirth** [Hawai'i]; **post partum** (flower, leaves) [Marshall Islands].
- **Groin swelling** [Hawai'i]; **swollen testicles** (juice from stem) [Tahiti]; "**fallen womb**" (uterine prolapse) [Hawai'i] (fruit internal)].
- **Vaginal discharge** [Hawai'i, Malaya].
- **Gonorrhea** (young leaves, bark) [Marshall Islands]; **syphilis** (fruit) [Marquesas].

RESPIRATORY

- **Asthma** (fruit) [Hawai'i]; **cough** [Java, Samoa]; **lung congestion** [Tahiti]; **chest problems** [Malaya]; **respiratory difficulties** (fruit) [Samoa].
- **Pulmonary tuberculosis** (root bark) [China].

URINARY

- **Bladder "disorder"** [Fiji (root infused), Hawai'i]; **painful urination, urinary tract infection** [Hawai'i (leaves infused), Java, Samoa (small crushed fruits infused)].
- **Kidney problems** [Fiji, Hawai'i].

OTHER MEDICINAL USES

- **Abdominal pain and swelling** [Polynesia (fruit boiled); Tahiti]; **abdominal problems** [Malaya]; **hernia** (juice from stem) [Tahiti].
- **Fatigue among the elderly** (fruit) [Hawai'i]; **low energy** (Bark and leaves pounded and infused) [Hawai'i].
- **Beriberi** [Java]; **Hansen's disease** (leprosy) (specific: old leaves heated, topical) [New Guinea]; **malarial fever** [Malaya, Samoa].
- **Inflammation** [Polynesia (leaf topical)]; **finger and toe inflammation** [Tahiti].

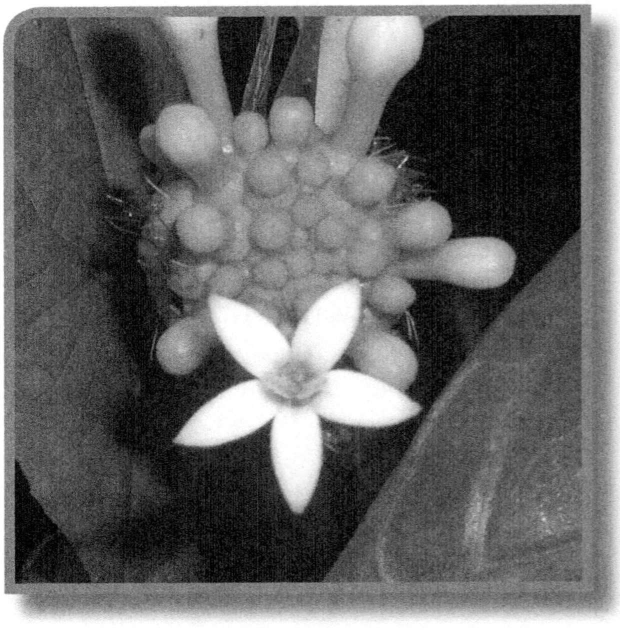

Morinda citrifolia: Noni flower

USE AS FOOD: Only in a pinch, although Barbara Fahs has written a wonderful booklet on cooking with Noni: Fabulous Noni Recipes. See http://hiiakas.com/.

OTHER USES: Yellow and red dyes were made from this plant.

CONSTITUENTS:
Acetic acid, acubin, alazarin, alizarin, anthroquinones & their glycosides, ascorbic acid, asperuloside, asperuloside, beta-carotene, beta-sitosterol, capoic acid, caproic acid, caprrylic acid, caprylic acid, citric acid, ethly caproate, ethly caprylate, flavonoids, glucose, gum, hexanoic acid, malic acid pectn, morindin, morindone, octanoic acid,

polysaccarides, rubiadin, scopoletin, sugar, ursolic acid.

POSSIBLE DRUG INTERACTIONS: Contraindicated with MAOIs (speculative) ~.

Noni
Local Combinations

Low energy: Add *Pandanus tectorius* (hala) fruit, *Trametes versicolor* (yun zhi), *Coix lacryma jobi* (pū'ohe'ohe / job's tears) leaf.
High blood pressure: Add *Cymbopogon refractus* (wāpine / lemongrass), *Verbena littoralis* (ha'uoi / vervain), *Pipturus albidus* (māmaki).

Noni
Cross-Cultural Combinations

Please note some of the ingredients in the following combinations are toxic! Do not self-administer without the supervision of a licensed practitioner or an experienced Elder.

Skin care: With lavender [Hawai'i - Ronnette Gonsalves].
Female abdominal tumor: With *Capsicum annuum* (pōpolo), *Thespesia populnea* (milo) fruit [Tahiti].
Ciguatera (fish poisoning): Green and ripe fruit juiced with coconut water [Tahiti].
Centipede bite: Scraped root topical with tobacco [New Guinea].
Ulcerated sores on the feet: With *Morus alba* (mulberry) fruit [Micronesia].
Eye infections: Shoots are crushed and inserted into baby coconuts. The liquid is used topically [Micronesia].
Asthma: With *Curcuma longa* ('ōlena / Turmeric), *Zingiber officinale* ('awapuhi pākē / ginger), and orange juice [Hawai'i].
As a purgative: *Morinda citrifolia* (green noni) mixed with roasted *Aleurites moluccana* (kukui) and pa'akai (Hawaiian salt) [Hawai'i].
Tuberculosis: With *Saccharum* spp. (kō'ele'ele / black sugar cane), and *Piper methysticum* ('awa) pounded, then boiled [Old Hawai'i].

RANGE: Polynesia to Southern China.

HABITAT: Likely native to the Northern Australia, New Guinea, and Indonesian areas. Does best at low elevations, but will grow up to 1300'. The best fruit in Hawai'i grows on hot dry lava flows near the ocean, but it does well both in the under-story and in full sun. Often found near *Aleurites moluccana* (kukui) and *Pandanus tectorius* (hala).

GATHERING: Fruit just as it begins to turn gray.

PROPAGATION: By seed or stem cutting. Seeds are better. Seeds should be scarified to reduce germination time (unless you are very patient). Keep germinating seeds very warm. Do not add fertilizer into the medium until true leaves have appeared. Stem cuttings may root in 30 - 60 days, but may not be as disease resistant as the mother plant. Fruit may be harvested as soon as 1 year after planting.

RESEARCH:
- Ethanol extract of the fruit is a COX-1 inhibitor, which may explain its use for inflammation [Li 2003].
- Antitubercular [Saludes 2002].
- Prevents cancer in lab animals [Hirazumi 1999; Wang 2001].
- Iridoid and flavonol glycosides in Noni leaves are antioxidant [Sang 2001].
- The root extract stops pain in mice and may be sedative [Younos 1990].
- The young leaf alcohol extract is anthelmintic in vitro against roundworm [Raj 1975].
- Extractions are cytotoxic against breast cancer cells in vitro, but does not kill lung carcinoma or sarcoma 180 cell lines. Noni anticancer mechanisms may include the activation of immunity and macrophage activity (probably due to polysaccharides) [Fiurusawa 2002; Johnson 2002].

NOTES 'N QUOTES
- In Hawai'i, some believe noni to be the original fruit of the tree of knowledge, the "golden apple." It is said that when Adam and Eve ate this fruit for the first time, God did not deny them its benefits, but instead modified it so that it might have an "interesting" flavor [Ronnette Gonsalves].
- "Aumiki 'awa" was a traditional noni drink used for tuberculosis. "Aumiki noni" was used to counter the unpleasant effects of *Piper methysticum* ('awa).
- One of my Hawaiian teachers, Auntie Nani Saffrey used to make her noni "apple sauce" and used it to treat her NIDDM (type II) diabetes.
- In Hawai'i, noni is one of the first dicots to colonize a lava flow.
- A truly handsome tree, Noni is very good medicine

for a multitude of ailments. The leaf is quite effective when heated (with prayer) and applied topically for acute injuries or chronic myalgia. The fruit is a useful detoxifier and makes a good general tonic for fatigue, dryness, and weak immunity if one doesn't mind the taste; I actually quite like it, especially after it has been refrigerated.

- Special thanks to Robert Newman for his research and translations.

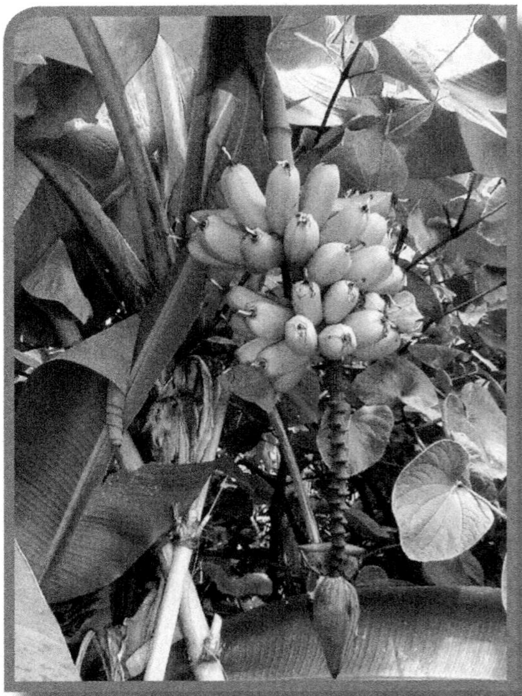

Musa spp. (Mai'a / Banana)

PLANT NAME: *Musa* spp.

SIMILARLY USED SPECIES: *Ensete glaucum, Musa paradisica, M. rubra, M. balbisiana, M. basjoo, M. coccinea, M. uranoscopos, M. fehi, M. lasiocarpa, M. nana, M. cavendishii, M. sinensis, M. sapientum, M. troglodytarum, M. wilsonii, Musella lasiocarpa.*

Status: Polynesian introduction. No pest factor.

Habitat: Wet, sunny. Likes phosphorous.

COMMON NAMES: **Mai'a** [Hawai'i], **banana**, plantain [English]; ba jiao, gan jiao, xiang jiao, ba jiao gen (stump), kan-lu (nectar), jiao yu (sap) [China]; guineo [Spanish], box haaz, mopan [Maya]; jaina [Fiji]; kera [Nepal]; mei'a [Tahiti]; meika [Cook Islands]; fa'i, soa'a [Samoa]; kadali [India].

NOMENCLATURE: Thought to be derived either from "mouz" (the Arab word for banana), or from Antonius Musa, a physician to Augustus Caesar.

FAMILY: Musaceae (banana family).

CATEGORY: Clear heat and poisons~.

PROPERTIES: Very cooling (fruit) [China]. Sap is cold~.

PLANT PART USED: All of it.

TOXICITY: None noted. There are reports of the stem juice used as arrow poison in Africa and Tahiti.

CAUTIONS AND CONTRAINDICATIONS: The sap stains (just TRY getting it off your clothes). Not to be used topically on infected sores, but it can be used on acute cuts and wounds before they become infected.

ENERGETIC CAUTIONS: Fruit should not be eaten in excess [China].

PREPARATION OF MEDICINE: Sap can be removed from the leaf (stronger) or from the trunk (milder), gathered in a container and refrigerated for future use. Fruit may be eaten raw or baked. Flower can be cut into sections and prepared for various ailments.

DOSAGE: Roots and stump 30 - 60 grams. Sap 1 / 4" in a small cup, 2-3 times per day.

MERIDIAN AFFINITIES: Lung, spleen, liver.

WESTERN FUNCTIONS REPORTED: **Alterative** (root); **anodyne** [China]; **antacid** [China]; **anthelmintic** (root); **antibilious** (root); **antidiabetic** (root); **antifebrile** (root internal) [China]; **antiflatulent** (powdered green fruits); **antiscorbutic** (root); **aphrodisiac** [China]; **astringent** (powdered green fruits); **astringent** (unripe fruit) [China]; **bacteriostat** [China]; **carminative**; **cicatrizant**; **demulcent**; **dentifrice**; **depurative**; **diaphoretic**; **diuretic** (leaves; stem juiced); **emollient**; **febrifuge**; **fungicide**; **hemostat**; **hypoglycemic** (flower); **intoxicant** (when properly prepared); **laxative** (ripe fruit) [China, Nepal, Universal]; **refrigerant**; **restorative** (root internal) [China]; **sialagogue**; **styptic** (root); **vermifuge** (human and animal use).

TRADITIONAL CHINESE ENERGETIC FUNCTIONS (~ = extrapolated):

Raw Fruit

1) Relieves thirst, moistens the lungs.
2) 'Purifies" the blood and heals wounds.
3) Relieves thirst and moistens the lungs (raw fruit).
4) Stabilizes and binds (unripe fruit).

Steamed Fruit

1) Invigorates blood and tonifies the jing.
2) Invigorates blood (steamed fruit, flower).
3) Tonifies the jing essence (steamed fruit).
4) Promotes bowel movement (ripe fruit).

Rhizome

1) Reduces heat, cools the blood and clears toxins.

Whole Plant

1) Clears heat (damp heat / toxins / fire).
2) Drains damp.
3) Speeds healing of wounds.

Mai'a (Banana) Cross-Cultural Medicinal Uses

BITES & STINGS

- **Insect and animal bites**, **centipede bites**, **scabies**, **scorpion bites** [China, Samoa]; **snake bite** (sap internal) [Asia].

COSMETIC

- **Balding in women** [China (sap)]; **dandruff** [India (ashes topical)]; **hair strengthener** [China (sap)]; **gray hair**.
- Choco tribe members believe the fruits **can cause blotches on the face** [Colombia].

Mai'a (Banana)
Common Medicinal Uses

- **Mild constipation (ripe fruit)**
- **Mild diarrhea (unripe fruit)**
- **Skin infections (sap internal)**
- **Bronchial infections (sap internal)**
- **GI protection from anti-inflammatory drugs (fruit internal)**

CARDIOVASCULAR

- **Bleeding**, **internal and external** (topical powdered green fruits / root internal [China, Colombia, Samoa]; **"blood disorders"** [Nepal (stems and root)]; **blood in the urine** [Nepal (ripe fruit)]; **nose bleed**.
- **Heart pain** [China (flowers)]; **heart disease** [Nepal (ripe fruit)].
- **High blood pressure** [China (fruit), Nepal (ripe fruit)].

DERMATOLOGICAL

- **Abscess**, **bacterial infections**, **boils**, **chronic sores and skin ulcerations** (ashes topical, leaves topical, stem juiced, root internal, bruised root topical) [Belize, China, Cuba, Hawai'i, Samoa]; **gangrene**.
- **Blisters** [Belize (leaves topical / stem juiced)].
- **Burns** (fruit juice, sap, stem juiced, and leaves mashed topical) [Belize, Bermuda, China, Fiji, Samoa, South America].
- **Rashes** (sap / fruit pulp topical) [Cook Islands, Hawai'i, Polynesia]; **hives** [China (root internal)];

psoriasis; **herpes**, **including shingles** (sap topical) [Cook Islands, Hawai'i, Polynesia]; **inflammation**, **eruption** (fruit pulp topical) [Polynesia, Samoa]; **ringworm**.

- **Itching**, **wrinkles**, **and sunburn** [USA (water extract of fruit peel)].
- **Warts**.

DIGESTIVE

- **Coated tongue from stomach trouble** [Hawai'i].
- **Constipation** (boiled ripe fruits / roots decocted) [Hawai'i, China].
- **Diarrhea** (unripe fruit, flower) [Belize, Nepal, Samoa]; **re-hydration after acute diarrhea** (banana flour); **dysentery** (flower juice, sap internal / ripe fruit) [Fiji (leaves) India, Nepal].
- **Flatulence due to "evil heat"** [China (root internal)].
- **Gastric acidity**, **heartburn** (ashes, fruit) [Belize, China]. **Gastric ulceration due to use of anti-inflammatory drugs** [USA (dried green fruit)].
- **Indigestion** (powdered green fruit); **stomach cramps** [Hawai'i (flower bud sap)]; **nausea**.
- **Intestinal disorders** [Nepal (powdered fruit)]; **enteritis**; **ulcerative colitis** [Nepal (fruit)].
- **Obesity**.
- **Rectal problems**; **hemorrhoids** [China (fruit), Fiji (stem)].
- **Thiamine deficiency** (beri-beri) [China (roots decocted)]; **scurvy**.

ENDOCRINE

- **Diabetes** (flower, fruit, root) [China, Nepal].
- **Thyroid troubles**.

HEAD AND THROAT

- **Headache** (root internal), **migraine** [China].
- **Toothache due to "wind"** [China (root internal)].
- **Dentifrice**.

HEPATIC

- **Bilious disorders** [China (ripe fruit)]; **jaundice** (fruit / roots decocted, juiced) [India, China].

INFECTION

- **Fever** (root) [China, Samoa]; **dry mouth**, **restlessness due to heat**, **fidgets** [China (root internal)]; **septicemia.**
- **Staph infection** [Hawai'i (sap internal)].
- **Smallpox**.

LYMPHATIC

- **Armpit swelling** [Fiji (stem)].

MUSCULOSKELETAL / TRAUMA

- **Back pain** [China].
- **Contusions** [USA (water extract of fruit peel)]; **fracture**; **spasm**, **strain**, **swelling**; **stalk used as splint** [Hawai'i]; **pain** [Samoa].
- **Gout** [Nepal (ripe fruit)].
- **Paralysis**.
- **Wounds** (bruised root topical, leaves mashed topical, unripe fruit) [China, Samoa].

NEUROLOGICAL

- **Epilepsy**, **convulsions** [China (sap), Fiji (root)].
- **Hallucinations** [Samoa].
- **Vertigo**, **dizziness** [China (sap)].

ONCOLOGY

- **Cancer** [China, Hawai'i]; tumor.

PARASITES

- **Malaria**.
- **Worms** [India (tuber)].

> **In Hawai'i, banana fruit was eaten after taking bitter medicine. Ripe banana fruit was also used by 'Awa drinkers to counter the taste of 'Awa. This is the first use of the term "pupu."**

PEDIATRIC

- **Carbohydrate intolerance in children** [Nepal (powdered fruit)]; **children who won't eat** [Samoa (sap internal)]; **infantile malnutrition**; **weak baby** [Hawai'i (flower sap)]; **as "vitamins" for infants** [Hawai'i (sap of flower)]. **Cuna infants are bathed in the juice of the young plants to give them strength**.
- **Childhood diarrhea** [Nigeria (fruit)]; **intestinal complaints of children** [Samoa]; **colic** (ashes)
- **Teething babies** (sap) [Cook Islands, Polynesia].
- **Thrush** (trunk and roots juiced) [Hawai'i, Samoa].

PSYCHOSPIRITUAL

Man is like a banana the day it bears fruit.
(A man dies when his work is done)
- - Hawaiian Proverb

- In some magickal traditions bananas are considered feminine and associated with the goddess Venus.

- In Western magick banana has been used for money and prosperity spells.

- Hawai'i: It is considered bad luck to dream of bananas or to meet a person carrying them, or to carry them on a fishing trip. And if you have a dream of an open hole in the ground it is a symbol of the grave and you should bury a young banana plant, a banana stalk, or a stone in the ground.
- In Hawai'i and Tahiti, banana stalks were sometimes substituted for human sacrifices and in recent times were substituted in coffins for the deceased.
- Bodies of Kings were wrapped in leaves of banana, wauke, and kalo (kapa lau- garment of leaves) in the first step of deification [Hawai'i].
- Banana is a symbol of the Gods in Voodoo, as both bananas and the dieties of Santaria dieties are hermaphroditic [Haiti].
- Banana fruits and leaves were made as offerings to the Gods, the leaves sometimes used to cover shrines called "Unu" [Hawai'i].
- Associated with the god Kanaloa and considered to symbolize fertitlity, potency, and prosperity [Hawai'i].
- A woman married under a banana tree is said to have good luck [Hawai'i].
- Mangaia: Swirling of banana leaves were used to predict hurricanes.

REPRODUCTIVE

- **Bleeding in childbirth** [Belize (root)]; labor pain [India (ripe fruit)]; **after childbirth** [China (juiced root internal)].
- **Groin swelling** [Fiji (stem), Hawai'i (leaf)]; **venereal diseases** (root powder), **gonorrhea**, **syphilis** (cooked fruit).
- **Menopausal bleeding** [India (sap internal)]; **uterine bleeding**, **painful menses** (flowers).
- **Vaginal discharge** [China (roots decocted)].

RESPIRATORY

- **Asthma** [Hawai'i (boiled ripe fruit), China (rhizome), Asia (sap or seedling juice)].
- **Cough**, **congestion**, **bronchitis** (dried leaves in syrup, leaves, sap) [Cuba, Hawai'i]. **Spitting up blood** [Cuba (root)]; **phlegm**.
- **Influenza** [China (juiced root internal)]; **chills**.
- **Pharyngitis**, **sore throat**, **tonsillitis**.
- **Tuberculosis**.

URINARY

- **Burning urination** [India (tuber chewed)]; **painful urination** [Fiji (leaf juice)]; **blood in the urine** [China (rhizome)].
- **Kidney infection** (ripe fruit) [Nepal].

OTHER MEDICINAL USES

- **Alcoholism** [China (fruit)].
- **Circumcision**.
- **Croton bean poisoning** (roots decocted) [China].
- **Debility**; **weakness of the body** [Hawai'i (flower sap)]; **consumption** [Fiji (leaves decocted)]; **as a tonic food** [Belize (fruit)].
- **Dengue fever**.
- **Opium and arsenic overdoses** (juice of the leaf and stem).
- **Navel pain** [Fiji (leaf in combination)].

USE AS FOOD:

- Most of the plant is edible and used as food but usually the unripe and partially ripe fruit is used in a way similar to potatoes or made into a type of "flour."
- Leaf buds as vegetable [Hawai'i].
- Flowers cooked and eaten [Philippines].
- Also used as "insurance against famine" [Hawai'i]. Unripe fruit used in curry [India].
- Ashes of the plants may be used as a substitute for salt.
- Green bananas are boiled in their skins, then removed, and made into a kind of "pancake" [Belize].
- Leaves used to wrap tamales [Belize].
- Used alternately as a delicacy and a famine food [Hawai'i].

Beverages

Smoothies [Universal among recovering hippies]. The fruit is used to make alcohol, vinegar, and wine. Banana wine is reputed to prevent malaria [Antilles, Congo]. Banana beer [Choco, Africa].

OTHER USES:

- Leaves and leaf sheaths (waterproof after scorching) are used as thatching for houses, gutters, umbrellas.
- Leaves are also used as plates, cattle food, cigarette papers, clothing, packing material, for stringing leis, and cordage [Hawai'i, Philippines].
- The banana plant was used to make aqueducts, plant pots, emergency sandals, and splints for broken limbs [Hawai'i].
- Fiber and paper made from the leaf stems [Japan].
- Ashes used for dyeing, tanning, in curries, and as a salt substitute [India].
- Dye made from juice of flower buds [Hawai'i, India].
- Splint for broken bones (hollow stalk) [Hawai'i].
- Banana trunks were used as rollers to move canoes [Hawai'i].
- The young plant was used as flag of truce in war [Hawai'i].

CONSTITUENTS: Alpha tocopherol (fruit peel),

ascorbic acid (fruit peel), beta-carotene (fruit peel), carbohydrates (fruit peel), delta tocopherol (fruit peel), iron (fruit peel), niacin (fruit peel), norepinephrine, protein (fruit peel), riboflavin (fruit peel), Vit A, B, C.
Forget Prozac: Bananas contain large amounts of serotonin (5-HT) [Garcia-Moreno 1980, Helander 1992], although it is not clear if it is broken down in the gut.

POSSIBLE DRUG INTERACTIONS: Bananas protect the gastric mucosa in laboratory animals against NSAIDs and other pharmaceuticals. Bananas also appear to stimulate growth of the gastric lining after damage has occured. In one study, ripe fruit bananas did not have the same effect [Best 1984], while in another "banana pulp powder" was used. It is not clear if the banana pulp powder was ripe or not [Goel 1986].

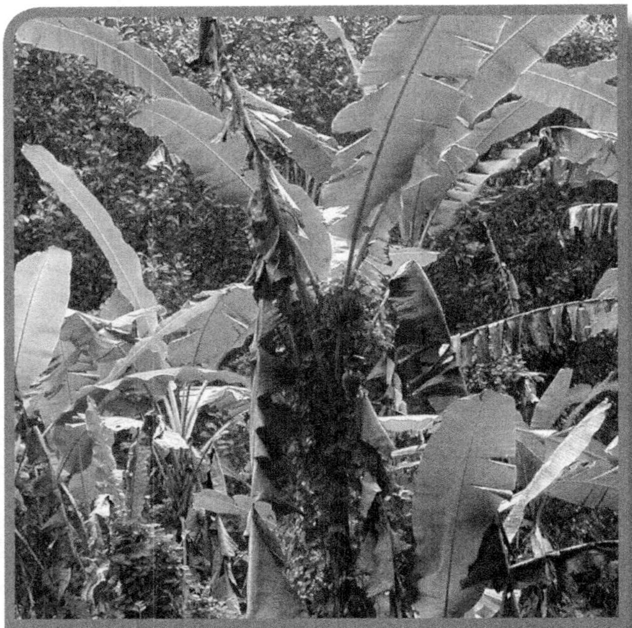

Musa spp.: Mai'a plant

Mai'a (Banana) Local Combinations

(all refer to *Musa* spp. sap)

Bronchitis: Add *Waltheria americana* ('uhaloa), *Sonchus oleraceus* (pualele / sow thistle).

Asthma: Add *Bidens pilosa* (kīnehi / spanish needle), *Curcuma longa* ('ōlena / Turmeric), *Piper methysticum* ('awa / kava).

Boils: Add *Plantago major* (laukahi / plantain).

Mai'a (Banana) Cross-Cultural Combinations

Please note some of the ingredients in the following combinations are toxic! Do not self-administer without the supervision of a licensed practitioner or an experienced Elder.

Stomach cramps: With dried squid ink, *Solanum nigrum* (pōpolo), *Colocasia esculenta* (taro leaf), *Bidens* spp. (ko'oko'olau), and with *Psilotum triquetrum* (moa) [Old Hawai'i].

Thrush: With *Aleurites moluccana* (kukui) sap or with half-ripe papaya fruit juice [Old Hawai'i].

Constipation: With *Aleurites moluccana* (kukui) nuts and flowers, *Hibiscus tiliaceus* (hau) *Syzygium malaccense* (mountain apple) bark, *Saccharum officinarum* (sugar cane), *Bidens* spp. (ko'oko'olau), and *Ipomoea cairica* (koali 'ai). [Old Hawai'i].

Asthma: With sweet potato, *Morinda citrifolia* (noni), *Saccharum officinarum* (sugar cane), *Cocos nucifera* (coconut), iron oxide ('alaea), and *Ipomoea cairica* (koali 'ai) [Old Hawai'i].

Asthma: Shoot with *Waltheria indica* ('uhaloa), Argemone glauca (puakala), *Syzygium malaccense* (mountain apple bark), *Aleurites moluccana* (kukui) bark, and *Eleocharis obtusa* (kohekohe) [Old Hawai'i].

Asthma: Flower juice with *Portulaca oleracea* ('ākulikuli / purslane), *Morinda citrifolia* (noni) fruit, *Syzygium malaccense* (mountain apple) bark, *Aleurites moluccana* (kukui) flowers, *Peperomia* spp. ('ala'alawainui), *Curcuma longa* (Turmeric) rhizome, Iron oxide ('alaea), *Saccharum officinarum* (sugar cane) and ashes of banana leaves [Old Hawai'i].

Pinworms: Fruit with *Ipomoea cairica* (koali 'ai), sweet potato, *Morinda citrifolia* (noni) fruit, *Hibiscus tiliaceus* (hau) bark, iron oxide ('alaea), *Syzygium malaccense* (mountain apple) bark [Old Hawai'i].

Cleansing: Sap with iron oxide ('alaea), Coral powder, and *Aleurites moluccana* (kukui) sap on tongue, forehead, temples, and navel [Old Hawai'i].

For "burning of chest and stomach" or for "excessive perspiration": Rotting banana stump, *Hibiscus tiliaceus* (hau) sap, iron oxide ('alaea), an "eating fern," and *Bidens* spp. (ko'oko'olau) [Old Hawai'i].

Jaundice: Fruit with "quicklime" [India].

Menopausal bleeding: Sap with curd [India].

Worms: Tuber with boiled rice, ghee, and molasses [India].

Anemia: Fruit with chicken eggs, wine, nutmeg, and salt [Choco: Colombia].

"Chiclero sore" (parasitic infection): Topical with

Piper nigrum (black pepper) [Belize].

RANGE: Pan tropical.

GATHERING: Timberrrrr.... Gather with reverence. Kinolau of Kāne.

PROPAGATION & CULTIVATION: Propagation by shoots. It really is self-propagating in the right environment. If one uses biodegradable soap, downhill from a washing machine works well.

RESEARCH:

- Flower extract reduces blood glucose in lab animals [Pari 1999, Pari 2000].
- Bananas can increase blood plasma levels of sulfate-conjugated norepinephrine and sulfate-conjugated dopamine. The sulfate-conjugated dopamine increase is enhanced by vitamin C [Dunne 1983]. Neurologically impaired patients often show lower levels of dopamine sulfate, norepinephrine sulfate, and epinephrine sulfate in their cerebral spinal fluid than in their blood plasma. While bananas can increase blood plasma dopamine levels, this is not reflected in cerebral spinal fluid levels. But, bananas effect on increased norepinephrine sulfate *is* reflected in cerebral spinal fluid levels [Kuchel 1985].
- The stem juice prevents and treats urinary stones in rats [Prasad 1993].

NOTES 'N QUOTES

- Sumatra: The god who was sent to earth to finish creation should have fasted or eaten crab (which gets a new shell every year), but instead he ate banana and so man's life is short like that of a banana stalk.
- In Europe and Asia banana was called "fruit of paradise" and "fruit of knowledge". The banana plant was said to be the source of good and evil and that the serpent was hiding in the banana plant before he tempted Eve.
- Tahiti: The first banana stem came from the windpipe of a man.
- It is uncertain if bananas were growing in America before European contact.
- The brother of Pele first brought bananas to Hawai'i.
- The most ancient people of Hawai'i, called the Mu, were said to be a tribe of wild banana eaters living in the hills.
- Fruits of certain bananas were fed to sharks by fishermen [Hawai'i].
- In old Hawai'i it was kapu (forbidden) for women to eat all but two varieties of bananas on penalty of death.
- In Hawai'i, he fruit was eaten after taking bitter medicine. Ripe banana fruit was also used by 'awa drinkers to counter the taste of 'awa. This is the first use of the term "pupu."
- When one wants to wrap a special gift in Hawai'i, a banana stalk is used.
- Legend has it that all bananas held their fruit erect until there was a battle between the upland and the lowland bananas. The lowland bananas lost and have ever since then held their heads in shame.
- Banana sap is one of the most accessible and useful medicinals in Hawai'i for infections.

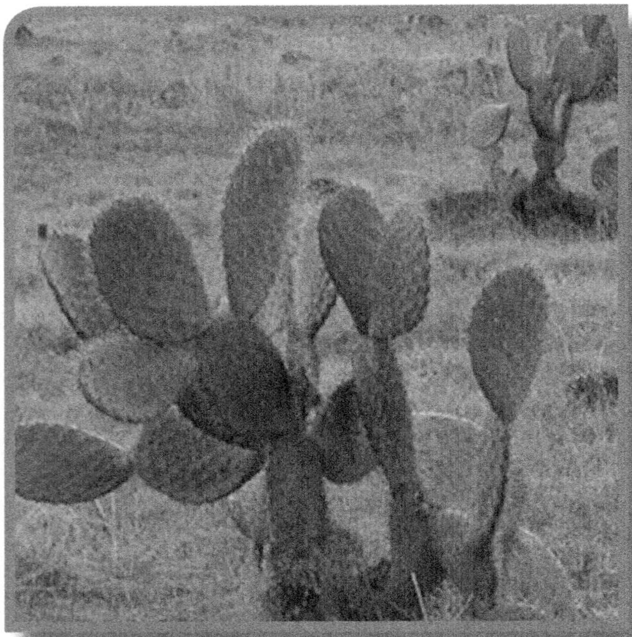

Opuntia spp. (Pānini / Prickly Pear)

PLANT NAME: *Opuntia* spp.

SIMILARLY USED SPECIES: Lots of them. *O. ficus-indica, O. vulgaris, O. decumana, O. compressa, O. leucotricha, O. streptacantha, O. stricta, Cactus opuntia.*

Status: Nasty, tasty, and painful alien.

COMMON NAMES: **Pānini**, pāpipi [Hawai'i]; **prickly pear**, barbary pear, indian pear [English]; **xian ren zhang** [China]; aathikan [Nepal]; cockineal [Bermuda]; nopal (whole plant), tuna (fruit) [Mexico]; nopal [South America]; rachette, cochineel [Carribean]; saptapheni [India]; scoggineal [Creole]; tuna, pa'kam [Mopal Maya].

Habitat: Dry and sunny.

NOMENCLATURE: "*Opuntia*" may have been taken from the name of a town in Greece. The Mexican name nopal, or nopalli was the Nahuatl name for prickly pear.

FAMILY: Cactaceae.

CATEGORY: Herbs that clear heat dry damp.

PROPERTIES: Bitter, cool to cold. Fruits are sweet.

PLANT PART USED: All of it.

TOXICITY: Oral administration of *O. streptacantha* is non-toxic to horses, humans, and mice [Ahmad 1996] While the aerial parts are safe, even if eaten in large amounts, the spines in one's skin are an acquired taste. **Some Chinese sources list the roots as mildly toxic.**

CAUTIONS AND CONTRAINDICATIONS: Not in pregnancy (root).

PREPARATION OF MEDICINE: It can be tinctured or cooked fresh. Medicine must be made from fresh materials, not dried. When cooked, keep the slimy material (pectin) and don't rinse it off, as it is medicinal. Please note: Pads are always used peeled or with the spines burned off.

DOSAGE: Fresh 30-60 grams.

STATUS IN HAWAI'I: Tasty and painful alien. Very high pest factor: terminate with extreme prejudice. *Opuntia* is native to the Americas. It was brought to Europe by the Spanish in the 1500s and was unfortunately introduced to Hawai'i from Acapulco by Don Francisco Paul de Marin before 1809.

WESTERN FUNCTIONS REPORTED: **Analgesic** (rhizome) [China]; **anti-diarrhea** (rhizome) [China]; **anti-inflammatory**; **antipyretic** (rhizome) [China]; **antiseptic**; **antitoxic** (rhizome) [China]; **antitussive** (rhizome) [China]; **astringent** (flowers poulticed) [Turkey]; **decongestant**; **demulcent** (decocted) [Central America]; **diuretic** [Mexico (juiced), Seri, Sicily (flower decocted), USA]; **emollient** [Spain (*O. ficus-indica)*]; **expectorant** [Africa, Bahamas]; **hallucinogen** [Sharanahua (Peru)]; **lactagogue** (pads peeled, cooked, poulticed) [USA]; **laxative** [Hawai'i]; **reduces swelling** (rhizome) [China]; **stop bleeding** (flowers).

TRADITIONAL CHINESE ENERGETIC FUNCTIONS (~ = extrapolated):

1) Regulates qi.
2) Invigorates blood.
3) Clears heat and toxin (rhizome).

Pānini (Prickly Pear) Common Medicinal Uses

- Diabetes
- Benign prostatic hypertrophy

Pānini (Prickly Pear) Cross-Cultural Medicinal Uses

COSMETIC

- **Balding** [Belize]; **hair conditioner** (fruit poulticed on hair then rinsed) [Barbados, Belize, Carribean, USA]; **increase hair growth** (roots).
- **Body lotion, hair gel, shampoo, and face cream** [Mexico]; **moisturizer & sunscreen** [Native American (leaves juiced)].
- **Moles** [Blackfoot]; **pimples** [India].

CARDIOVASCULAR

- **Arteriosclerosis; high blood pressure** [Belize (pad decocted)]; **high cholesterol** [Mexico (pads)].
- **Bleeding** [Kiowa (pads topical)].

DERMATOLOGICAL

- **Hematoma** [China (rhizome)].
- **Inflammation** [Barbados, Carribean, Mexico, Sri Lanka].
- **Rashes, sunburn** (juice topical)
- **Skin ulcers** [Belize (pad topical)].
- **Warts** [Blackfoot, Nanticoke (topical fruit juice), Shoshone].

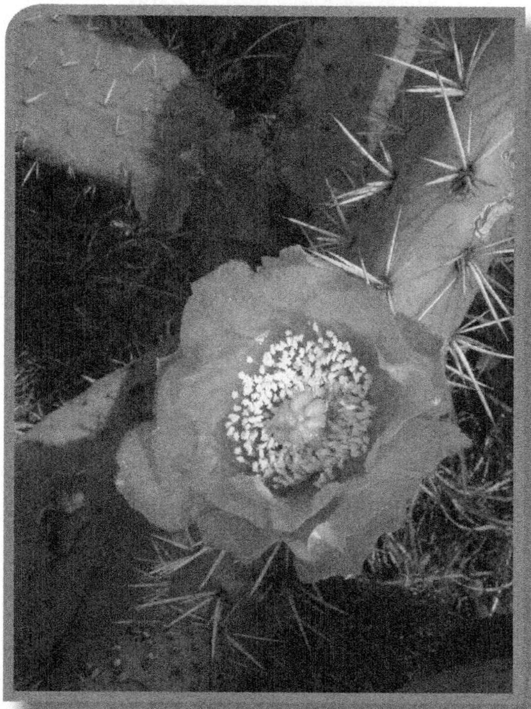

Opuntia ficus-indica: Pānini flower

DIGESTIVE

- **Colitis** (dried flowers); **diarrhea** (flower as tea, root chewed, or stem infused) [China, Flathead, Hopi, Seri, Turkey, USA]; **dysentery** [China, Colonial USA, Turkey], **irritable bowel syndrome** (flower as tea).
- **Gastric and duodenal ulcer** [China]; **gastric pain** [Barbados (pads peeled and boiled in seawater)].
- **Diverticulosis** (dried flowers).
- **Dyspepsia** [Kickapoo]; **gastrointestinal complaints** (pads eaten or flower as tea) [Canary Islands, Pima].
- **Hemorrhoids** [China]; **obesity** [Mexico (pads)].

ENDOCRINE

- **Diabetes** [Mexico (pads ingested broiled, blended or as juice)].

HEAD AND THROAT

- **Canker sores** (pads poulticed); **sore throat** [China, Costanoan, Dakota, Pawnee, Shoshone, Shuswap]; **epidemic parotitis** [China (pads topical)]; **toothache** [Seri (Mexico)].
- **Headaches** (pad poulticed or decocted topical) [Barbados, Belize, Native American].
- **Eye problems** [Native American (pads, decocted topical)]; **ophthalmia**.

INFECTION

- **Boils** [Bahamas, India (latex topical), Navaho, Sri Lanka].
- **Fever** [Belize (pads topical, decocted)].
- **Popliteal abscess** [China (pads topical)].

MUSCULOSKELETAL / TRAUMA

- **Arthritis** [Belize]; **back ache** [Flathead]; fruit used as heating pads for **muscle pain and to reduce swelling, joint pain** (pad topical) [Costanoan, Dakota, Pawnee, Shoshone, Shuswap]; **rheumatic conditions** (heated pad topical) [USA].
- **Bruises** (Veterinary) [Kickapoo]; **pain** (pad poulticed) [Barbados]; **spasms; swelling** (pad poulticed) [Barbados, Kickapoo, USA].
- **Burns** [China]; **cuts and burns** [Cahuilla (pad ash topical)]; **wounds** (flowers poulticed or pad topical) [Bahamas, Blackfoot, Costanoan, Dakota, Pawnee, Shoshone, Shuswap].
- **Dog bites** (pads topical) [China]; **snake bite** [China, Native American (indigestible seeds reclaimed and ground... yum!)]; **tarantula bites** (poultice)
- **Fractures** [Mexico].
- **Gout** (pads topical) [Bahamas].

ONCOLOGY

- **Tumors** [Chile, Haiti, Mauritius, USA].

PARASITES

- **Favus** (a scalp parasite) [China].

PEDIATRIC

- **Measles** [Sicily].
- **Mumps** [Kickapoo].
- **Pertussis**.

PSYCHOSPIRITUAL

- Used in magickal traditions for **protection against negativity, unwanted intrusions, burglaries, and to induce chastity**. (I bet!)
- **Insomnia** [Native American (pads, decocted)].
- **Malaise** [Belize (pad decocted)].

REPRODUCTIVE

- **Benign prostatic hypertrophy** [British Herbal Pharmacopeia (flowers)].
- **Chronic vaginitis** (dried flowers)
- **Excess menstruation** [Barbados (pads peeled and boiled in seawater)].
- **Gonorrhea** [USA]; **syphilis** [India].
- **Mastitis** [China]; **sore breasts from nursing** (topical) [Sri Lanka]; **to increase lactation** [Shoshone (heated pad tropical)].
- **To facilitate childbirth** [Belize, Lummi (pads infused)].
- **Used by Navaho midwives to lubricate their hands before removing the placenta.**

RESPIRATORY

- **Asthma** [USA (dried flowers or heated pad topical)].
- **Bronchial problems** [Africa, Canary Islands]; **cough** [Africa]; **lung ailments** (pad in tea); **mild bronchiectasis** (dried flowers).
- **Lung abscess** [China].
- **Pulmonary tuberculosis** [Bahamas, China].

URINARY

- **"Bladder conditions"** [Belize]; **dysuria** [Bahamas]; **male urinary discomforts** [Native American]; **urinary tract infections** [Mexico (juiced)].
- **Kidney problems** [Sicily]; **kidney stones** (pads juiced)

OTHER MEDICINAL USES

- For **"organ pain"** a mold of the patient's foot is cut from the skinned pad and dried over a fire [Belize].
- **Calluses** [South Africa]; corns [Argentina].
- **Leprosy** [Ethiopia].
- **Radiation burns**.
- **Shortwindedness** [Seri (Mexico)].
- **Thirst**.

USE AS FOOD:

- The use of cactus as food has been carbon dated to 65 B.C.
- In Mexico, *Opuntia* fruit ("tuna") is made into jam, marmalade, syrup, and a paste called queso de tuna.
- Eaten during lent in Mexico, when Catholics don't eat meat.
- One of Hawai'i's tastiest psychopaths, *Opuntia* fruit is marvelous. They can be eaten fresh or dried for storage [Cahuilla]. They can be boiled like greens, pickled, cooked like eggplant, or put in scrambled eggs.
- Young pads are despined, peeled, boiled and eaten. They can be breaded with seasonings and fried, sauteed, or boiled. They can also be used as a container in which to boil water.
- Flowers roasted and eaten [Pima].
- Dried seeds are used as a soup thickener.
- In Mexico, a beverage called Tecuin is made with *Opuntia* fruit and Acacia bark.
- A Central American beer, Colonche, (reputed to be over 2,000 years old) is made from *Opuntia* fruit. The fresh juice of pānini can be blended with orange or grapefruit juice, or made into wine (which reportedly ferments in a day). Interestingly, in a double blind crossover clinical trial, *Opuntia ficus-indica* was shown to be moderately effective against hangover [Wiese 2004]. Perhaps a "net-sum-game" dandelion / pānini wine is waiting to be born.
- The annual amount of Nopalitos eaten in Mexico is the same as the annual amount of cauliflower eaten in the US.

OTHER USES:

- Dye (fruit) [Barbados, Mexico].
- Hunting poison (?) [Navaho].
- The Pima tribe makes the dried plant into, napkin rings, canes, and souvenirs. Some tribes added the juice to mortar or whitewash [Native American].

CONSTITUENTS:

Plant: 17 amino acids (8 essential), B vitamins, calcium, magnesium, iron, and insoluble fiber (cellulose and lignin).
Fruit: 83% water, 10% sucrose, tartaric acid, citric acid, mucilage & mucopolysaccharides,
Seed: Fixed oil, fatty acid, albumen and starch.

Pānini (Prickly Pear) Local Combinations

NIDDM (type II) diabetes: Add *Morinda citrifolia* (noni), *Momordica charantia* (ka'ukama / bitter melon), *Cocos nucifera* (coconut) water.

Pānini (Prickly Pear) Cross-Cultural Combinations

Urinary obstruction: Flowers with *Hordeum vulgare* (barley seeds) & *Zea mays* (yu mi xu / corn silk) [North Africa].
Respiratory infections: With honey.
Dysentery: Root boiled with milk.

RANGE: Semi-tropical and tropical areas. North, Central, and South America to Southern Europe, Mediterranean, India, & Australia.

HABITAT: Where ever it pleases, but likes it dry and sunny. On Maui it grows in drier areas of Kula and Omaopio. Also on the Big Island on Kohala mountain.

The Aztecs, after wandering for 157 years, one day saw an eagle perched on a prickly pear cactus. It had a snake in its talons and its wings were opened and embraced the rising sun. They took this as an omen that this was to be the place where they were to build their city. That city was called Tenochtitlan ("Place of the Prickly Pear") and it is now known as Mexico City.

GATHERING: With gloves or a special coffee-can gathering device. The pads used for diabetes can be gathered year round [Meckes-Lozoya 1989]. While the fruit is a favorite and delicious food at luaus, gathering it may prove to be an interesting experience. The short barbed hairs that protect *Opuntia* spines (as if they *need* any protection) are called "glochids" and are living proof that evolution does indeed adore a psychopath. After harvest the tiny biological reminders can continue their imbedded lessons for days. Hawaiians call this "Ho'opa'ana'au."... "Remembering in the body."

PROPAGATION & CULTIVATION: Do not propagate in Hawai'i. *Opuntia* spp. can be tenacious invaders, both in the Hawaiian Kingdom and elsewhere. In Australia alone they took over 24 million hectares and had to be eradicated: a predator moth, (*Cactoblastus cactorum*), was used to keep the *Opuntia* from spreading. However, in Arizona *Opuntia* are protected, as they are native to North America.

RESEARCH:

- The effectiveness of *Opuntia* for experimentally induced diabetes in lab animals is well documented, but its use for diabetes in humans has not been established [Frati-Munari 1992; Veronin 2000]. Results, however, are promising [Frati-Munari 1989(a), 1989(b), 1990; Wolfram 2002]. Some of the effects of *Opuntia* may vary with its preparation. Broiled *Opuntia* stems decreased serum glucose in patients with type II diabetes mellitus, whereas crude extracts did not [Frati-Munari 1989(a)].
- Improves benign prostatic hypertrophy [Palevitch / Earon / Levin 1994].
- *O. ficus-indica* increases gastric mucus [Galati 2002(b)] and prevents ulcers in rats [Galati 2003], possibly due to its own mucilage content [Galati / Monforte 2001] or its' anti inflammatory effect [Park / Kahng 1998]. The anti inflammatory effect may be due to beta-sitosterol [Park / Kahng 2001]. In addition to being anti inflammatory, it is also analgesic in rats and mice [Loro 1999].
- *Opuntia* cladodes (leaf pads), flowers, and fruit are diuretic, with the fruit having the strongest effect [Galati 2002(a)]. In laboratory rats, *Opuntia* modulates renal sodium and fluid processing [Bwititi 2001].
- *Opuntia ficus-indica* var. saboten contains neuroprotective flavonoids [Dok-Go 2003]. Many *Opuntia* species are anti-oxidant [Budinsky 2001; Butera 2002; Galati 2003], possibly due to phenolic compounds [Lee / Kim 2002]. Prickly pear fruit reduced oxidative stress better than vitamin C in a human clinical trial [Tesoriere 2004].
- Lowers LDL cholesterol in lab animals [Fernendez 1994], possibly through LDL receptor supression [Fernendez 1992; Palumbo 2003]. *Opuntia* has ingredients such as pectins and mucilage that are helpful to digestion [El Kossori 1998].
- *O. ficus-indica* may inhibit Monoamine oxidase-B (MAO-B) [Han 2001].
- *O. streptacantha* is antiviral against equine herpes,

herpes simplex, influenza, respiratory syncytial virus, pseudorabies virus, and HIV [Ahmad 1996].

- In a small human clinical trial, *Opuntia* improved platelet function [Wolfram 2003]. Speeds the healing of wounds in lab animals [Park / Chun 2001].

NOTES 'N QUOTES

- Juan de Zumarraga, the first archbishop of Mexico, spent much of his spare time trying to eliminate all remnants of native culture. In his zeal to "cleanse" the New World of pagan ways, he managed to destroy most of the information as to how cacti were used as food, medicine, housing, dyes, glue, tools, and as spiritual implements.
- There are 87 genera in the Cactaceae family and 2000 species. In the *Opuntia* genus alone there are 300 species. This includes a cultivated variety, *Opuntia ficus-indica* cv., which has no spines.
- A useful upcountry medicine, pānini tends to take a back seat to other medicinals as the process of gathering is time consuming and somewhat prohibitive. Stabilizing the juice in alcohol can help extend its shelf life.

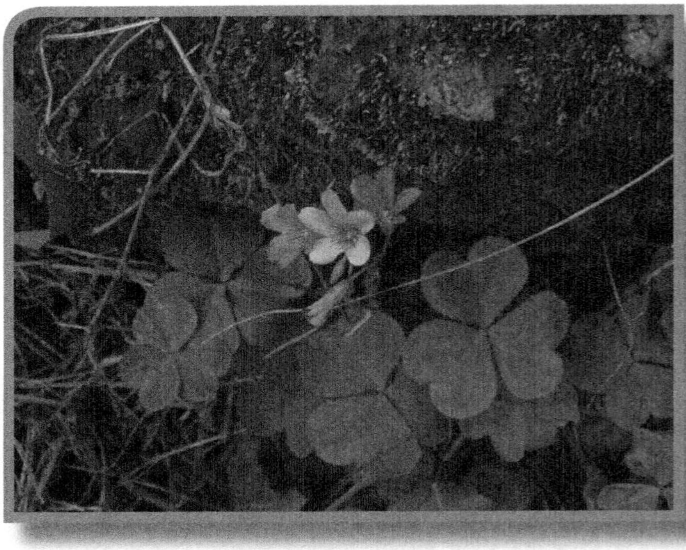

Oxalis corymbosa: 'Ihi Pehu

Oxalis spp. ('Ihi Mākole / 'Ihi Pehu / Sorrel)

PLANT NAME: *Oxalis* spp.

SIMILARLY USED SPECIES: *Acetosella corniculata; O. acetosella; O. amplifolia; O. convexula; O. corniculata; O. corniculatus; O. crassicaulis; O. decaphylla; O. depressa; O. dichondraefolia; O. drummondi; O. hedysaroides; O. langloisii; O. latifolia; O. martiana; O. montana; O. obliquifolia; O. otaviensis; O. pes-caprae; O. pusilla; O. repens; O. stricta; O. trilliifolia; O. villosa; O. violacea; Xanthoxalis corniculata; X. langloisii; X. repens; X. rufa.*

Status: Uncertain. Possibly native.

Habitat: Wet and shady.

COMMON NAMES: **'Ihi**, **'ihi pehu** [*O.* martiana], **'ihi mākole** [*O. corniculata*] [Hawai'i]; **sorrel**, cuckoo bread, fairy bells, green sauce, hallelujah, shamrock, sour trefoil, stickwort, stubwort, surelle, three-leaved grass, wood sour [USA]; biahd nan coinean [Gaelic]; cangeri, puliyaral [India]; chari amilo [Nepal]; cuckoos meat [Scotland]; gaukesyre, gaukesyra / gjøkesyre[Norway]; hain-sauerklee / sauerklee / wald-sauerklee [Germany]; harsyra [Sweden]; 'i'i [Samoa]; ketunleipā / kāenkaali [Finland]; kihikihi [Tonga]; koi'i [Rapa]; kok'i [Cook Islands]; malgoj [Dominica]; pa'ihi [Austral Islands]; pakihi [Marquesas]; patoa 'awa' awa [Tahiti]; skovsyre, surkløver [Denmark]; sursmæra [Iceland]; szczawik zajeczy [Poland]; wood sorrel [Great Britain]; gowkemeat[Scotch]; pain de coucou [French]; seamsog [Ireland]; iuliole [Italy].

NOMENCLATURE:
- "*Oxalis*" comes from "Oxys" the Greek word for "sour" or "acidic." One taste tells you why.
- The specific epithet "*corniculata*" means "horned."
- 'Ihi means "sacred" or "holy." Mākole means "inflamed" or "reddish," sometimes a reference to blood-shot eyes. This may be a reference to the uses of 'ihi mākole, or to its' pink flowers.
- Pehu means "swollen," sometimes as a reference to edema or water retention. This may be a reference to *Oxalis*' use as a diuretic.

FAMILY: Oxalidaceae.

CATEGORY: Herbs that calm the spirit.

PROPERTIES: Sour, cool. In Indian texts *Oxalis* spp. are listed as both cool and hot. Go figure....

PLANT PART USED: The aerial parts.

TOXICITY: *Oxalis* spp. are used as a poison in Australia, India, Spain, & Turkey. Large doses can cause oxalate poisoning. Overdose in animals results in coma and death. Oxalates can bind with calcium causing physiological problems. The oxalates in Sorrel can be minimized by properly decocting the herb.

CAUTIONS AND CONTRAINDICATIONS: *Oxalis* spp. should be avoided by those with gout, arthritis, kidney stones, or hyperacidity. Not in pregnancy.

PREPARATION OF MEDICINE: Decocted or poulticed fresh.

WESTERN FUNCTIONS REPORTED: **Analgesic; anodyne; anthelmintic; anti inflammatory; antidote; antiemetic; antiphlogistic; antipyretic; antiscorbutic; antiseptic; antithelmintic; aperitif; appetizing; arsenic antidote; astringent; beverage; bilious; bitter tonic; cleanses the blood; cyanogenetic; datura antidote; decoagulant; depurative; detergent; diaphoretic; digestive stimulant; diuretic; emmenagogue; expectorant; febrifuge; hypotensive; increases appetite; irritant; lithontriptic; mercury antidote; refrigerant; removes obstructions of the viscera; resolvent; scorpion antidote; soporific; stomachic; stomachic; stops vomiting; strengthens a weak stomach; styptic; suppurative; tonic; vermifuge.**

TRADITIONAL CHINESE ENERGETIC FUNCTIONS (~ = extrapolated):

1) Clears heat and toxins.
2) Calms the spirit.
3) Lowers blood pressure.

OTHER ENERGETIC FUNCTIONS: Alleviates vata and kapha. [India]

'Ihi (Sorrel)
Common Medicinal Uses

- **Topical for sprains, broken bones.**
- **Internal "blood cleansing" for skin conditions.**
- **Internal for urinary tract infections.**
- **Irritability, insomnia**

'Ihi (Sorrel) Cross-Cultural Medicinal Uses

BITES & STINGS
- **Snake bites**, **bug bites**, **stings** [China (poulticed); Lesotho].

CARDIOVASCULAR
- **Anemia** [*O. corniculata*] [General]; **as a blood tonic, after a "winter without greens"** [USA].
- **Bleeding** (juiced topical) [Eclectic, Peru]; **internal bleeding** [Cook Islands]. Please note that *Oxalis* is also used as a decoagulant in China.
- **Hypertension** [China]; **sclerosis** [*O. acetosella*].

DERMATOLOGICAL
- **Eczema** [China (poulticed)]; **itching** [Philippines].
- **Skin sores**, **eruptions** [China, Native American]; **"scrofulous and indolent ulcers"** [Eclectic (juice topical)].
- **Warts**, **corns** [India (poulticed)].
- **Athletes foot** [China (poulticed)].

DIGESTIVE
- **Stomatitis**.
- **Diarrhea** [China, Kickapoo, Nepal, Panama]; **dysentery** [India, Philippines]; **enteritis** [China].
- **Indigestion** [India]; **nausea** [USA (leaves chewed)]; **vomiting** [Cherokee]; **stomach ache**.
- **Hemorrhoids** [India, Nepal]; **prolapsed rectum** [Nepal].
- **Mild constipation** [Hawai'i].

HEAD AND THROAT
- **Eye problems**; **conjunctivitis** [Java]; **opacities of the cornea** [India].

- **Mouth problems** [Guatemala, Panama]; **mouth sores** [Native American, USA (leaves chewed)]; **sore gums and teeth** [Phillipines (leaf juice)]; **mouth ulcers** (juice as a gargle or eaten) [Scotland]; **gum inflammations**; **gingivitis** [Java]; **oral cysts** [Tahiti].
- **Sore throat** (infusion or leaves chewed) [Caribbean, Tahiti, USA]; **streptococcal tonsillitis** [UK].
- **Increased thirst**.
- **Nosebleed** [Panama].
- **Tympanitis**.

HEPATIC

- **Bilious headaches** [India].
- **Liver problems** [Haiti]; **hepatitis** [China, Kickapoo (Mexico)].

INFECTION

- **Abscess** [Haiti]; **boils** [China (poulticed)].
- **Fever** [China, Dominican Republic, Eclectic, India, Philippines, Scotland, Turkey, USA, Venezuela].

MUSCULOSKELETAL / TRAUMA

- **Body aches** [Cook Islands].
- **Inflammation & pain** [Haiti, India (poulticed), Mexico].
- **Sprains**, **swelling**, **traumatic injuries**, **bruises**, **and wounds** [China, Hawai'i, Scotland (poulticed) Tahiti].
- **Burns** [China (poulticed)].

NEUROLOGICAL

- **Convulsions** [Tonga].

ONCOLOGY

"*This herb, freshly gathered, is well bruised in a mortar... this extract makes a powerful application in the treatment of cancer.... The extract of these plants [Oxalis & Rumex] constitutes the basis of probably three-fourths of the marvelous "cancer-cures" with which such a large portion of mankind is steadily humbugged...*"
- - Kings Dispensatory, William Cook, M.D., 1869

- **Cancer** [Eclectic (topical), Native American, USA (poulticed)].
- **Armpit cancer** [USA].
- **Abdominal tumors**.

PARASITES

- **Intestinal worms** [USA].

PEDIATRIC

- **Children's ailments** [Hawai'i].
- **Thrush** [Cook Islands]; **mouth infections in infants** [Tonga (crushed leaves topical)].
- **Navel problems in children** ("Tapitopito") [Tonga].
- **Delayed closure of the fontanel** [Tonga (crushed leaves topical)].
- **Hook worms** [Cherokee (infused & topical)].

PSYCHOSPIRITUAL

- **Neurasthenia**, **emotional distress** [China].
- Venus rules *Oxalis*. **It is said to bring luck**, **protect the heart from disease**, **and to enable one to see fairies**.

REPRODUCTIVE

- **Gonorrhea** [Eclectic, Kickapoo, Peru (juiced].
- **Childbirth**.
- **Urogenital problems**.

RESPIRATORY

- **Respiratory trouble** [Hawai'i].
- **Asthma** [Hawai'i]; **cough** [Java]; **phlegm in the lungs** [Eclectic, Hawai'i, Peru (juiced)].
- **Colds and flu** [China].
- **Tuberculosis** [Hawai'i].

URINARY

- **Problems with urination** [Eclectic, India]; **bladder infections** [China, Scotland, USA].
- **Urinary stones** [China] (not recommended).

VETERINARY

- **Hoof and mouth disease** [Haiti].
- **Medicine for dairy cows** [India].

OTHER MEDICINAL USES

- **Debility** [Hawaii].
- **Pain** [India].
- **Intoxication** [India].
- **Prickly-heat** [Java].
- **Scurvy** [Eclectic, India, Scotland, USA].

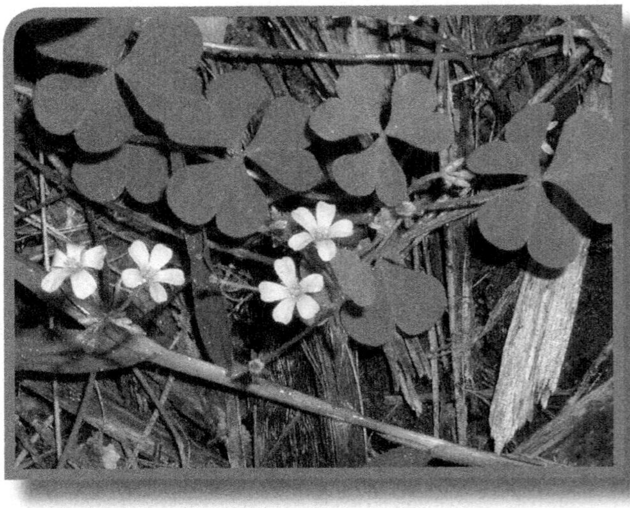

Oxalis corniculata: 'Ihi Mākole

USE AS FOOD:
- Small amounts are used in salads and sauces.
- In soup while recovering from diarrhea [India].
- *Oxalis* is juiced and made into a sherbet for thirst, dysentery, or rectal prolapse [India].
- In the time of Henry VII, *Oxalis* was commonly used as a pot-herb, but lost its popularity when it was replaced by French Sorrel (*Rumex scutatus*).

OTHER USES:
- Flowers can be used to dye cotton.
- Dried herb can be used to curdle plant milks.
- The juice is said to remove "iron mould" stains from linens. [Haiti]

CONSTITUENTS: The leaves contain 7-12% oxalates. Beta carotene, calcium, iron, phosphorus, niacin, vitamin C.

POSSIBLE DRUG INTERACTIONS: None noted.

DOSAGE: 10-15 grams in combination. Topical as needed.

'Ihi (Sorrel) Local Combinations

Irritablity: Add *Verbena littoralis* (ha'uoi / vervain), *Pipturus albidus* (māmaki).
Hepatitis or high blood pressure: Add *Prunellla vulgaris* (xia ku cao / self heal), *Vernonia cinerea* (iron weed).
Urinary tract infection: Add *Desmodium* spp. (pua-pilipili), *Bidens pilosa* (kīnehi / spanish needle).

'Ihi (Sorrel) Cross-Cultural Combinations

Urinary infections: Decocted with *Lygodium japonicum* (jin sha teng), *Desmodium styracifolium* (jin qian cao) and *Cayratia japonica* [China].
Agitation, emotional distress, and insomnia: With *Pinus massoniana* [China].
Indigestion and diarrhea in children: With buttermilk [India].
Enteritis, chronic dysentery, rectum prolapse, hemorrhoids or thirst: Boiled as a tea with yogurt water (lassi), or blended with honey [India].
Skin eruptions: Juiced with ghee and pepper [India (topical)].
"Bilious headaches": Topical with onions [India].
"Blood cleanser": With *Phymatosorus scolopendria* (laua'e fern) [Hawai'i].
Urinary infection: With *Lygodium japonicum*, *Desmodium styracifolium* and *Cayratia japonica* [China].
Scurvy and malignant fevers: "Conserva Ligulae," a beverage for scurvy and malignant fevers, used to be made with mashed *Oxalis* spp. ('ihi / sorrel) leaves, sugar, and orange peel.

RANGE: *Oxalis* spp. are globally pandemic.

GATHERING: 24 / 7.

PROPAGATION & CULTIVATION: Self propagating.

NOTES 'N QUOTES

"*Greene Sauce... is good for them that have sicke and feeble stomaches... and of all Sauces, Sorrel is the best, not only in virtue, but also in pleasantness of his taste.*"
- - Gerard

"*The apothecaries and herbalists call it Alleluya and Paniscuculi, or Cuckowes meat, because either the Cuckoo feedeth thereon, or by reason when it springeth forth and flowereth the Cuckoo singeth most, at which time also Alleluya was wont to be sung in Churches.*"
- - Author Unknown

- Saint Patrick's shamrock was actually an *Oxalis*. It was a Druid symbol associated with the Celtic Sun Wheel. The Celtic name "seanrog" became "shamrog" and finally "shamrock." Saint Patrick (390 - 464 A.D.) used this pagan symbol to represent the Trinity.
- Some "Dock" (Rumex) species are known as the "Sour Docks" or "Sorrels." The generic name "Sorrel" is common to many plants that contain binoxalate of potash.
- Because the *Oxalis* leaves trigger a mucilaginous film when chewed, magicians have used them to protect their mouthes while they eat glass.
- Possibly as a counter-irritant, Uncle Kalua Kaiahua commonly used 'ihi for broken bones and sprains. It is useful in combination for eczema and skin rashes.
- Universally munched on by children for its sour taste, this pleasant creeper makes its home in the shady areas near Hawaiian homes. Arguably the most common medicinal herb seen in Hawai'i, 'ihi functions as a mild diuretic and sedative.

Oxalis spp. ('Ihi / Sorrel)

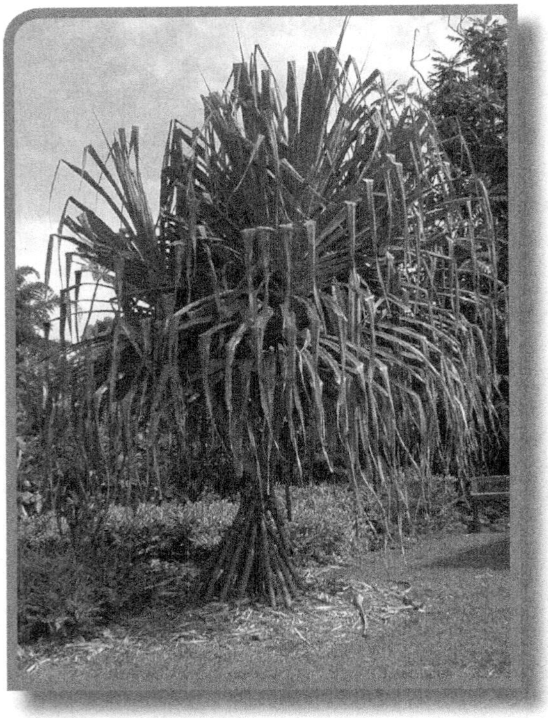

Pandanus tectorius (Hala)

PLANT NAME: *Pandanus tectorius* S. Parkinson ex. Z.

OTHER NAMES: *P. chamissonis, P. douglasii, P. odoratissimus,*

Status: Indigenous.

Habitat: Wet coastal areas to 1000'.

SIMILARLY USED SPECIES: *P. aurantiacus, P. furcatus, P. klossii, P. odorus, P. polycephalus, P. utilis*

COMMON NAMES: **Hala** [Hawai'i]; **screwpine** [English]; fa [Tonga]; ketaki, kewra [India]; palma de tornillo [Colombia]; toei-hom (*P. odorus*) [Thailand].

FAMILY: Pandanaceae (screwpine family).

CATEGORY: Cool acrid release the exterior.

PROPERTIES: Sweet, bland, cool.

PLANT PART USED: Fruit, flowers, leaf buds, aerial roots. Leaves for non-medicinal uses.

TOXICITY: The LD50 of water extracted *P. odorus* in rats is 1.18-2.76g / kg for intraperitoneal injection, and 8g / kg for oral administration [Peungvicha 1996].

CAUTIONS AND CONTRAINDICATIONS: Not in pregnancy.

PREPARATION OF MEDICINE: Aerial roots infused or decocted. Seeds decocted. Pollen sprinkled on bedding. Leaf buds decocted.

DOSAGE: Aerial root: 15-30 grams; Fruit: 30-90 grams.

STATUS IN HAWAI'I: Indigenous.

WESTERN FUNCTIONS REPORTED: **Anodyne** [Hawai'i]; **antidote** (*P. furcatus, P. tectorius*) [Java]; **aphrodisiac** (*P. utilis*); **cosmetic** (*P. odorus*) [Malaya]; **depurative**; **diaphoretic** [China]; **laxative** [Hawai'i]; **sedative** (*P. latifolius*) [Java]; **stimulant**; **sudorific** [France].

TRADITIONAL CHINESE ENERGETIC FUNCTIONS:

Leaf buds

1) Clears heat, cools the blood.
2) Relieves toxins.

Flowers

1) Clears heat and disinhibits water.
2) Dispels damp heat.
3) Stops heat with diarrhea.

Aerial roots

1) Relieves the surface.
2) Clears heat, frees water & transforms dampness.

Fruit / seeds

1) Tonifies the spleen & stomach; supports a weak spleen.
2) Strengthens the source qi.
3) Subdues rising yang; benefits the head and eyes.
4) Reduces phlegm.
5) Benefits & increases the blood.
6) Relieves toxins from alcohol; stops thirst after drinking alcohol.
7) Strengthens the mind & spirit; makes one happy and benefits the mind.
8) Releases & resolves abdominal lumps.

Hala Common Medicinal Uses

- **Colds and flu (aerial root)**
- **Urinary tract infection / fluid retention (aerial root)**
- **Red eyes (aerial root)**
- **Low energy (fruit)**
- **Aphrodisiac (pollen)**

Hala
Cross-Cultural Medicinal Uses

CARDIOVASCULAR
- **Anemia** (*P. odorus*) [Malaya].

DERMATOLOGICAL
- **Erysipelas** [China (root)].

DIGESTIVE
- **Constipation** [Samoa].
- **Diarrhea** [Java (*P. furcatus*), Samoa]; **dysentery** [China (fruit decocted), Java (*P. furcatus*), Samoa].
- **Hemorrhoids** [China (fruit or seeds decocted)].
- **Stomach ache** [Tonga].

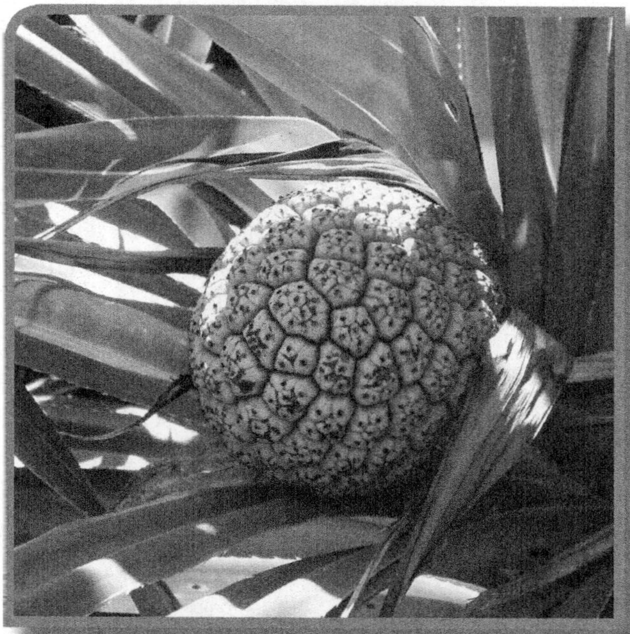

Pandanus tectorius: Hala fruit

ENDOCRINE
- **Diabetes** (roots juiced internal)

HEAD AND THROAT
- **Conjunctivitis** [China (root decocted)]; **macular eruptions** [China (root)]; **visual obstruction** [China (fruit)].
- **Earache**.
- **Bleeding gums** [China (root)]; **gingivosis** [Panrang (*P. polycephalus*)].
- **Headache**.

HEPATIC
- **Ascites** [China (root decocted)]; **cirrhosis** [China (root decocted)]; **hepatitis** [China (root decocted)].

INFECTION
- **Fever** [China (root decocted)].
- **Sores** [China (root); India]; **boils on nape of the neck** [China (flower)].
- **"Foot rot"** [China (root)].
- **Smallpox**.

LYMPHATIC
- **Elephantiasis** [Samoa].

MUSCULOSKELETAL / TRAUMA
- **Arthritis**; **rheumatism**.
- **Fractures** [Fiji]; **swelling** [Samoa].
- **Spasms** [Iran].

PEDIATRIC
- **Children's coughs** (roots juiced internal).
- **Measles** [China (root), Malaya (*P. odorus*)].
- **Thrush** [Hawai'i].

PSYCHOSPIRITUAL
- A lei made from the seeds, while beautiful, is said to bring bad luck.
- **Giddiness** [Arabia].

REPRODUCTIVE
In Hawai'i, pollen from the male flower (hinano) is sprinkled on beds as an aphrodisiac: "*Put some of that on your pillow tonight! You and your sweetie have plenty good time!*" - - Auntie Nani Saffrey
- **Coitus captivus** (ouch!) [Marshall Islands].
- **Difficult childbirth** [Hawai'i (aerial roots)]; **childbirth** (*P. aurantiacus, P. klossii, P. odorus*) [Pahang, Malaya].
- **Gonorrhea** [Malaya (*P. odorus*)]; **syphilis** [Malaya (*P. odorus*)]; **venereal disease** (*P. utilis*).
- **Inflamed or infected testicles** [China (seeds decocted)].

RESPIRATORY
- **Common cold with fever** [China (flower, fruit, or root decocted)].
- **Cough** [China (fruit decocted), Java (*P. furcatus*)].

URINARY
- **Edema** [China (root decocted)]; **nephritis with swelling / edema** [China (root)].
- **Urinary tract infection** [China (root decocted)]; **cloudy or difficult urination** [China (flower)]; **urinary stones** [China (root decocted)].

OTHER MEDICINAL USES
- **Chest pain** [Hawai'i (aerial roots)].

- **Debility** [Hawai'i].
- **Dizziness** [Java].
- **Hernia** [China (flower)].
- **Leprosy**.
- **Blood poisoning from bad food**. (*P. odorus*) [Malaya].
- **"Summer heat" conditions** (root) [China].

USE AS FOOD:

- Although *Pandanus* is used as food all over Polynesia, the varieties that grow in Hawai'i are waxy and not terribly edible. In a pinch the tips of the ripe seeds may be eaten raw or cooked and stored for later use. Some varieties have calcium oxalate crystals that are destroyed through cooking. Some species of *Pandanus* contain significant amounts of provitamin A carotenoids [Englberger 2003]. The orange seeds contain more than the yellow ones.
- *P. odorus* has 131.5 g / kg of alpha-tocopherol (vit E) [Ching 2001].

OTHER USES:

- Used in Hawai'i for everything from floor mats to hats to canoe sails. Trunks of the female tree were hollowed out and used to channel water in wetland kalo patches (lo'i), and the male tree parts were used as building materials.
- Australian Aboriginals used to lash together *Pandanus* to make a small frame with *Melaleuca* bark tops as river rafts during the wet season.
- The leaf skin has been used as cigarette papers.
- Allied forces in the Gilbert Islands used *Pandanus* as building material in World War Two.
- On Maui, the dried seeds were used as paint brushes to decorate kapa cloth.

Pandanus tectorius: Hala aerial roots

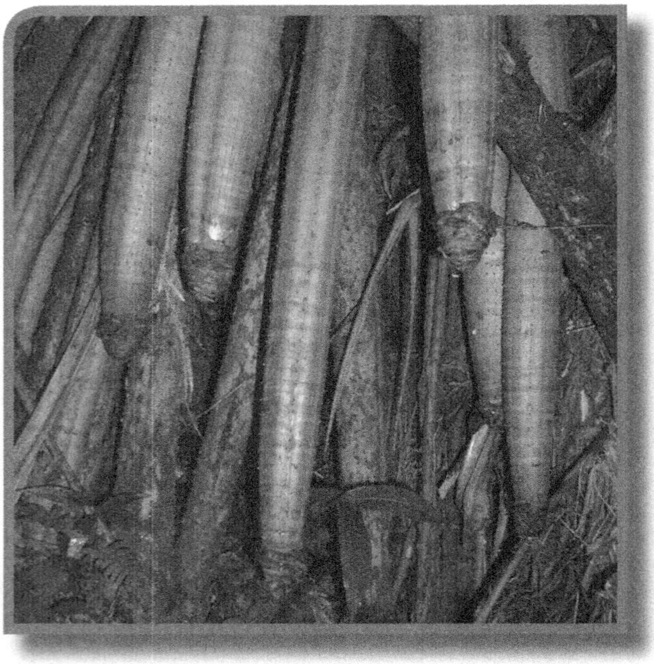

Hala Local Combinations

Common cold: Aerial root internal. Add *Eucalyptus* spp. (nuhōlani) in a pūlo'ulo'u (steam bath).
Urinary tract infection: Add *Coix lacryma jobi* (pū'ohe'ohe / jobs tears) kernals or roots.
Low energy: Add *Coix lacryma jobi* (pū'ohe'ohe / jobs tears) leaves and *Morinda citrifolia* (noni) fruit.
Red eyes: Add *Vitex rotundifolia* (pōhinahina seeds).

Hala Cross-Cultural Combinations

Difficult childbirth: Tips of aerial roots with *Hydrocotyle verticillata* leaves (pohe), *Eleocharis* spp. (kohekohe), *Peperomia* spp. stems ('ala'alawainui), *Oxalis corniculata* leaves and fruit ('ihi makole / sorrel), *Myoporum sandwicense* leaf buds (naio), and *Saccharum* spp. (kō kea / sugar cane) [Hawai'i].
Nephritis or edema: Root with lean pork [China].
Skin sores: Juiced aerial roots with *Cocos nucifera* (niu / coconut) and *Curcuma longa* ('ōlena / Turmeric), topical for [Tonga].
Chest pain: Tips of aerial roots and base of leaves with *Rorippa sarmentosa* leaves (Pā'ihi), *Solanum americanum* roots (pōpolo), *Waltheria indica* whole plant ('uhaloa), *Peperomia* spp. stems ('ala'alawainui), *Syzygium malaccense* bark ('ōhi'a 'ai mountain apple), *Morinda citrifolia* ripe fruit (noni) and *Saccharum* spp. (kō kea / sugar cane) [Hawai'i].
Other: Hala seeds are one of the main ingredients in the "Resurrection Tea" formula for low energy and hangover. Other ingredients include *Glycyrrhiza glabra* (licorice), *Pueraria lobata* (ge gen / kudzu), *Zingiber officinale* ('awapuhi pākē / ginger), and *Astragalus membranaceus* (huang qi) [Hawai'i].

RANGE: Tropics world-wide.

GATHERING: Kinolau of Kamapua'a. Hala leaves, fruit, aerial roots, and branches have sharp protrusions, so take care when gathering.

RESEARCH:

- Get out your vines! DMT has been found in *Pandanus* fruit growing in New Guinea [Barrau 1958, 1962].

- A saline extract of *Pandanus amaryllifolius* produces the lectin Pandanin, which has been shown to be antiviral against *Herpes simplex* virus type-1 and influenza virus [Ooi 2004].
- Water extracted *Pandanus odorus* lowers plasma glucose in diabetic, but not non-diabetic, rats [Peungvicha 1996].

NOTES 'N QUOTES

- New Caledonian crows (*Corvus moneduloides*) have been shown to use *Pandanus* plant materials as three distinct types of tools. Oddly enough, they also demonstrate " species-level laterality" i.e. they have a right and left-handedness, with one side strongly predominating. The crows that is, not the plants [Hunt 2000, 2004].
- In a Chinese medicine clinical context, the aerial roots are sweet and cool and rather pleasant tasting. They release the exterior and drain dampness. They are similar to *Chrysanthemum morifolium* (ju hua), in that they also clear heat in the upper part of the body and seem to smoothe the flow of liver qi.
- A reliable friend that lives by the ocean, *Pandanus* has the advantage of being easy to find and accessible as the need arises, although the hinano (male flower) can be hard to come by. The taste of the aerial root is surprisingly pleasant, as is the fruit in decoction. Acupuncturists will find the aerial roots useful as a diaphoretic and diuretic. The ripe fruits, while sometimes difficult to find, are well placed in formulas for qi deficient low energy and blood deficient irritability and insomnia.

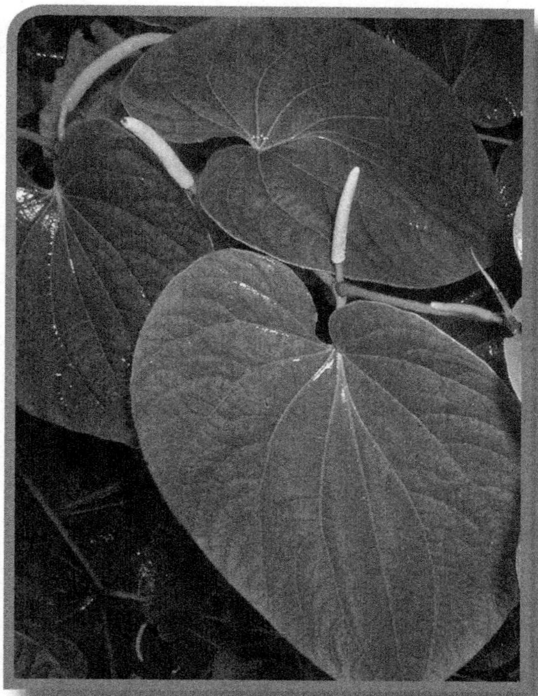

Piper methysticum ('Awa / Kava)

PLANT NAME: *Piper methysticum*, Forst.

COMMON NAMES: **'Awa**, **kava** [Hawai'i], Mönch pfeffer (monk pepper) [Germany]

NOMENCLATURE: 'Awa was given its botanical name by Johann Georg Forster, a botanist with Captain Cook on his second voyage to the Pacific from 1772 to 1775. He called it "*Piper methysticum*" which means "pepper that intoxicates." "Methy" means "wine" in Greek. The word "awa" means "bitter" in Hawaiian.

Status: Polynesian introduction.

Habitat: 150-1500'. Wet and shady.

FAMILY: Piperaceae.
The family Piperaceae has within it five genera comprised of more than 2000 species, more than 1000 of which are in the genus *Piper*.

CATEGORY: Expel wind dampness~.

PROPERTIES: Acrid warm~. One source lists it as hot, aromatic, bitter.

PLANT PART USED: Rhizome.

TOXICITY: Kava resin is non-lethal given orally to

mice at 600 mg / kg (heavy kava users consume roughly 133 mg / kg of kava resin per day) [McKenna 2002]. The oral LD50 of kavalactones for mice has been reported in the range of 920 - 1,050 mg / kg, and the injection LD50 at 300-400 mg / kg. 50 mg / kg doses given three times a week for 90 days caused no toxicity in rats. However, alcohol (ethanol) injections in mice can increase the toxicity of kava resins given orally, with small increases in alcohol resulting in large increases in toxicity [McKenna 2002].

CAUTIONS AND CONTRAINDICATIONS:

"*Subjects receiving kava reported subjective feelings of intoxication that was also reflected in a higher level of body sway.*"

- - Dennis McKenna

- Safe and non-addictive at moderate doses. Recent warnings of liver failure from kava are due to use of the leaf or stem and not the root [Dragull 2003, Nerurkar 2004]. So... don't use the leaves or stems. As Mark Twain once said "*Reports of my death are greatly exaggerated.*"
- Do not use in pregnancy or when nursing. (Hawaiians traditionally considered 'awa to cause miscarriage. Although it is used in pregnancy in other parts of Polynesia, I would still discourage its use in pregnancy.)
- 'Awa is known to cause a reversible scaly skin disorder among chronic users called "kani kani" in Fiji or "ichthyosiform eruption" in medicalese. It is thought to be due to interference in cholesterol metabolism. In order to acquire this condition, one would have to ingest a lot of kava for many months. I have never seen this condition, even in Hawai'i where there are numerous kava bars.
- Most side effects involve gastrointestinal discomfort or skin allergies. Some varieties of kava will cause stomach discomfort after only two or three servings. Even with some experimenting I've found no way to counteract this, although mixing with coconut water and eating ginger can sometimes help. Varieties to be avoided include "Tudei" (so named because one can feel its effects for two days) and *P. wichmannii.* Because kavain turns to dihydrokavain with age, fresh 'Awa may be less disturbing to the digestion than dried.
- Continued chewing of the root is reported to damage tooth enamel.
- Not with endogenous depression.
- Do not use in Parkinson's disease. There have been case reports of possible dopamine antagonism from kava extracts. Until more information becomes available, Parkinson's patients should avoid using kava [Schelosky 1995].
- In one Australian study, kava users were more likely to complain of poor health. Users showed increased HDL cholesterol and red cell volume, decreased platelet volume and lymphocyte count, and a higher incidence of hematuria than non-users. Very heavy users were 20% underweight [Mathews 1988].
- Do not use large doses while driving, skydiving, performing neurosurgery, competing in a chainsaw toss, or with any piece of equipment more difficult to operate than a spoon. I've met Polynesians who have told me of "driving home by Braille" (using the highway bumps to keep them in their lanes) after a long night of ingesting too much kava.

PREPARATION OF MEDICINE: Decocted, pounded, chewed, cold infused.

- Tincture fresh 1:2, dried 1:3-5, 60% alcohol. Commercial hot alcohol extractions are very potent.
- Among Polynesians 'awa is often cold infused (i.e. soaked at room temperature) in a large collective drinking bowl with each participant dipping their cup into the bowl. Properly prepared 'awa looks (and tastes) like dishwater. Sometimes it is mixed with coconut milk or lecithin to emulsify it prior to drinking. Lipid soluble extractions of kava have a greater range of effects in mice than water-soluble extractions [Jamieson 1989]. This would seem to validate the Hawaiian tradition of mixing 'awa with coconut milk.
- A traditional Hawaiian method of preparing 'awa involved chewing the rhizome and spitting the resultant sludge into the collective bowl before mixing it with water. (Yum!)
- 'Awa was traditionally strained through *Cyperus laevigata* ('ahu'awa / makaloa), an endemic sedge.
- Traditionally drunk before dinner, so that food will not impede the effects.

DOSAGE:

- If standardized: 50-70 mg kava lactones three times per day for anxiety, or 150-210 mg kava lactones before bed for mild insomnia. Kavalactones to 300mg daily.
- Dried root internal to 4 g. daily.
- Cold infusion 1-4 coconut cups, as desired.

Decocted to 10 grams in combination

MERIDIAN AFFINITIES: Heart, liver, kidney~.

WESTERN FUNCTIONS REPORTED: **Anaesthetic**; **analgesic**; **anodyne**; **anticonvulsant**; **antifungal** (not with *Candida* spp.); **antiseptic**; **antispasmodic**; **anxiolytic**; **aphrodisiac**; **blennostatic**; **circulatory**

stimulant; **diaphoretic**; **diuretic**; **expectorant**; **intoxicant**; **local anesthetic**; **myorelaxant**; **narcotic**; **pacifier**; **reduces sex drive**; **rubefacient** (topically); **sedative**; **sialagogue**; **soporific**; **stimulant**; **stomachic**; **sudorific**; **tonic**; **urinary-antiseptic**.

TRADITIONAL CHINESE ENERGETIC FUNCTIONS (~ = extrapolated):

1) Calms the sprit~.
2) Expels wind dampness~.
3) Regulates qi and stops pain~.
4) Clears damp stagnation in the lower burner~.

OTHER ENERGETIC FUNCTIONS: Increases pitta, decreases vata and kapha.

'Awa (Kava)
Common Medicinal Uses

- **Muscle spasm**
- **Stress**
- **Insomnia**
- **Pain**
- **Urinary dysfunction**

'Awa (Kava) Cross-Cultural Medicinal Uses

BITES & STINGS

- **Fish stings, insect and centipede bites** [Tonga (yellow leaves)].

DERMATOLOGICAL

- **Fungal skin diseases**.
- **Skin conditions**.

DIGESTIVE

- **Low appetite** [Eclectic].
- **Diarrhea** [Germany].
- **Digestive pain** [Eclectic].
- **Duodenal ulcers, with navel pain** [Michael Moore].
- **Hemorrhoids** [Eclectic].

HEAD AND THROAT

- **Canker sores**; **tooth pain** (not from a cavity) [Eclectic]; **sore throat** [Fiji].
- **Headache, severe and migraine headache** [Hawai'i, Polynesia (poulticed)]; **nerve pain of the branches of the 5th cranial nerve** [Eclectic].
- **Neuralgia of middle ear** [Michael Moore].

INFECTION

- **To induce sleep during fever** [Hawai'i (root cold infused)].

LYMPHATIC

- **Elephantiasis** [Samoa].

MUSCULOSKELETAL / TRAUMA

- Unlike so called "muscle relaxants," 'awa actually does directly relax the muscle rather than blocking neurotransmitters. I've found 'awa more effective than many Chinese or Western herbs for **back and neck pain with attendant spasm**.
- **Back pain** [Samoa]; **rheumatism** [Eclectic, Germany, Polynesia]; **pain**, **sore muscles** [Hawai'i (root cold infused)].
- **Wounds** [Polynesia (leaf juice topical), Samoa].
- **Gout** [Germany].
- **Leaves were used as a "band aid"** [Polynesia].

NEUROLOGICAL

- In 1950 'awa was listed in the US Dispensary as a treatment for **nervous disorders** under the name Neurocardin.

PARASITES

- **Worms** [Polynesia].

PEDIATRIC

- **Children who were weak and recovering from illnesses** [Polynesia].
- **For child's fever or agitation** [Hawai'i (flower buds chewed and given to children).
- **Thick white tongue coat in children** [Hawai'i (ashes rubbed on the stomach].
- **Used in weaning rituals** [Hawai'i].
- **Digestive problems in children** [Hawai'i (ashes rubbed on the stomach].

PSYCHOSPIRITUAL

"*Low [and] accessible is the day whereby knowledge is gained, knowledge from the source, knowledge by hearing, like the flourishing 'awa plant is the knowledge of the gods, hear me.*"

- - Hawaiian chant offering pig and 'awa to Laka, the goddess of hula

"*E hānai 'awa a ikaika ka makani*"
Carry 'awa to strengthen the wind (one's spirit)
- - Hawaiian proverb

- Kahuna would sometimes use 'awa bubbles as a divination tool to diagnose illness, predict the future, or determine the gender of an unborn child. This was one way that a Kahuna could gain access to hidden knowledge ("Huna"), particularly through contact with the ancestors or the gods. In old Hawai'i, 'awa was a common choice for making offerings to the gods. Laka, in particular, (the hula goddess and sister of Pele) was fond of 'awa.
- A Samoan legend tells of the Sun god and his wife Ui, who had a stillborn child named Tangaloa Ui. The fetus was raised by a hermit crab and when Tangaloa grew up he taught humans the 'awa ceremony.
- 'Awa constituents are said to produce brain wave patterns similar to anti-anxiety medications without the attendant dependence or tolerance.
- **Phobias**.
- **Chest pain from nervous indigestion** [Eclectic].
- **Insomnia** [Hawai'i (root cold infused)], **sleep disorders**.
- **Stress and nervous anxiety** [Germany].
- **Used to help focus during meditation**; **dream enhancement** [USA].

REPRODUCTIVE

"*It does not occasion priapism, but, on the contrary, antagonizes it.*"
-- King's Dispensatory, 1898

"[It] *is also held to be a certain cure for venereal infection. I have known many white men who go through a course of this powerful medicine.*"
-- P. Corney, 1818

- Used in Europe in the late 1800s as a remedy for **gonorrhea**, and in the U.*S.* as late as 1950 in a medication called Gonosan.
- In combination for "**weaknesses arising from virginity**" or for "**displaced uterus**" [Hawai'i].

- **Contraceptive** [Polynesia (leaves chewed or inserted into the vagina)].
- **Gonorrhea** [Eclectic, 19th century Germany, India, New Guinea, Samoa], **syphilis-like sores** [Samoa].
- **Painful menses** [Eclectic, Hawai'i (root)], **womb displacement** [Hawai'i], **uterine problems** [New Guinea].
- **Inflamed vagina**, **vaginal discharge** [Eclectic, India].
- **Prostate infections**.
- **Lactation problems**.

> **Probably the second-most unfairly maligned herb on the planet, 'awa adds a powerful tool to any pharmacy for anxiety, muscle spasm, fatigue, or mild insomnia.**

RESPIRATORY

- **Lung troubles** [Hawai'i].
- **Asthma** [Hawai'i, Polynesia]. Native Hawaiians have a higher mortality from asthma than any other ethnic group in Hawai'i [Hope 1993]. King Kamehameha IV (Alexander Liholiho) died from an asthma attack.
- **Bronchitis** [Germany, New Caledonia]; **chronic bronchitis** [Eclectic]; **cough** [Fiji, Samoa].
- **Common cold** [Fiji Hawai'i (with chills)]; **diaphoretic - to induce sweating during colds or fevers** [Polynesia].
- **Tuberculosis** [Samoa].

URINARY

"*The patient is pale, the urinary product inconstant in quality; the tissues, especially of feet and legs, are edematous; patient is indisposed to exertion, and has the general appearance of one with Bright's disease, yet there is no albumen nor evidence of any particular disease. Such symptoms clear up quickly under this remedy, and the appetite is quickly restored.*"
-- The Eclectic Materia Medica
by Harvey Wickes Felter, M.D., 1922

- 'Awa was a favorite of the Eclectic physicians, particularly for **conditions of the urinary tract**.
- **Urogenital problems** [19th century Germany, Oceania]; **bladder inflammation** [Eclectic, Germany]; **urethral discharge** [Eclectic].
- **Painful urination** [Eclectic (with pus); Michael Moore (from sexual activity)]; **kidney pain** [Germany].
- **Edema** [Eclectic (from kidney disease), Germany].
- **Kidney problem**s [Fiji, Samoa].
- **Bedwetting from weakness** [Eclectic]; **nocturnal incontinence** [India].

OTHER MEDICINAL USES

- Some cultures would reserve the use of 'Awa for those who were healthy rather than those who were sick. Hawaiians would drink it the evening **before a day of anticipated physical labor**.
- **General weakness**, **fatigue** [Polynesia], **debility** [Hawai'i].

- **Inflammation** [New Guinea].
- **Chills** [Hawai'i].
- **Hansen's disease** (leprosy).

AS AN INTOXICANT:

"*In sufficient quantities it is mildly paralyzing and creates a euphoric but clear-minded state in which the drinker cannot be annoyed.*"
- - Dr. W. Arthur Whistler

"*... in large doses it produces an intoxication, which, unlike that from alcohol, is of a reserved, drowsy character, and attended with confused dreams.*"
- - King's Dispensatory, 1898

Used throughout Polynesia as an intoxicant. From the outside looking in, Captain James Cook reported that the symptoms of 'awa intoxication looked to him to be similar to opium intoxication.

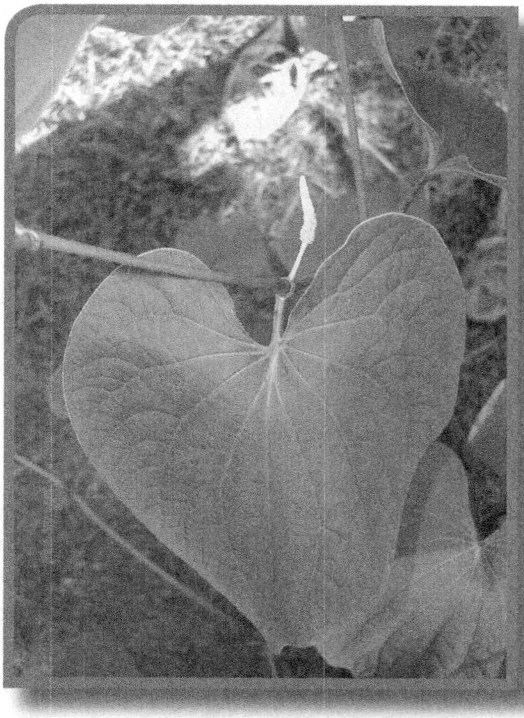

Piper methysticum: 'Awa leaves

OTHER USES:
- Used during tattooing for pain [Fiji (root internal and topical)].
- In Fiji, an anti-smoking campaign was successful with one of the strategies being a kava ceremony declaring tobacco taboo.
- 'Awa was traditionally used socially, to resolve differences, to welcome guests and dignitaries, during life changes, during important meetings and in burial ceremonies,

CONSTITUENTS:
- Kava lactones (pyrones): Demethoxyyangonin, dihydrokavain, dihydromethysticin, kavain (the numbing of the mouth is caused by kavain), methysticin, yangonin.
- Different varieties of 'awa have different mixtures of kava lactones. Varieties with a high percentage of kavain are preferred, while those with high proportions of dihydrokavain and dihydromethysticin are avoided due to their tendency to make one feel nauseous. All parts of *Piper methysticum* contain the active kava-lactones, but the root tips are the safest to use and contain the highest concentration.
- Kava lactones are similar in structure to myristicin, an ingredient found in nutmeg.

POSSIBLE DRUG INTERACTIONS:
- There are numerous (probably accurate) reports of kava potentiation of benzodiazepines and barbiturates, but I could not verify the original sources.
- Naloxone is ineffective for reversing the effects of kava [Jamieson 1990(a)].
- Err on the side of safety: Do not use with anti-Parkinson's medications, sedatives, anti-psychotics, antidepressants, hypnotics, or alcohol (unless in a tincture, and then not in large amounts).

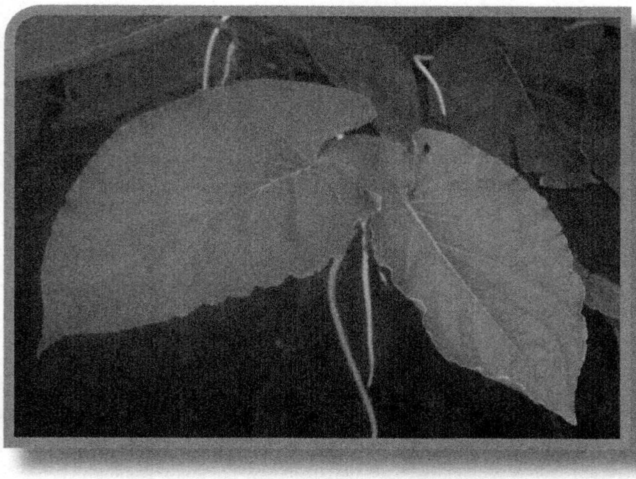

Photograph by Stacy Domer

False Kava: *Piper auritum*.

Note that the leaf veins emerge from the mid-rib and not from the attachment of the stem.

'Awa (Kava) Local Combinations

Bladder infections: Add *Bidens pilosa* (spanish needle).

Back pain and spasm: Add *Desmodium* spp. (pua pilipili), *Siegesbeckia orientalis* (xi xian cao).

Menstrual cramps: Add *Cyperus rotundus* (nutgrass rhizome), *Mimosa pudica* (hilahila).
Anxiety: Add *Pipturus albidus* (māmaki).

'Awa (Kava) Cross-Cultural Combinations

Please note some of the ingredients in the following combinations are toxic! Do not self-administer without the supervision of a licensed practitioner or an experienced Elder.

Asthma: With *Curcuma longa* (Turmeric) [Old Hawai'i].
Lung problems: With *Portulaca oleracea* ('purslane), *Morinda citrifolia* (noni), and *Syzygium malaccense* (mountain apple) buds and bark [Old Hawai'i].
Common cold with chills and fever: With *Syzygium malaccense* ('ōhia 'ai / mountain apple), *Bidens* spp. (ko'oko'olau), *Aleurites moluccana* (kukui), and *Saccharum officinarum* (kō / sugar cane) [Old Hawai'i].
After a day of hard labor: With coconut milk [Old Hawai'i].
Difficult urination: With *Curcuma longa* ('ōlena / Turmeric) [Old Hawai'i].
Bladder infections: With *Thespesia populnea* (milo), *Morinda citrifolia* (noni) [Cook Islands].
Irritable bladder: With pumpkin seed.
Inflammation: Leaves used with grated *Zingiber officinale* (ginger) [Tonga].
Bladder disorders: With *Althaea officinalis* (marshmallow) root, *Apium*, *Agropyron desertorum* (wheat grass).
Rheumatoid arthritis: With *Menyanthes*, *Cimcifuga*, *Apium*.

RANGE: Pan-tropical. Indigenous to the Pacific Islands: Melanesia, Micronesia, and Polynesia.

GATHERING:
- Along riverbeds, found in some of the more remote valleys in Hawai'i. Often a remnant of old settlements. Take only what you need. Keep the location a secret, 'lest the whole plant grow legs and crawl away. Or, better yet, grow your own.
- Be aware that there is an 'awa "imposter" about known as *Piper auritum* that smells like root beer due to its high saffrole content. On a true kava (*Piper methysticum*) leaf, the veins all emerge from the stem attachment ("palmate venation"), while on a *Piper auritum* leaf some of them emerge from the spine of the leaf ("pinnate venation").

PROPAGATION & CULTIVATION:
- Propagate by nodes. Sometimes just sticking a stem along a riverbed will work. Coffee grinds make 'awa plants particularly happy once they have gotten above 16" tall. If you're patient enough, you can harvest after 6 years.
- Technically called a "cultigen," 'awa does not produce seeds. Humans first usurped its reproductive function as long as 3000 years ago, probably in Vanuatu. Its wild ancestor is known as *Piper wichmannii*. The female plants are known only in Vanuatu, where residents currently differentiate more than 247 different types of kava.
- Kava from Vanuatu is reported to be the most potent.
- **For more information** on growing 'awa see "Super Simple Guide to Creating Hawaiian Gardens" by Barbara Fahs. http://www.hiiakas.com.

RESEARCH:
- In double blind clinical trials kava has been shown to reduce anxiety [Kinzler 1991, Volz 1997], with the effects more pronounced after eight weeks of use [Volz 1997]. The mechanism is unclear. It may be through the modulation of serotonin-1A receptors [Walden 1997], although one study did not find kava constituents altering dopamine or seratonin levels in rats [Boonen 1998(b)]. In any event, a meta-analysis of double blind, randomized, placebo-controlled studies has verified that kava outperforms placebo for symptomatic treatment of anxiety [Pittler 2000]. It does not induce tolerance in mice [Duffield 1991].
- In animals, kava works as a hypnotic through mechanisms unrelated to benzodiazepines or tricyclic thymoleptics [Holm 1991]. One study reports that its effects may be unrelated to any actions on GABA or benzodiazepine binding sites [Davies 1992], but others report GABA activity [Jussofie 1994, Boonen 1998(a)].
- Methysticin reduces seizure activity in rats [Schmitz 1995], and muscle contractions (and presumably spasms) in frogs [Singh 1983]. There is evidence that 'awa reduces current though voltage-activated sodium (Na+) and calcium (Ca2+) channels [Schirrmacher 1999]. It reduces amphetamine-induced excessive movement in rats, but much less than haloperidol or chlorpromazine [Duffield 1989].
- As an analgesic it works through non-opiate pathways [Jamieson 1990(a)].
- The extract prevents ischemic brain damage in mice [Backhau 1992] and in rats [Gleitz 1996].

- Kava lactones may inhibit MAO-B in human platelets [Uebelhack 1998]. Kavain reduces human platelet aggregation through suppression of arachadonic acid and inhibition of cyclooxygenase (COX) [Gleitz 1997].
- The extract is mildly anti-fungal [Locher 1995].
- One study showed an inverse correlation between kava consumption and cancer in Pacific Island Nations [Steiner 2000].
- In a small double-blind placebo-controlled study menopause symptoms were alleviated by kava extract [Warnecke 1991].
- Interestingly enough, in spite of my caveats (See *CAUTIONS AND CONTRAINDICATIONS*), clinical trials indicate that *Piper methysticum* does not impair the ability to concentrate or reaction time. In one double blind clinical trial kava was shown to improve cognition [Munte 1993]. At therapeutic doses it may actually improve performance [Heinze 1994]. In another study, people taking kava with alcohol had better cognitive function than those taking alcohol alone, [Herberg 1993], although a study in mice showed alcohol potentiated kava and increased its toxicity [Jamieson 1990(b)].

NOTES 'N QUOTES

"*For a white man to ignore the etiquette followed at kava parties would be considered the height of ill-breeding.*"
- - Anthony Andoh

"*... a disgusting drink is prepared by the natives, and even by the whites, of these islands.*"
- - King's Dispensatory, 1898

- In 1616, the Dutch explorers Jacob Le Maire and Willem Schouten arrived at Wallis-Futuna and probably were the first Europeans to encounter kava.
- While there is some controversy regarding the historical existence of a Hawaiian 'awa ceremony, other Polynesian cultures have used 'awa ceremonies for centuries. These ceremonies are important as a means to welcome guests and to create social bonding in Polynesian societies.

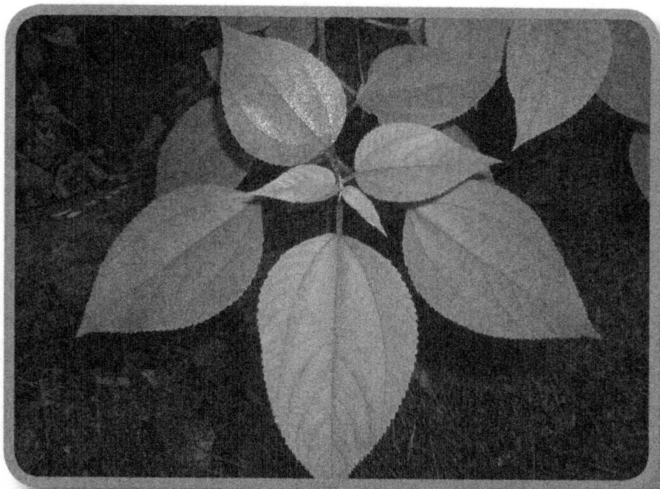

Pipturus spp. (Māmaki)

PLANT NAME: *Pipturus* spp.

Status: Endemic.

Habitat: Likes it wet.

SIMILARLY USED SPECIES: *P. albidus, P. forbesii, P. kauaiensis, P. ruber.*

COMMON NAMES: **Māmaki, māmake**, waimea [Hawai'i]; ro'a [Tahiti].

NOMENCLATURE: The name *Pipturus* means "tail that drops."

FAMILY: Urticaceae (nettles family).

CATEGORY: Regulate qi~.

PROPERTIES: Sweet cool ~.

PLANT PART USED: Usually leaves, sometimes fruit.

TOXICITY: None noted.

CAUTIONS AND CONTRAINDICATIONS: Ironically, in some people, māmaki can cause mild agitation or insomnia.

PREPARATION OF MEDICINE: Infused.

DOSAGE: 30 – 60 grams (1 – 2 oz) as a single herb. Up to 20 grams in combination.

STATUS IN HAWAI'I: Endemic. Māmaki is an endemic plant appropriate for use because it is not rare or endangered.

WESTERN FUNCTIONS REPORTED: **Laxative** [Hawai'i (fruit)].

Māmaki Common Medicinal Uses

- **Insomnia, irritability**
- **Tissue cleansing**
- **Syndrome X (diabetes / hypertension / obesity)**

TRADITIONAL CHINESE ENERGETIC FUNCTIONS (~ = extrapolated):

1) Regulates liver qi ~.
2) Harmonizes the middle burner~.
3) Clears damp heat in the lower burner ~.

Māmaki Cross-Cultural Medicinal Uses

CARDIOVASCULAR

- **High blood pressure** [Hawai'i (leaves infused)].
- **High cholesterol** [Hawai'i (leaves infused)].

DIGESTIVE

- **Constipation** [Hawai'i (fruit)].
- **Stomach, colon, and digestive problems** [Hawai'i (leaves infused)].

HEPATIC

- **Liver problems** [Hawai'i (leaves infused)].

PEDIATRIC

- **Colic in children** [Hawai'i (leaves infused)].
- **Thrush** [Hawai'i (fruit)].

PSYCHOSPIRITUAL

- In Hawai'i, māmaki was used in **love potions**. Today it is sometimes given as part of a **wedding gift**.
- **Depression** [Hawai'i (leaves infused)].
- **Insomnia** [Hawai'i (leaves infused)].
- **Irritability** [Hawai'i (leaves infused)].

REPRODUCTIVE

- **PMS** [Hawai'i (leaves infused)].
- **Used to relax the muscles for childbirth** [Hawai'i].

URINARY

- **Bladder problems** [Hawai'i (leaves infused)], **bladder infections**.

OTHER MEDICINAL USES

- **Syndrome X (diabetes / hypertension / obesity)** [Hawai'i (leaves infused)].
- **Fatigue, debility of the body** [Hawai'i (leaves)].
- **For cleansing the body and as a "blood cleanser" or "spring tonic"** [Hawai'i (leaves infused)].

USE AS FOOD: The leaves are reportedly edible, but they seem a bit fibrous. The fruits are tasty, but are used as a laxative.

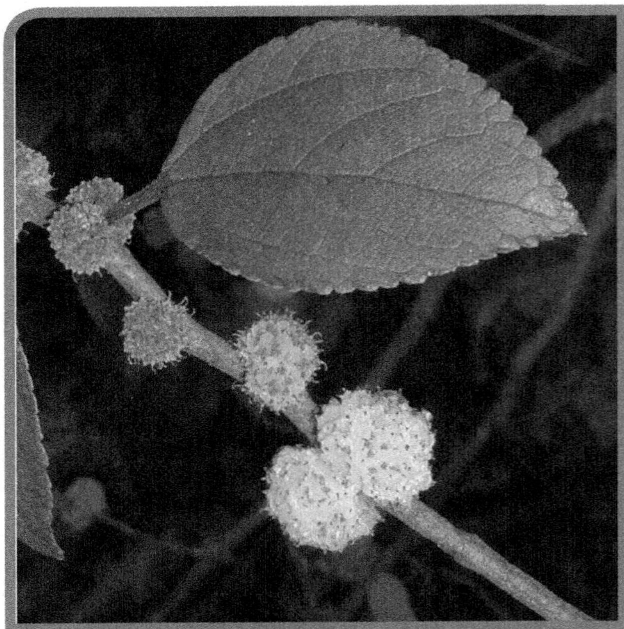

Pipturus spp. (Māmaki fruiting bodies)

OTHER USES:

- Bait for cowries [Hawai'i (branches)].
- Nets and ropes [Tahiti]. Fishing lines on the Marshall Islands were made from different *Pipturus* species.
- In old Hawai'i māmaki was used to make kapa (fiber cloth). In a well-known Hawaiian collection, it is estimated that more than one third of the kapa samples are made from *Pipturus* spp. The kapa produced was brown and was sometimes oiled with *Aleurites moluccana* (kukui) oil.

Māmaki Local Combinations

Anger: Add *Cyperus rotundus* (xiang fu / nutgrass rhizome), *Mimosa pudica* (hilahila).
Irritability: Add *Oxalis* spp. ('ihi / sorrel), *Verbena littoralis* (vervain), *Passiflora edulis* (liliko'i / passion fruit).
"Tissue cleansing": Add *Phymatosorus scolopendria* (laua'e fern), *Oxalis* spp. ('ihi / sorrel).

Māmaki Cross-Cultural Combinations

Constipation: With *Hernandia* spp. (pua) inner bark, *Wedelia* spp. (ateate) [Samoa].
Dysentery: Root decocted with *Pandanus tectorius* (hala) root [Samoa].
Abdominal pain: With *Hernandia* spp. (pua), *Artocarpus communis* ('ulu), *Cocos nucifera* (niu) leaf stalks, all with "over-ripe" coconut water [Samoa].
Fatigue: With *Ipomoea* spp. (sweet potatoes) and *Broussaisia arguta* (kanawao) leaves and fruit.

RANGE: Polynesia.

HABITAT: Likes it wet. Often occurs as part of the under-story in native or mixed forest, particularly along streambeds.

GATHERING: Going makai (down stream), pick younger leaves and watch for hō'ailona (signs) such as leaves that naka (quiver).

PROPAGATION & CULTIVATION: By seed.

RESEARCH:
In vitro, the extract is anti-viral in vitro against *Herpes simplex* 1 & 2; anti-bacterial against *Streptococcus pyogenes* & *Staphylococcus aureus*, and anti-fungal [Locher 1995].

NOTES 'N QUOTES
- Two endemic butterflies, the Kamehameha butterfly and the Blackburn butterfly feed on māmaki.
- There are four species of māmaki in Hawai'i, although all are very similar, both in appearance and in medicinal use. What is sometimes referred to as "green māmaki" is not māmaki at all but 'ākōlea (*Boehmeria grandis*), whose medicinal uses are different than that of māmaki.
- A remarkable friend, māmaki has a soothing effect on the nervous system in a similar way to jasmine tea. It works well for irritability or just to decompress after a day in Babylon.

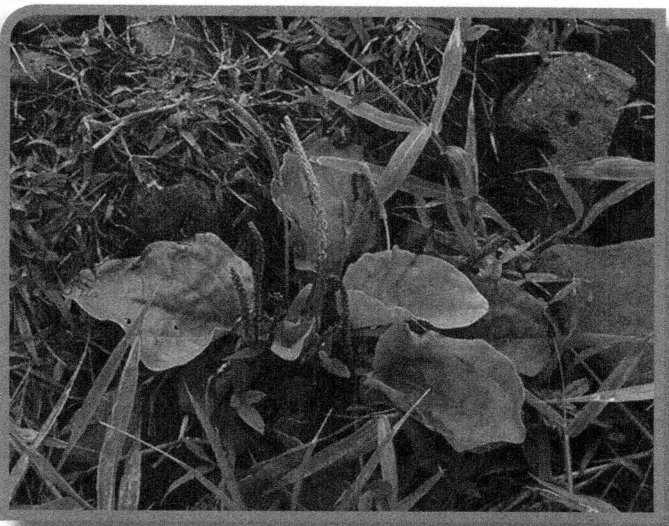

Plantago major: Laukahi
Photograph by Marco Biancardi

Plantago spp. (Laukahi / Plantain)

PLANT NAME: *Plantago* spp.

SIMILARLY USED SPECIES: *P. amplexicaulis; P. arenaria; P. asiatica; P. ciliata; P. cordata; P. coronopus; P. cynops; P. depressa; P. erosa; P. griesebachii; P. insularis; P. ispaghula; P. ispagula; P. lagopus; P. lanceolata; P. macrostachys; P. major; P. media; P. mexicana; P. minor; P. ovata; P. psyllium; P. rocae; P. rugelii; P. sericea; P. tomentosa; P. ureades* (whew!).

Status:
3 of our 7 species are endemic.

Habitat:
Where ever you walk. Likes disturbed areas.

COMMON NAMES: **Laukahi**, kuhekili [Hawai'i]; **che qian zi**, **che qian cao** ("beside-the-cart-grass") [China]; **plantain**, white man's foot [US]; breitwegerich [German]; curl doddy (*P. lanceolata*), healing blade (*P. major*) [Scotland]; llantén [Spanish]; millet [Martinique]; sat isabgol (*P.* ovata) [India]; slan lus (healing plant) [Gaelic]; tanchagem [Portuguese]; tha ram [Tibet]; waybread [Anglo-Saxon].

NOMENCLATURE:
- The name "*Plantago*" means "sole of the foot." "Laukahi" can be translated as "first cut" or "first leaf," a reference to its topical uses.
- *Plantago lanceolata* was once called "costa canina"or "quinquenervia" a reference to the long lateral veins on the leaves. Today it is still referred to as ribwort plantain.
- The Chinese name "che qian cao," meaning, "be-

side-the-cart-grass," is a reference to plantain's habit of growing in disturbed and well-traveled areas.

- Plantain was once referred to as "kemps," named after the Anglo-Saxon word "cempa" which meant "soldier." This was a reference to a children's' game which was played by banging plantain stalks against each other.
- In the Ireland the Gaelic name for *Plantago* spp. is "slan-lus," or the "healing plant."

FAMILY: Plantaginaceae.

CATEGORY: Drain damp.

PROPERTIES: Sweet, cold [China], bitter cool [India].

PLANT PART USED: The whole plant. The seeds are used more as a diuretic and the leaves more for respiratory infections, as a demulcent, and for liver problems.

TOXICITY: None noted.

CAUTIONS AND CONTRAINDICATIONS: Not in pregnancy.
The pollen may trigger allergies.
Psyllium seed powder can trigger asthma attacks if inhaled.

ENERGETIC CAUTIONS: Caution in severe Qi deficiency.

PREPARATION OF MEDICINE:

- I much prefer to use this fresh, unless the dried seeds are called for in a bladder infection. The seeds should be put in a muslin bag before decocting.
- If the plant is to be dried for later use, it should be dried as quickly as possible to avoid leaf discoloration. Some of my Hawaiian teachers will freeze fresh herbs rather than drying them, for future use.
- Laukahi can be prepared as an ointment for hemorrhoids and skin ulcers.
- Topical for infections, the fresh plant is better than an infusion or decoction as heat may kill some of the antibacterial properties.

DOSAGE: Seeds to 15 grams. Whole plant used alone up to 30 grams.

STATUS IN HAWAI'I: Worldwide there are 265 species of *Plantago*. In Hawai'i, three of our seven local species are endemic. However, the native ones are rare. It's more than likely that the ones on your lawn are alien.

WESTERN FUNCTIONS REPORTED: **Analgesic**; **anodyne**; **antibacterial**; **antidiarrheal**; **antidote**; **antiemetic**; **anti-inflammatory**; **anti-microbial**; **antioxidant**; **antiphlogistic**; **antirheumatic**; **antiseptic**; **antitussive**; **aperitif**; **aperitif**; **aphrodisiac**; **astringent**; **bactericide**; **bacteriostatic**; **blood**; **burn dressing**; **cold remedy**; **decongestant**; **demulcent**; **deobstruent**; **depurative**; **dermatological aid**; **diaphoretic**; **disinfectant**; **diuretic**; **ear medicine**; **emollient**; **expectorant**; **eye medicine**; **febrifuge**; **gast-intestinal aid**; **gynecological aid**; **heals wounds**; **heart medicine**; **hemostatic**; **immunostimulatory**; **kidney aid**; **laxative**; **mild expectorant**; **ophthalmic**; **orthopedic aid**; **pain-relieving**; **pediatric aid**; **poultice**; **protisticide**; **psychological aid**; **pulmonary aid**; **purgative**; **refrigerant**; **sedative**; **snake bite remedy**; **spasmolytic**; **stimulant**; **stops bleeding** (topically); **strengthener**; **styptic**; **suppurative**; **throat aid**; **tonic**; **urinary aid**; **uterine tonic**; **vermifuge**; **vulnerary**.

TRADITIONAL CHINESE ENERGETIC FUNCTIONS (~ = extrapolated):

1) Clears heat and relieves toxicity.
2) Drains dampness.
3) Clears the eyes.
4) Stops cough & removes phlegm.

OTHER ENERGETIC FUNCTIONS: Benefits vata.

Laukahi (Plantain) Common Medicinal Uses

- **Urinary infections (seeds)**
- **Topical for wounds, bites, stings (aerial parts)**
- **Bronchial infections (aerial parts)**
- **Hepatitis, jaundice (aerial parts)**

Laukahi (Plantain) Cross-Cultural Medicinal Uses

COSMETIC

- Laukahi has been used as **a rinse for dandruff**, and as hair-set. (Haoles take note: *Plantago* spp. can turn blond hair green!)
- Used in night cream for **wrinkles**.
- **To promote healing of wounds without scarring** [Paiute].
- **Eye shadow** [Dominican Republic, Trinidad].

CARDIOVASCULAR

"*It is good to stay spitting of blood and other bleedings at the mouth, or the making of foul and bloody water, by reason of any ulcers in the reins or bladder, and also stays the too free bleeding of wounds.*"

-- Nicholas Culpepper

- **Difficult breathing from chest pain** [Iroquois (in combination)].
- **"Blood medicine"** [Western herbalism].
- **Bleeding** (topical) [Eclectic].
- **Hypertension**.
- **High cholesterol**.

DERMATOLOGICAL

"*The same also with the juice of Houseleek is profitable against any inflammations and breakings out of the skin, and against burnings and scaldings by fire and water.*"

-- Nicholas Culpepper

- **Bee stings, cuts, blisters, bruises, skin ulcers, boils and open sores** [Appalachia, Cherokee, Eclectic, Hawai'i, Iroquois, Kwakiutl, Mohegan, Nitinaht, Shuswap, Thompson, Yurok].
- **To draw out inflammation from "sore spots"** [Chippewa, Shinnecock]; **malignant or varicose ulcers**.
- **Eczema**; **erysipelas** [Eclectic]; **impetigo**; **poison ivy**; **itching**; **warts**; **sunburn**; **nail disease**, **finger lesions.**
- **Skin disorders resulting from "depraved blood"**.
- **Leaf rubbed on the body to produce sweating** [Shuswap].

DIGESTIVE

"*... prevails wonderfully against all torments or excoriations in the intestines or bowels...*"

-- Nicholas Culpepper

"*... for cankers and sores in the mouth or privy parts of man or woman; and helps also the pains of the piles in the fundament.*"

-- Nicholas Culpepper

- **Vomiting** [England (seeds powdered)].
- **Digestive problems**, **stomach trouble**, **bowel complaints** [Cherokee, Iroquois; Isleta, Meskwaki, Shoshoni].
- **Diarrhea** [China (seeds), Eclectic, Iraq, Japan, Turkey]; **constipation** [Costanoan].
- **Stomach pain**, **gastritis**, **gastric ulcers** [Eclectic, Europe, Martinique, Mexico, Nitinaht, Russia, US].
- **Enteritis**, **chronic colitis** [Russia]; **dysentery** [China, Eclectic, Europe, Cherokee, Iroquois]; **dysentery associated with "cold" diseases** [Tibet]; **irritable bowel syndrome.**
- **Hemorrhoids** [Eclectic, Thompson].

ENDOCRINE

- **Blood sugar control**; **diabetes** [Hawai'i, Java].

HEAD AND THROAT

"*The clarified juice, or distilled water, dropped into the eyes, cools the inflammations in them, and takes away the pain and web; and dropped into the ears, eases the pains in them, and heals and removes the heat.*"

-- Nicholas Culpepper

- **Headache** [Cherokee]; **trigeminal neuralgia** [Eclectic].
- A distilled water made from *Plantago* spp. is said to be used as an **eye wash. Eyelid inflammation** [Haiti]; **conjunctivitis**, **blepharitis**, **ophthalmia**, **cataracts** [China (seeds internal and as a wash)]; topical for **dry or sore eyes** [Cherokee (juice), China (seeds), Shinnecock]; **red swollen eyes**, **sensitive to light** [China (seeds internal), Cherokee, Shinnecock, Trinidad, Carribean]; **inflammation of the retina**; **eye tumor**.
- **Ear ache** [Eclectic, Kawaiisu (infusion topical)]; **congested sinuses affecting middle ear.**
- **Throat problems**; **sore throat**; **laryngitis & hoarseness** (as a gargle); **voice loss**; **toothache from dental cavities** [Eclectic]; **cancer of the mouth** [Canary Islands, Germany]; **to lubricate the throat to remove a lodged bone** [Potawatomi]; used in Ghana **to clean the teeth**.

HEPATIC

"*The herb (but especially the seed) is held to be profitable against the dropsy, the falling-sickness, the yellow jaundice, and stoppings of the liver and reins.*"

-- Nicholas Culpepper

- **Jaundice**, **liver dysfunction**, **hepatitis** [China, Bolivia, England (seeds powdered), USA]; **obstruction of the liver** [England (seeds powdered)].

IMMUNITY

- **Lowered immunity**.

INFECTION

- **Fever** [Cheyenne, Costanoan, Rappahannock]; **intermittent fever.**
- **Infections and boils**, **abscesses** [Iroquois, Nitinaht, Okanagan-Colville, Shoshoni]; **to draw out pus from infections**, **topical for blisters** [Hesquiat, Kwakiutl].
- **"Lightning infection."** [Navajo, Ramah].

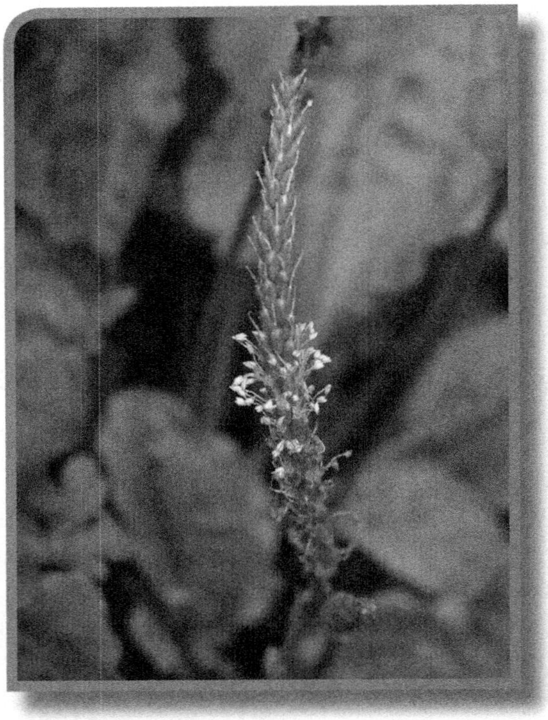

Plantago major: Laukahi flowers

LYMPHATIC

- **Glandular disease**, **scrophula** [Eclectic].

MUSCULOSKELETAL / TRAUMA

"*... is profitably applied to all hot gouts in the feet or hands, especially in the beginning. It is also good to be applied where any bone is out of joint, to hinder inflammations, swellings, and pains that presently rise thereupon.*"

-- Nicholas Culpepper

- **Wounds**, **bruises**, **sprains and contusions** [Algonquin, Delaware, Eclectic, Ireland, Mexico, Ojibwa, Ontario, Shoshoni, Tete-de-Boule, UK, USA]; **battle bruises** [Shoshoni]; **broken bones**; **swelling and inflammations** [Meskwaki, Potawatomi].
- **Rheumatism** [Abnaki, Chippewa, Shoshoni]; **orthopedic ailments**. In China, a *Plantago* spp. seed extract is injected into joint spaces for **hypermobility**. This is even done to the temporomandibular joint.
- **Burns** [Algonquin, Cherokee, Meskwaki, Mexico, Ojibwa, Tete-de-Boule]; **snakebite** [Cherokee, Mohegan, Ojibwa]; **the "bites of mad dogs"** [Europe].
- As a "drawing poultice" **to remove thorns and splinters** [Mahuna, Ponca].

NEUROLOGICAL

- **Convulsions**, **epilepsy** [England (seeds powdered)].

ONCOLOGY

- **Cancer** [Algeria, Ecuador, Iran, Native American, Panama, Poland, Wales].
- **Cancer of the uterus** [Europe].
- **Tumor of the foot** (neuroma?).

PARASITES

"*The powder of the dried leaves taken in drink, kills worms of the belly; and boiled in wine, kills worms that breed in old and foul ulcers.*"

-- Nicholas Culpepper

- **Amoebas** [Iraq].
- **Malaria** [Africa].

PEDIATRIC

"*In the nocturnal incontinence of urine, in young children, accompanied with a large flow of colorless urine, this agent has produced curative results in many cases.*"

-- Ellingwood

- **Bedwetting in children** [Eclectic]; **incontinence in children.**
- **Infantile jaundice** [Bolivia].
- **Cholera infantum** ("summer complaint")[Eclectic]; infusion given **to check babies' bowels** [Cherokee].
- **Uncomplicated indigestion in children** [China (powdered seeds)]; **colic** [Eclectic].
- **Used to strengthen a child learning to walk** [Cherokee (in combination)].
- **Pertussis**.
- **Adrenal tumors in childhood**.
- **Thrush** [Eclectic]. Sometimes made into syrup for **childhood thrush**.

PSYCHOSPIRITUAL

"*It is true, Misaldus and others, yea, almost all astrology-physicians, hold this to be an herb of Mars, because it cures the diseases of the head and privities, which are under the houses of Mars, Aries, and Scorpio. The truth is, it is under the command of Venus, and cures the head by antipathy to Mars, and the privities by sympathy to Venus; neither is there hardly a martial disease but it cures.*"

-- Nicholas Culpepper

"*The juice mixed with oil of roses, and the temples and forehead anointed therewith, eases the pains of the head proceeding from heat, and helps lunatic and frantic persons very much; as also the biting of serpents, or a mad dog.*"

-- Nicholas Culpepper

- In the Chippewa & Ojibwa tribes the ground root was carried **to repel snakes**.
- Early Christians thought plantain **symbolized the path of those who sought Christ.**
- *Plantago lanceolata* was **used by lovers in Scotland as divination to tell if they would marry**.

REPRODUCTIVE

"*... and stays all manner of fluxes, even women's courses, when they flow too abundantly.*"
- - Nicholas Culpepper

- **Female disorders** [Delaware (in combination), Eclectic]; **lack of menses** [Martinique]; **excessive menstrual bleeding** [Eclectic]; **to regulate and shorten menses** [Iroquois].
- **Infusion to "check discharge" and used as a douche** [Cherokee]; **vaginal discharge**, **yeast infections** [Eclectic].
- **Malpositioned fetus** [China (seeds)].
- **"Syphilitic, mercurial, and scrofulous diseases"** [Eclectic]; **gonorrhea**.
- **Prostatitis** [China (seeds)].
- **Male sterility** [China (seeds)].
- **Contraceptive**.

RESPIRATORY

"*It is held an especial remedy for those that are troubled with the phthisic, or consumption of the lungs, or ulcers of the lungs, or coughs that come of heat.*"
- - Nicholas Culpepper

- **Common cold** [Paiute].
- **Hay fever**; **rhinitis**; **sinusitis**; **middle ear congestion**.
- **Asthma** [Hawai'i]; **chest congestion**.
- **Cough** [China, Malaya]; **chronic cough**; **nervous & dry coughs**; **coughing blood** [Eclectic].
- **Acute & chronic bronchitis** [India, Spain]; **cough with yellow phlegm** [China, Hawai'i, Europe]; **upper respiratory catarrh.**
- **Emphysema**; **pleurisy** [Hawai'i]; **pneumonia** [Paiute]; **tuberculosis**; **to strengthen the lungs after serious pulmonary diseases**.

URINARY

- **Bladder problems** [China, Panama].
- **Urinary tract infections**, **painful urinary dysfunction**, **urinary stones** [Cherokee, China (seeds), Eclectic, England (seeds powdered), Iroquois, Java]; **blood in the urine** [Cherokee, Eclectic].
- **Kidney inflammation**; **edema from kidney dysfunction** [China (seeds)]; **dropsy** [England (seeds powdered), Shoshoni].
- **Excessive urination**; **bed wetting** [Eclectic].

VETERINARY

"*If a woodhound (mad dog) rend a man, take this wort, rub it fine and lay it on; then will the spot soon be whole.*"
- - Old English Herbal Text

- Most small birds enjoy the seeds. **Fed to caged birds** in England.
- **A food plant for caterpillars** of many types of butterflies

OTHER MEDICINAL USES

"*And of Plantaine he hath his herb sovereine.*"
- - Gower (1390)

- Root used as a **"life medicine"**. [Navajo, Ramah]; **debility** [Hawaii]; **lethargy** [England (seeds powdered)]; **loss of body mass** [China, Eclectic].
- **Leprosy** [Europe].
- **Nettles** (*Urtica dioica*) **sting**.
- **Pain** [Abnaki].
- **To "purify the blood"** [Iroquois].
- **Mercury poisoning** [Eclectic].

USE AS FOOD:

- The young fresh leaves can be juiced, used in salads, or steamed. However, while plantain is often described as "edible"... that might depend on what one is willing to eat.
- Combined with pigweed, mustard, dock and nettle and used as mixed greens [Mohegan].
- Leaves cooked and eaten as greens [Cherokee].
- Used as a coagulating enzyme (rennet) to make cheese.

OTHER USES:

- Used in a transdermal patch created by Dr. Mary Cody for nicotine addiction. It is said to cause an aversion to tobacco.
- With an alum mordant, used to make yellow and brown dyes for wool.
- A seed extract was once used in France to stiffen woven fabrics.

POSSIBLE CONSTITUENTS (depending on the species): Acteoside; allantoin (vulnerary); anthraquinones; apigenin; ascorbic-acid; aucubin (an anti-inflammatory glycoside / hepatoprotective / anti-venom); baicalein; benzoic-acid; carotenoid; chlorogenic and neochlorogenic acids (vulneraries); cistanoside F; citric-acid; cubin and catapol (iridoid glycosides); erucic acid; fatty acids; ferulic-acid; flavonoids; sugars; hispidulin; homoplantaginin; isoacteoside; lavandulifolioside; lutelin; monoterpene alkaloids; mucilage; nepetin; nitrates; oleanolic-acid; phenylethanoids; plantagoside; plantamajoside; polysaccharides; potassium; salicylic-acid; scutellarin; silica; silicic acid; tannins; triterpenes; ursolic acid; verbascoside; vitamin C; vitamin K; volatile oils; zinc.
The glycoside Aucubin occurs in numerous *Plantago* spp. It is thought to help the plant ward off pathogens and predators [Biere 2004], and yet may also be responsible for many of its healing properties in humans [Chiang 2003(a)].

POSSIBLE DRUG INTERACTIONS: Laukahi is high in vitamin K so theoretically it could act as a warfarin antagonist. [Brinker 2001]

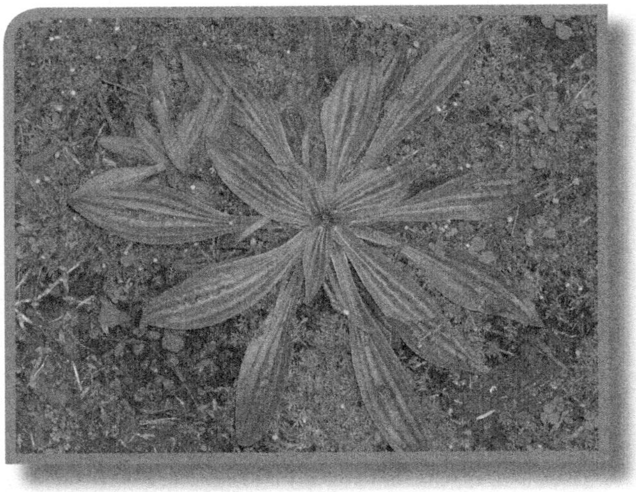

Plantago laneolata: Laukahi

Laukahi (Plantain) Local Combinations

Jaundice: Add *Taraxacum officinale* (laulele / dandelion), *Sonchus oleraceus* (pualele / sow thistle), *Bidens pilosa* (kīnehi / spanish needle).

Boils: Topical. Add *Hibiscus rosa-sinensis* (aloalo / red hibiscus), *Hibiscus tiliaceus* (hau).

Acute bronchitis: Add *Waltheria indica* ('uhaloa).

Chronic bronchitis: Add *Usnea* spp. ('umi koa), *Zingiber officinale* ('awapuhi pākē / ginger), *Trametes versicolor* (yun zhi), *Morinda citrifolia* (noni).

Urinary tract infections: Seeds. Add *Bidens pilosa* (kīnehi / spanish needle), *Piper methysticum* ('awa).

Red eyes: Add *Pandanus tectorius* (hala).

Laukahi (Plantain) Cross-Cultural Combinations

"*One part of Plantain water, and two parts of the brine of powdered beef, boiled together and clarified, is a most sure remedy to heal all spreading scabs or itch in the head and body, all manner of tetters, ring-worms, the shingles, and all other running and fretting sores.*"
-- Nicholas Culpepper

Rattlesnake bite: Root with *Marrubium vulgare* (horehound).

Wounds: Raw leaves poulticed with *Clematis* spp. [Shoshoni].

GI bleeding and hemorrhoids: With *Symphytum officinale* (comfrey) roots.

Shock: With *Mentha* spp. (mint), *Thymus vulgaris* (thyme), and salt. [Carribean]

Diarrhea: With *Coix lachryma jobi* (yi yi ren / jobs tears) [China].

To benefit the eyes: With *Cuscuta* (tu si zi), *Chrysanthemum morifolium* (ju hua) [China].

Chronic cough in children: With *Citrus reticulata* (chen pi / tangereen peel) [China].

Inflammation: Topical with *Nepeta cataria* (catnip) leaves, *Trigonella foenum-graecum* (fenugreek) seeds.

Slow healing wounds: With *Prunella vulgaris* (xia ku cao / self heal), *Symphytum officinale* (comfrey), *Achillea millefolium* (yarrow).

Toothache: Topical with *Anacyclus pyrethrum* (pellitory of spain) (both roots powdered).

Burns and abrasions: An ointment can be made with *Plantago* leaves, clarified butter, *Artemisia abrotanum* (southernwood), *Ribes nigrum* (black currant) leaves, *Sambucus nigra* (elder) buds, *Angelica archangelica* and *Petroselinum crispum* (parsley). Another ointment includes *Ranunculus ficaria* (celandine), *Sambucus nigra* (elder) buds, *Sedum acre* (houseleek) and *Plantago major* leaf.

Spitting of blood: With *Symphytum officinale* (comfrey) roots, juice of plantain and sugar.

Diuretic: Juiced leaves with lemon juice.

RANGE: Native to Europe and Asia, but globally pandemic.

GATHERING: Away from the road, uphill (mauka) if possible. This herb is often gathered along busy roadsides in Hawai'i. This is a bad idea. Oil, (among other things), flows downhill. Unless you have a craving for used motor oil, you should find other areas from which to collect herbs.

In Japan, reseach has shown midfall to be the optimum time to harvest *Plantago* spp. [Tamura 2002].

PROPAGATION & CULTIVATION: No need.

RESEARCH:

- In one study, water-soluble constituents were shown to be mildly antileukemic in human leukemia and lymphoma cells; while water-insoluble constituents (triterpenoids such as ursolic acid and oleanolic acid; the monoterpene linalool; and the flavonoid luteolin) were shown to be strongly antileukemic [Chiang 2003(c)]. This may point to an alcohol extraction or ingestion of the whole plant for leukemia.
- Acteoside & plantamajoside (*P. lanceolata*) inhibited arachidonic-induced edema in mice.
- Arachidonic-induced mouse ear edema is inhibited by acteoside & plantamajoside from *P. lanceolata*

- *P. psyllium* reduces serum cholesterol in humans [Jenkins 2002].
- Induces interferon [Chiang 2003(a); Chiang, 2003(b)].
- May reduce mammary tumor formation in mice [Lithander 1992].
- May reduce carcinogenic liver damage in rats [Karpilovskaia 1989].
- Ethanol extracts of *P. major* may be immune enhancing [Gomez-Flores 2000].
- Catalpol in plantain increases appetite in caterpillars [Bernays 2000].
- There is some evidence in mice and rats that the polysaccharides in *P. major* stimulate the innate and not the adaptive immune system. While counter-intuitive to many TCM practitioners, what this means is that fresh *Plantago major* extract may have adaptogenic functions in mammals [Hetland 2000].

Arguably the most commonly wildcrafted plant medicine in the world, laukahi is definitely one of the top ten. I am hard-pressed to find a place where it doesn't grow. On Maui it can be found from the beaches of Kihei or Pāi'a to the top of Haleakala at 10,000 feet. I have seen *Plantago* spp. in Europe, Asia, South America and Hawai'i. Our endemic Hawaiian species are fascinating.

NOTES 'N QUOTES

- In the Lacnunga (an old Saxon herbal) "weybroed" (plantain) is said to be one of the nine sacred herbs of the Saxons.
- Chaucer refers to plantain in the prologue of "Chanounes Yeman," and Longfellow mentions it in "Hiawatha."
- Legend has it that plantain was once a young woman who spent so much time by the roadside waiting for her lover that she was eventually transformed into a plant.
- Both Native Americans and the Maori of New Zealand have called plantain "white-man's-foot' because it seemed to sprout up wherever White people stepped. It certainly follows me around.
- It is said that a Native American was once given a reward from the South Carolina Assembly for discovering that plantain was "the chief remedy for the cure of the rattlesnake."
- In Scotland in 1623 a woman named Bessie Smith was accused of witchcraft for using *Plantago major*. She confessed to giving the leaves to people with "heart fevers". She instructed them to eat the leaves for nine mornings in a row while reciting a specific charm.
- *Plantago* spp. are hermaphroditic, having male and female flowers on one plant.
- Keoki Sousa tells of struggling for a month with a mysterious and stubborn respiratory illness. After treating it himself without success, he finally went to see a Western doctor. Three hundred dollars and many lab tests later, the doctor sent him away with a prescription for a bottle of pills and a "diagnosis": Pleurisy. Not being a pill-taker, he went to see one of our Hawaiian teachers for a second opinion. After describing the symptoms, the Kupuna looked at him and said, "Keoki, you've got pleurisy." He laughed to himself: "I just paid $300 for the exact same diagnosis!" The Kupuna then said, "You need laukahi." As is our tradition, he awoke before dawn the next day, and set out to gather laukahi. After drinking the medicine, the pleurisy disappeared.
- Shakespeare referred to plantain in plays such as Love's Labour's Lost, Two Noble Kinsmen, Troilus and Cressida, Schoolmistress, and Romeo and Juliet:

Romeo: *Your plantain leaf is excellent for that.*
Juliet: *For what I pray thee?*
Romeo: *For your broken shin.*
- - William Shakespeare

Plantago spp. (Laukahi / Plantain)

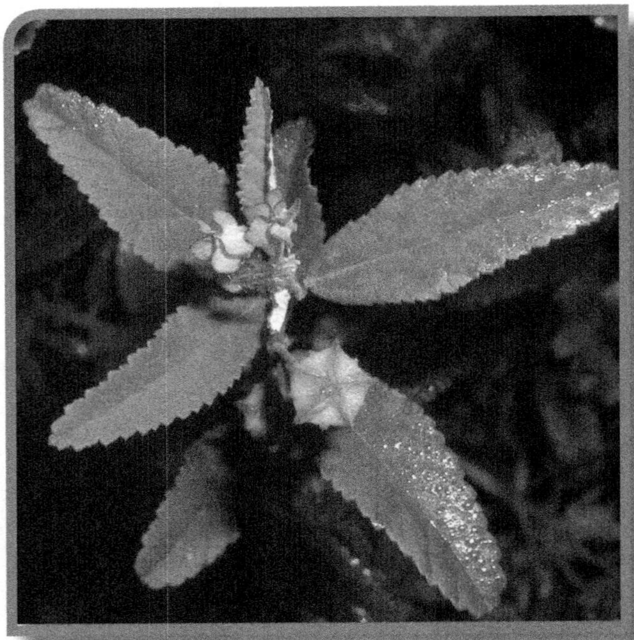

Sida rhombifolia (Huang Hua Mu)

PLANT NAME: *Sida rhombifolia* L.

OTHER NAMES: *Sida hondensis, Sida ruderata.*

COMMON NAMES: **Huang hua mu** [China] country mallow [English]; bala, mahabala [India]; chittamadi [Srilanka]; escobilla [Panama]; mautofu [Samoa]; petoria-bossie [Africa].

Status: Unknown. Possibly indigenous.

NOMENCLATURE: The name "*Sida*" was originally from Theophrastus who used it for Nymphaea alba. Linneaus applied it to this genus.

Habitat: Sea level to 3600'.

FAMILY: Malvaceae (mallow family).

CATEGORY: Clear damp heat.

PROPERTIES: Sweet bland cool.

PLANT PART USED: All of it. Stems are rich in mucilage. Root contains ephedrine

TOXICITY: No toxicity of the water extracted aerial parts in rats, even at doses of 10 g / kg, p.o. The LD50 for the root water extraction was 8.5g / kg p.o [Rao 1997].

CAUTIONS AND CONTRAINDICATIONS: *Sida rhombifolia* has recently been declared illegal by the federal government due to its ephedrine content. Because this plant is now illegal, it should not be used. If you see this plant growing anywhere, please contact the appropriate authorities.

PREPARATION OF MEDICINE: Decocted.

DOSAGE: 15 grams in combination. Up to 30 grams (1 oz.) alone.

WESTERN FUNCTIONS REPORTED: **Antibiotic**; **anti-inflammatory** [China]; **abortive**; **analgesic** [China, India]; **antidiabetic** [India]; **anti-inflammatory** [India]; **aphrodisiac** [India (roots)]; **beautifies** [India]; **demulcent** [India (stems), Panama (seeds)]; **diuretic** [China, India (whole plant), Panama]; **emmenagogue**; **emollient** [India (stems), Panama (seeds)]; **febrifuge** [India (stems)]; **hypoglycaemic** [India]; **lactagogue**; **nutritive** [India]; **sedative** [Panama]; **strengthens the body** [India]; **tonic** [India].

TRADITIONAL CHINESE ENERGETIC FUNCTIONS (~ = extrapolated):

1) Clears heat.
2) Benefits dampness.
3) Stops pain.

Huang Hua Mu Common Medicinal Uses

- Depression
- Bronchitis, cough, wheezing
- Urinary tract inflammation.

Huang Hua Mu Cross-Cultural Medicinal Uses

BITES & STINGS

- **Scorpion sting** [India (mucilage)].
- **Snake bite**.
- **Wasp sting**.

COSMETIC.

- **Alopecia**.

DERMATOLOGICAL.

- **Skin diseases** [India (stems)]; **dermatosis**; **itching**; **eczema of the scrotum** [China]; **impetigo**.
- **Sores**; **boils** [China (poultice or a wash)].
- **Burns**.
- **Herpes**.
- **Warts**.

DIGESTIVE

- **Stomach disorders** [Panama]; **stomach pain** [China]; **indigestion** [Australian Aborigines (root eaten raw)]; **flatulence** [India].
- **Diarrhea** [Australian Aborigines (root decocted), India]; **dysentery** [China, India (roots infused)]; **irritable bowel syndrome**.
- **Gastritis**; **enteritis** [China].
- **Hemorrhoids** [India (roots and leaves)].
- **Constipation**.

ENDOCRINE

- **Diabetes insipidus**, **diabetes mellitus**.

HEAD AND THROAT

- **Facial paralysis**.
- **Headache and migraine headache** [India (fruit)].
- **Eye problems** [India]; **conjunctivitis**; **ophthalmia**; **sty**.
- **Sinusitis** [India].
- **Tonsillitis** [China]; **toothache**.

HEPATIC

- **Bilious conditions**; **jaundice** [China].

IMMUNITY

- **Lupus**.

INFECTION

- **Fever**, **chills with fever.**

LYMPHATIC

- **Cervical tuberculous lymphadenitis** [China].
- **Elephantiasis**.

MUSCULOSKELETAL / TRAUMA

- **Cramps**; **joint pain** [India]; **rheumatism** [India (roots)].
- **Sciatica**.
- **Fracture**; **swelling** [India (leaves poulticed)].
- **Cuts** [Asia (leaves)]; **wounds**.

NEUROLOGICAL

- **Parkinson's disease** [India].
- **Hemiplegia**.

ONCOLOGY

- **Abdominal tumors**.

PARASITES

- **Malaria** [China].

PEDIATRIC

- **Colic** [India].
- **Chickenpox**.
- **Whooping cough** [India].
- **Thrush** [Samoa].

PSYCHOSPIRITUAL

- Phenelethylamine (PEA) is a neuroamine that is sometimes used for depression. It is also associated with people in love. It occurs in chocolate and is secreted by the brains of athletes when they are in "the zone." ***Sida rhombifolia* contains both PEA and ephedrine, hence its use as a mood enhancer.**
- **Depression**.
- **Mental instability**; **delirium**; **insanity**.
- **Irritability**.

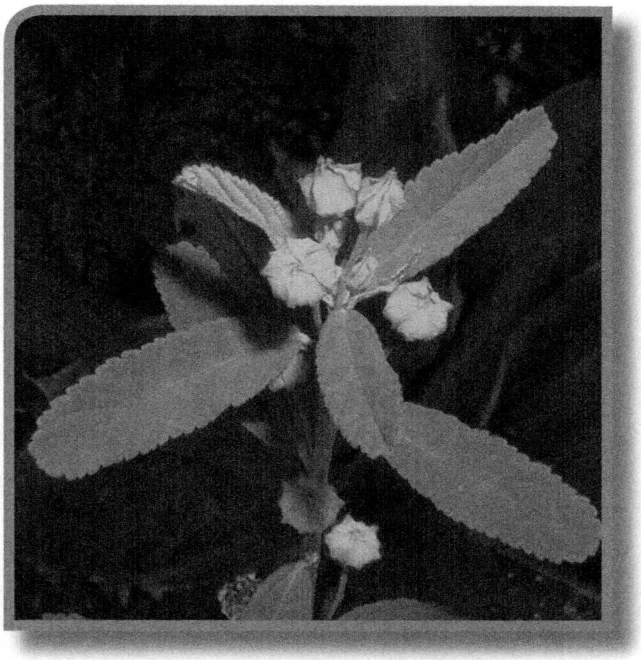

Sida rhombifolia: Huang Hua Mu

REPRODUCTIVE

- In India, bala root is prepared with oil and boiled milk, and then used room temperature as **a douche for sterility**. It is also taken internally for the same purpose.
- **Uterine disorders** [India]; **dysmenorrhea**; **vaginal discharge** [India (roots)].
- **Gonorrhea** [India (roots, seeds, leaves)].
- **Sexual weakness**; **impotence** [India].
- **During delivery** [India (root infusion internally)].
- **PMS**

RESPIRATORY

- **Respiratory complaints** [Eclectic]; **respiratory inflammation**.
- **Wheezing**; **shortwindedness.**
- **Common colds** [China].
- **Bronchitis**; **bronchial asthma** [India]; **cough**.
- **Pulmonary tuberculosis** [India]; **tuberculosis** [Europe]; **consumption** [India].

URINARY

- **Bladder ailments**; **urinary tract infections**; **blood in the urine.**
- **Urinary stones** [China].
- **Frequent urination.**

OTHER MEDICINAL USES

- **Burning sensation in the body.**
- **Emaciation** [India].

OTHER USES:

- Stems used as cordage.
- Brooms.
- Used as soap.
- The bark has been used for making rope.
- Brought to the US in the late 1800's for fiber.
- *Sida rhombifolia* leaves are smoked in Mexico.
- Edible. Contains up to 25% protein. Toxic to goats.

CONSTITUENTS: Alkaloids (root), ascorbic-acid (leaf), ash (leaf), beta-carotene (leaf), beta-phenethylamine, calcium (leaf), carbohydrates (leaf), choline, cobalt, copper, cryptolepine, ephedrine (root), fat (leaf), fiber (leaf), flavonoids (& their glycosides), gums, hipaphorine, indole alkaloids, iron (leaf), magnesium, mucilage (stem), niacin (leaf), phenolic compounds, phosphorus (leaf), potassium, protein (leaf), pseudoephedrine, riboflavin (leaf), saponin (leaf), sodium, steroids (& their glycosides), tannins, thiamin (leaf), triterpenoids (& their glycosides), vascin, vasicine, zinc. No cardiac glycosides have been found.

Huang Hua Mu Local Combinations

Depression: Add *Morinda citrifolia* (noni).
Bronchial asthma: Add *Waltheria indica* ('uhaloa).
Urinary tract infections: Add *Bidens pilosa* (kīnehi / spanish needle), *Plantago* spp. (laukahi / plantain).
With blood in the urine: Add *Capsella rubella* (shepherds purse).
To increase empathy (?): Add *Hibiscus rosa-sinensis* (aloalo) petals or *Passiflora incarnata* (passion flower) leaves as a tea.

Huang Hua Mu Cross-Cultural Combinations

Dysentery or enteritis: With *Plantago major* (laukahi / plantain) or *Polygonum hydropiper* [China].
Jaundice: Decocted with *Desmodium styracifolium* (jin qian cao) and *Saururus chinensis* [China].
Cervical tuberculous lymphadenitis: With meat as food [China].

RANGE: Temperate, tropical and subtropical areas in over 70 countries. Native to Europe.

PROPAGATION & CULTIVATION: By seed. Scarify (acid, heat, or cold storage) and plant at 1 to 2 cm. One *Sida rhombifolia* can produce more than 11,000 seeds.

RESEARCH:

- Water extracts of the whole plant were liver protective in rats [Rao 1997].
- Methanol extracts of the aerial parts suppressed edema in rats [Rao 1997].
- Stops pain and is anti- inflammatory [Venkatesh 1999].
- Weakly antibacterial and cytotoxic to cancer cells [Islam 2003].

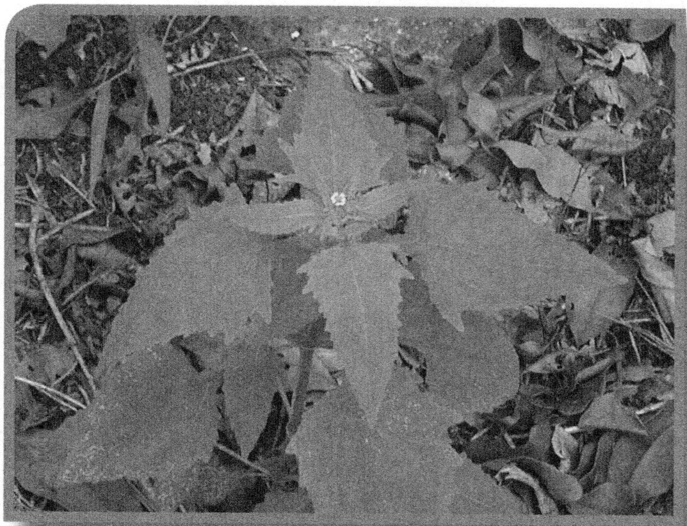

Siegesbeckia orientalis (Xi Xian Cao / Crown beard)

PLANT NAME: *Siegesbeckia orientalis* L.

SIMILARLY USED SPECIES: *S. pubescens* Mak., *S. glabrescens* Mak.

COMMON NAMES: **Xi xian cao** [China]; **small yellow crown beard** [English]; colle colle ("stick stick") [Creole]; hay lim cho [Canton]; kakamika [Tonga]; kirenso [Japan]; oech'umch'o [Korea]; st. paulswort [English]; trompetilla (*S. cordifolia*) [Colombia].

Status: Alien. Moderate pest potential.

Habitat: Disturbed areas to 3600'.

NOMENCLATURE: Carl Linnaeus (1707-1778) was the "father" of modern plant nomenclature, having invented the basis for the system we currently use today. He was a controversial character who insisted on using an organizational system based on plant sexuality. Among his critics was a botanist named Johann Siegesbeck (1686–1755). Objecting to Linnaeus' system of sexual classification, Siegesbeck referred to Linnaeus' work as "loathsome harlotry." Undisturbed, Linnaeus had the last laugh. He selected the ugliest little weed he could find and named it *Siegesbeckia*. I don't know anything about Mr. Siegesbeck, but I find the plant quite lovely.

FAMILY: Asteraceae.

CATEGORY: Expel wind dampness.

PROPERTIES: Bitter, cold, slightly toxic.

PLANT PART USED: Aerial parts.

TOXICITY: Some Chinese sources list *Siegesbeckia* as slightly toxic.

CAUTIONS AND CONTRAINDICATIONS: Not in pregnancy.

ENERGETIC CAUTIONS: Caution in blood or yin deficiency.

Xi xian cao is useful as a mild sedative and specific for joint and back pain. It can be used for insomnia due to physical discomfort

PREPARATION OF MEDICINE: Decocted or juiced fresh. I use it fresh or dried. In China it is sometimes prepared with wine.

DOSAGE: 6 to 15 grams. Up to 60 grams for malaria.

MERIDIAN AFFINITIES: Liver, kidneys.

WESTERN FUNCTIONS REPORTED: **Anti-inflammatory**; **antioxidant**; **parasiticide**.

TRADITIONAL CHINESE ENERGETIC FUNCTIONS (~ = extrapolated):

1) Dispels wind damp.
2) Strengthens the tendons, clears the channels.
3) Calms the spirit.
4) Clears damp heat.
5) Cleans heat and dispels toxins.
6) Clears liver heat.
7) Invigorates blood and stops pain.
8) Dispels gas and opens the luo channels.

OTHER ENERGETIC FUNCTIONS: Sedates kapha.

Xi Xian Cao (Crownbeard) Cross-Cultural Medicinal Uses

COSMETIC

- Used in cosmetic moisturizers for it's **anti-oxidant properties.**

CARDIOVASCULAR
- **Cerebral thrombosis** [China (decocted)].
- **High blood pressure** [China (internal)].

DERMATOLOGICAL
- **Skin disease and inflammation** [China, Mauritius Islands, Tonga (infusion topical)].
- **Boils, carbuncles, furuncles** [China (decocted)].
- **Itching and eczema, oozing dermatitis** [China (decocted)].
- **Ringworm** [19th Century England (juice internal)].
- **Wounds, burns** [Creole (juice topical)].

HEAD AND THROAT
- **Headache from high blood pressure** [China (internal)].

Xi Xian Cao (Crown Beard) Common Medicinal Uses
- Joint pain
- Hypertension
- Insomnia
- Skin disorders

HEPATIC
- **Acute infectious hepatitis** [China (whole plant)].

INFECTION
- **Leprosy** [Mauritius Islands].

MUSCULOSKELETAL / TRAUMA
- **Arthritis, including acute & chronic rheumatoid arthritis** (esp. of knees), **weakness & pain in the low back & legs, sciatica** [China (decocted, internal)].

NEUROLOGICAL
- **Dizziness** [China (internal)].
- **Hemiplegia and facial paralysis** [China (decocted, internal)].

PARASITES
- **Malaria** [China (whole plant decocted)].

PEDIATRIC
- **Measles** [China (decocted)].

PSYCHOSPIRITUAL
- **Forgetfulness, insomnia, irritability, "neurasthenia"** [China (whole plant decocted)].

REPRODUCTIVE
- **Antifertility**.
- **Syphilis** [Mauritius Islands].
- **Mastitis** [China].

RESPIRATORY
- **Allergies**.
- **Asthma**.

URINARY
- **Painful urination** [19th Century England].
- **Kidney pain** [China].

Xi Xian Cao (Crownbeard) Local Combinations

Neck pain: Add *Xanthium strumarium* (cang er zi), *Piper methysticum* ('awa / kava).

High blood pressure: Add *Cymbopogon refractus* (wāpine / lemongrass), *Prunella vulgaris* (xia ku cao).

Mild insomnia: Add *Oxalis* spp. ('ihi / sorrel), *Pipturus albidus* (māmake).

Moderate insomnia: Add *Piper methysticum* ('awa / kava), *Mimosa pudica* (hilahila).

Acute hepatitis: Add *Desmodium* spp. (pua pilipili), *Bidens pilosa* (kīnehi / spanish needle), *Plantago major* (laukahi / plantain).

Xi Xian Cao (Crownbeard) Cross-Cultural Combinations

Ringworm topical with:
- Glycerine [19th Century England].

Sinusitis with:
- *Magnolia liliflora* (xin yi hua), *Xanthium strumarium* (cang er zi), *Angelica dahurica* (bai zhi), *Chrysanthemum morifolium* (bai ju hua), *Mentha arvensis* (bo he) [China].

Joint pain with:
- *Clerondendron trichotomum* (chou wu tong) [China].
- *Clematis chinensis* (wei ling xian) [China].

High blood pressure with:
- *Clerondendron trichotomum* (chou wu tong), *Uncaria* (gou teng) [China].
- *Alisma plantago-aquatica* (ze xie); *Salvia miltiorrhiza* (dan shen); *Paeonia rubra* (chi shao); *Ligusticum chuanxiong* (chuan xiong), *Carthamus tinctorius* (hong hua) [China].

To prevent cerebral thrombosis with:

- *Angelica sinensis* (dang gui), Borneolum, *Carthamus tinctoruis* (hong hua), *Hirudo nipponica* (leaches), *Ligusticum wallichi* (gao ben), *Moschus moschiferus* (she xiang), *Panax notoginseng* (tien qi), *Prunus persica* (tao ren) [China].

RANGE: Native to tropical areas of North and South America.

GATHERING: Any time in Hawai'i, but it's best just before flowering

RESEARCH:
Shows strong anti-anaphylactic activity as an antihistamine (presumably in lab animals) in a dose-related manner [Kang 1997]. This appears to be through the suppression of immunoglobulin (Ig)E [Kim 2001, Hwang WJ]. A constituent (darutoside) in *Siegesbeckia glabrescens* is abortifacient in lab animals [Dong 1989].

NOTES 'N QUOTES

- The uses of xi xian cao were first recorded in China in 659 A.D.
- The flowers are sticky, as are the seeds, which spread via animal contact.
- There are six species in the genus *Siegesbeckia.*
- Xi xian cao treats an unusual constellation of symptoms, giving it uncommon flexiblity as a medicinal. It is a common roadside weed on windward sides.

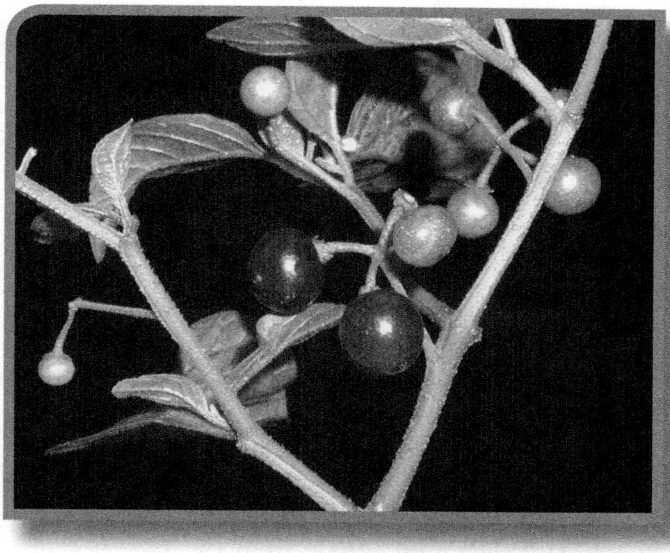

Solanum americanum (Pōpolo / Black Nightshade)

PLANT NAME: *Solanum americanum* Mill.

OTHER NAMES: *S. caribaeum, S. nigrum, S. nodiflorum, S. fauriei.*
(Please note: *S. americanum* is very closely related to *S. nigrum* and are sometimes considered synonyms. Much of the following information refers to *S. nigrum.*)

Status: Uncertain. Possibly native.

Habitat: Warm, wet, and sunny. To 4000'.

SIMILARLY USED SPECIES: *S. rubrum, S. incertum, S. incompletum* (pōpolo kū mai)

COMMON NAMES: **Pōpolo** [Hawai'i]; **black nightshade** [English]; long kui [China (*S. nigrum*)]; 'enab edh dhi'b, 'enab eth tha'lab, ribriq [Arabic]; guaraquinha [Brazil]; ghamai, handiguli, kakamachi [India]; hierba mora, yerba mora [Spanish]; hulablub [Visayan]; inu hôzuki.[Japanese]; kaburgia [Cuna]; kambai [Kashmir]; kanti, Lubi lubi [Tagalog]; kōpek memesi, kōpek ūzūmū, tilki ūzūmū [Turkish]; leunca ayam, leunca manuk [Indonesia]; mnavu [Swahili]; morella, solano nero [Italian]; morelle commune, morelle des jardins, morelle à fruits noirs, morelle noire [French]; mustakoiso.[Finnish]; nattskatta [Sweden]; pinatmora [Panama]; psianka czarna [Poland]; ranti [Malay]; schwarzer nachtschatten, nachtkraut.[German]; sort natskygge [Denmark]; svartsøtvier [Norway]; zwarte nachtschade [Dutch].

NOMENCLATURE: The name "*Solanum*" is from 'Solor' ("I ease"), a reference to the healing power of this genus. A plant in this genus with the common name "*Solanum*" was long ago used to treat epilepsy.

FAMILY: Solanaceae. (For twisted information about the family solanaceae visit www.tomatoesareevil.com)

CATEGORY: Clear heat and toxins ~.

PROPERTIES: Bitter, slightly sweet. Cool to cold.

PLANT PART USED: All of it.

TOXICITY: **Toxic**, but the levels of toxicity are uncertain. There are reams of conflicting research surrounding the toxicity of this plant. **The green berries are almost certainly more toxic than the ripe berries.** Toxicity may well result from a combination of factors including variety, plant part used, ripe or unripe fruits, size of fruit, water, soil, other plants in the area, etc.
The toxic principle is thought to be a saponic glycoalkaloid called solanine, which breaks down into an alkamine (solanidine), and a sugar (solanose). The LD50 of solanine in mice is 42 mg / kg.
The fruits have been made into preserves, jams, and pies with no ill effects. Boiling may break down solanine but drying does not. The fruit may be more toxic to children than adults. Three kilograms of green *Solanum nigrum* were once fed to a horse without any hazardous results. Symptoms of solanine overdose include nausea, vomiting and diarrhea. Dehydration may result from continued vomiting and diarrhea. Larger doses may cause cardiac arrhythmia, respiratory failure, and circulatory failure, leading to paralysis, convulsion, and coma. [All sources for toxicity are websites.]

CAUTIONS AND CONTRAINDICATIONS: THIS PLANT MAY BE *TOXIC.* DO NOT USE EXCEPT UNDER PROFESSIONAL SUPERVISION. See *Notes 'N Quotes*, and toxicity. In places where *Solanum nigrum* leaves and berries are used as food, epidemiological studies have linked this to cancer.

ENERGETIC CAUTIONS: Caution with cold deficient spleen stomach ~.

DOSAGE: Dosage of the dried plant in China is 10 - 30 grams in decoction.

STATUS IN HAWAI'I: Status uncertain. Possibly native. There are endemic species of *Solanum* that look very similar to *S. americanum.*

WESTERN FUNCTIONS REPORTED: **Alexiteric** [China (*S. nigrum*)]; **alterative** (fruit, juice) [India, Pakistan]; **analgesic**; **anodyne** [India, Pakistan]; **anthelmintic** [Houma]; **anti-inflammatory** (topical); **antiperiodic**; **antiphlogistic**; **antispasmodic**; **astringent** (herb decocted) [China (*S. nigrum*)]; **bactericide**; **cathartic** (juice) [Dominican Republic, India, Pakistan]; **ceremonial medicine** [Ojibwa]; **CNS-depressant**; **cyanogenetic** [USA]; **depurative** (herb decocted) [Haiti, Trinidad]; **dilates the pupils** (fruit); **diaphoretic** (syrup, leaf, herb infused) [India, Iraq, Pakistan]; **diuretic** (juice, fruit, leaf, herb decocted) [China (*S. nigrum*), India, Pakistan, Turkey]; **emetic** [Cherokee]; **emollient** [Haiti]; **expectorant** [India, Pakistan]; **febrifuge** [India (fruit)]; **heart tonic** [India, Pakistan]; **hydragogue** [India, Pakistan, Turkey]; **increases virility** (young shoots cooked and eaten) [China (*S. nigrum*)]; **jaundice** (herb decocted); **laxative**; **molluscicide**; **narcotic** [Haiti, Spain]; **nervine** [Turkey]; **opium antidote** [India]; **promotes perspiration** [India (fruit)]; **psychological aid** [Cherokee]; **purgative** [Sudan]; **refrigerant** [China (*S. nigrum*)]; **sedative** [China (*S. nigrum*), France (leaves poulticed), Haiti, India, Mexico, Pakistan, Rappahannock, Turkey]; **stimulant** [India (fruit)]; **tonic** (leaves) [Hawai'i]; **vasodilator**; **vulnerary** [Mexico].

TRADITIONAL CHINESE ENERGETIC FUNCTIONS (~ = extrapolated):

1) Clears heat and toxin.
2) Drains damp.
3) Reduces swelling.

Pōpolo (Black Nightshade)
Common Medicinal Uses

- Common cold with fever
- Chronic bronchitis
- Urinary tract infection
- Calming children (topical)
- Eye diseases

Pōpolo (Black Nightshade) Cross-Cultural Medicinal Uses

CARDIOVASCULAR

- **Heart disease** (fruit, with leg and foot swelling) [India].
- **Hypertension**.

DERMATOLOGICAL

- **Chancre** (poultice).
- **Cold sores** [China (*S. nigrum*)]; **shingles** [Trinidad]; **herpes** (green berries, poulticed).
- **Skin diseases** (leaves, herb juiced, ointment, poulticed) [Central America, Houma, India, Mexico, Venezuela]; **dermatitis** [China (*S. nigrum*)], **eczema & eruptions** [Venezuela (tea topical)]; **itching** [Venezuela]; **tinea** [Venezuela]; **leucoderma** [Philippines]; **pruritis** [Haiti].

DIGESTIVE

- **Bloating** (leaves eaten) [Hawai'i]; **stomach complaints**; **stomach ache** [Haiti]; **toning up digestive tract** [Hawai'i].
- **Constipation** [Trinidad].
- **Diarrhea** [China (*S. nigrum*)]; **dysentery** (herb infused).
- **Hemorrhoids** (fruit, herb juice, internal) [Dominican Republic, India].

HEAD AND THROAT

- **Inflammation of the amygdala** [Dominican Republic]; **loose teeth** (topical); **mouth ulcers** (leaf chewed); **mouthwash** [Trinidad]; **sore throat** (leaves chewed or brewed) [China (*S. nigrum*), Hawai'i]; **tongue problems**; **toothache** (fruit juice topical) [Costanoan (smoked)].
- **Eye problems** [Hawai'i (leaves poulticed), India]; **eye wash** (leaves decocted) [Native American]; **cataracts**, **glaucoma** (ripe berries cold infused, topical) [Hawai'i], **inflamed eyes** [Hawai'i]; **sore eyes** (decocted topical) [Miwok].
- **Headache** (leaves poulticed) [India].

HEPATIC

- **Cirrhosis**; **enlargement of the liver** (herb decocted, herb juice, internal, fruit) [India]; **hepatitis** [Haiti, Sudan]; **hepatoma** [China (*S. nigrum*)].

INFECTION

- **Abscess** [China, General (ointment)]; **boils** [Bahamas, Costanoan (heated leaves poulticed), Hawai'i, Trinidad]; **corroding ulcers** (poulticed); **sores** [China (*S. nigrum*), Haiti, Houma (fresh leaves poulticed)].
- **Fever** (fruit, leaves juiced, syrup in beverage) [China (*S. nigrum*), India].

LYMPHATIC

- **Enlarged spleen** (fruit) [India].
- **Scrofula** [Iraq].

MUSCULOSKELETAL / TRAUMA

- **Bruises** [Dominican Republic]; **cuts**, **abrasions**, **wounds** [China (herb decocted), Hawai'i (leaves poulticed with salt)]; **pain** (leaves poulticed) [France]; **relapse from injury** [Iroquois]; **sprains** [Hawaii]; **swelling** [China (*S. nigrum*), India].
- **Burns** [General (poultice), Haiti].
- **Pain and inflammation** [China (*S. nigrum*), India (fruit)]; **lumbago** [Lesotho]; **rheumatic**, **arthritic**, **and gouty joints** [Cuba (leaf and fruit with almond oil), Dominican Republic, India (poultice)]; **spasms** [Haiti].

NEUROLOGICAL

- **Epilepsy**.

ONCOLOGY

- **Cervical cancer** [China (*S. nigrum*)]; **cancer** [Belgium, China (*S. nigrum*), Guiana, Indochina]; **cancerous sores** (herb decocted), **digestive cancer**, **and lung tumors** [China (*S. nigrum*)]; **tumors** [Egypt, France, Morocco, Pakistan, Potawatomi, Tunisia]; **uterine cancer** [Italy].

PARASITES

- **Roundworms** (fruit).

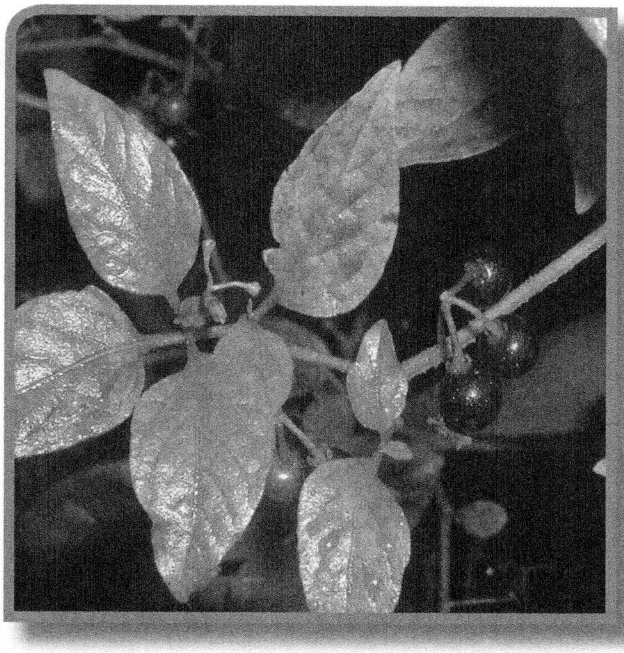

Solanum americanum: Pōpolo

PEDIATRIC

- **Colic** [Haiti]; leaves placed in the cradles **to help babies sleep** [Bohemia].
- **Pertussis** [Haiti].
- **Worms in children** (roots infused or decocted) [Houma].
- Fruit rubbed on the fontanel **to calm children and**

to keep the fontanel open [Hawai'i].

PSYCHOSPIRITUAL

- **Hydrophobia**.
- **Insomnia** (weak infusion) [Rappahannock].
- **Medicine ceremonies** [Ojibwa].
- Taken as an emetic and **to relieve loneliness due to death in family** [Cherokee].

REPRODUCTIVE

- **Painful menses** [China (*S. nigrum*)]; **female problems & menstrual disorders** [China (*S. nigrum* young shoots cooked and eaten), Panama].
- **Gonorrhea** (herb juice, internal) [India (fruit); **venereal disease** (root) [Delaware].
- **Inflammation of the testicles** [(hot compress), India (topical)].
- **Vaginal discharge** (douche) [China (*S. nigrum*)]; **vaginal discomfort** (decoction diluted douche); **vaginitis & vulvitis** [Haiti].
- **Pregnancy** (bath).

RESPIRATORY

- **Asthma** [Trinidad].
- **Common cold** (leaves chewed or brewed) [China (*S. nigrum*), Hawai'i].
- **Coughs** [Hawai'i (leaves as tea or chewed), India (fruit)].
- **Bronchitis** [Hawai'i (leaves chewed)], **chronic bronchitis** [China (*S. nigrum* decocted)].

URINARY

- **Bladder and kidney pain or inflammation** [China (*S. nigrum* decocted), General (juice), Haiti].
- **Edema** [India (fruit), Java, Sudan].

VETERINARY

- **Cattle either will or will not eat it**, depending on whom you ask.

OTHER MEDICINAL USES

- *Solanum nigrum* is used experimentally in Egypt to help control **schistosomiasis**, a tropical disease transmitted via snails.
- **Anthrax** (don't try this at home); **bubonic plague** (leaves as food) [Central America]; **Hansen's disease** (leprosy) (juice); **scarlet fever** [Costanoan]; **scurvy** (leaves).
- **Cramps** [Haiti].
- **Fatigue** [Trinidad].
- **Spitting of blood** (herb juice, internal).
- **Yaws** (a tropical disease caused by a spirochete) [Malaya].

USE AS FOOD: **Toxic**. See *Cautions and Contraindications.*

- Leaves are eaten in place of spinach [Bourbon, Mauritius].
- As a pot herb (leaves and stems) [Cherokee, Lesotho].
- Ripe fruit used as food [Mendocino, Tubatulabal].
- As a vegetable (leaves) [Central America].

OTHER USES: Used to detoxify soil contaminated with PCB's. Plants infected with *Agrobacterium tumefaciens* are more effective at detoxifying soil.

CONSTITUENTS: The leaves contain almost 7g of beta carotene per 100g and 5% protein.

Pōpolo (Black Nightshade) Cross-Cultural Combinations

Please note some of the ingredients in the following combinations are toxic! Do not self-administer without the supervision of a licensed practitioner or an experienced Elder.

Herpes: With *Mellisa officinalis* (lemon balm) & *Hypericum perfoliatum* (st. johns wort) as a cream.
Eye wash: With *Curcuma longa* ('ōlena / Turmeric), *Cordyline fruticosa* (lā'ī / ti), *Aloe vera* (aloi), and rose water [Old Hawai'i].
Swelling: Juice with butter as an ointment [Kashmir].
Hansens disease (leprosy): The fruit and leaf are used with almond oil [Cuba].

RANGE: Pandemic.

GATHERING: Anytime in Hawai'i. Autumn elsewhere. My teacher, Kawika Ka'alakea, always said that pōpolo is best gathered from plants standing on their own rather than from a large group. If one gathers from a large group the others will become jealous for not having been chosen.

PROPAGATION & CULTIVATION: By seed. Grows well with clover. When grown near *Artemesia* (wormwood) or *Brassica alba* (white mustard), *Solanum nigrum* reportedly will become more toxic.

RESEARCH:

- Antineoplastic [Hu 1999].

- Alcohol extract of *Solanum nigrum* reduces gastric ulcer formation in rats [Akhtar 1989].
- Fruit produces acetylcholine-like activity [de Melo 1978].
- Mildly hepatoprotective [Sultana 1995].
- Use of *Solanum nigrum* (pōpolo) as food has been correlated to an increased risk of esophageal cancer [Sammon 1992].
- Anti-fungal in vitro against *Epidermophyton floccosum*, *Microsporum canis*, and *Trichophyton rubrum* [Locher 1995].
- Ethanol extract of *Solanum nigrum* fruit may induce CNS depression. It prolongs pentobarbital-induced sleeping time & suppresses aggressive behavior in lab animals [Perez 1998].

NOTES 'N QUOTES

"*Do not mistake the deadly nightshade for this, if you know it not, you may then let them both alone.*"
- - Nicholas Culpepper

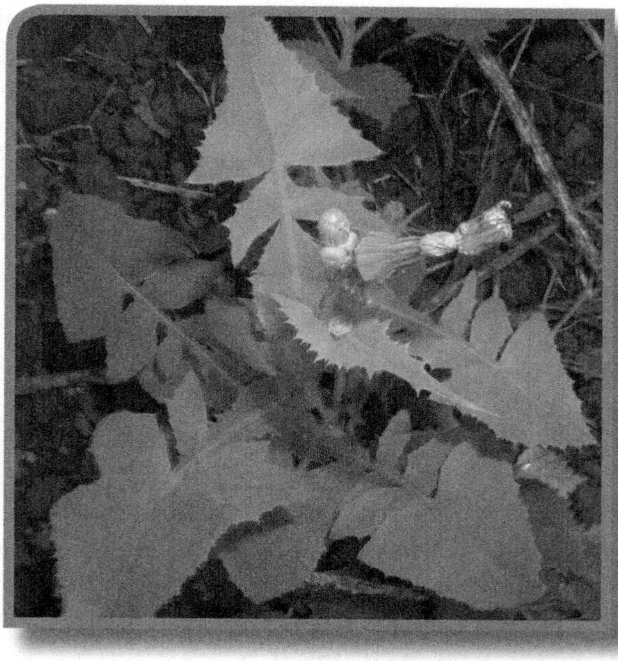

Sonchus oleraceus (Pualele / Sow Thistle)

PLANT NAME: *Sonchus oleraceus* L.

SIMILARLY USED SPECIES: *Sonchus alpinus, S. arvensis, S. asper, S. brachyotus, S. kirkii, S. palustris, S. tenerrimus, S. uliginosus, S. wightianus.*

Status: Alien. Moderate pest factor.

COMMON NAMES: **Pualele** [Hawai'i]; **sow thistle**, hare's thistle, hare's lettuce [USA]; rauriki, pororua, puwha, puha [Maori]; cerraja, serraja, diente de leon lechoso [Colombia]; leche [Bolivia]; llamp'u [Aymara]; qarasapi [Quechua].

Habitat: Upcountry. Wet and dry sides.

NOMENCLATURE: *Sonchus oleraceus* was named by Carolus Linnaeus in 1753 in his "Species Plantarum." "*Sonchus*" is the Greek name for sow thistle and means "hollow." This is a reference to the hollow stems. The epithet oleraceus means "kitchen vegetable."

FAMILY: Asteraceae (Daisy family).

CATEGORY: Clear heat and toxins~.

PROPERTIES: Bitter, cool to cold, mildly toxic.

PLANT PART USED: Leaves, stems, juice, root.

TOXICITY: **Possibly mildly toxic. May contain large quantities of nitrates**. See *Use as Food.*

CAUTIONS AND CONTRAINDICATIONS: Not in pregnancy. Overuse of stem juice as a cathartic can cause anal irritation and GI cramping.

ENERGETIC CAUTIONS: Caution with cold deficient spleen / stomach~.

PREPARATION OF MEDICINE: Infused or decocted.

DOSAGE: 15 - 30 grams. 10 - 15 grams in formulation.

STATUS IN HAWAI'I: Alien. Moderate pest factor. Get rid of it. *Sonchus* has the questionable distinction of being considered one of the world's worst weeds, a pest in more than 55 countries. In Hawai'i, however, I have never seen it out of control.

WESTERN FUNCTIONS: **Abortifacient** [Houma]; **anticancer** (sap); **antidiarrheal** [Houma]; **anti-inflammatory** [China]; **"blood purifier"**[Hoama]; **calms the nerves** (leaves); **cathartic** [Pima (stem juice), Turkey]; **clears infections** [China]; **cure for opium addiction** [China, Pima]; **digestive purgative** [Pima]; **diuretic** [Turkey]; **emmenagogue**; **emollient** [Haiti]; **febrifuge** (leaves and roots infused); **gynecological aid** [Potawatomi (*S. arvensis*)]; **heart medicine** [Navaho (*S.* asper)]; **hepatic**; **hydrogogue** (stem juice) [Turkey]; **insecticide**; **lactogogue** [Turkey]; **mild laxative** [New Zealand]; **narcotic** [China]; pectoral; **pediatric aid** [Houma, Iroquois (*S.* asper)]; **poison** [Navaho (*S. asper*)]; **poultice**; **refrigerant** [Spain, Turkey]; **sedative** [China, Iroquois (*S.* asper)]; **stop bleeding** [China]; **to prevent infection** (topical) [New Zealand]; **tonic** [Sudan, Turkey]; **toothache remedy** [Houma]; **vermicide** [Tanzania].

TRADITIONAL CHINESE ENERGETIC FUNCTIONS (~ = extrapolated):

1) Clears heat and toxin.
2) Invigorates blood and stops bleeding.
3) Clears heat and fire ~.
4) Clears damp heat ~.
5) Cools the blood ~.

Pualele (Sow Thistle)
Common Medicinal Uses

- Liver imbalances
- Poor digestion (as a bitter)
- Infections

Pualele (Sow Thistle) Cross-Cultural Medicinal Uses

COSMETIC

"*It is wonderful good for women to wash their faces with, to clear the skin, and give it a lustre.*"
- - Nicholas Culpepper

CARDIOVASCULAR

- **Heart disorders** [England]; **high blood pressure** [England].
- **Hemorrhage** [China].

DERMATOLOGICAL

"*The juice or distilled water is good for all hot inflammations, wheals, and eruptions or heat in the skin, itching of the hæmorrhoids.*"
- - Nicholas Culpepper

- **Dermatitis**
- **Warts** (sap topical) [China, New Zealand, USA].

DIGESTIVE

"*Sow Thistles are cooling, and somewhat binding, and are very fit to cool a hot stomach, and ease the pains thereof. The herb boiled in wine, is very helpful to stay the dissolution of the stomach, and the milk that is taken from the stalks when they are broken, given in drink, is beneficial to those that are short winded, and have a wheezing.*"
- - Nicholas Culpepper

- **Appendicitis** [China].
- **Burning stomach** [New Zealand]; **dyspepsia**; **stomach problems** [Peru, New Zealand].
- **Diarrhea** [Houma (infused)]; **dysentery**, **enteritis** [China]; **tenesmus** [Dominican Republic].
- **Hemorrhoids** [China, Europe].

HEAD AND THROAT

"*The juice boiled or thoroughly heated in a little oil of bitter almonds in the peel of a pomegranate, and dropped into the ears, is a sure remedy for deafness, singings, etc.*"
- - Nicholas Culpepper

- **Ear infections** [China, New Zealand]; **earache** (leaves).
- **Sore throat**, **tonsillitis** [China].
- **Toothache** [Houma].

HEPATIC

- **Ascites**, **hydrothorax**.
- **Infectious hepatitis**, **cirrhosis**, **jaundice** [China]; **liver dysfunction** [China, USA].

INFECTION

- **Abscess** [China]; **boils**, **carbuncles** [China, New Zealand]; **fever** [China, England, Sudan, Turkey]; **infections** [China, New Zealand].

MUSCULOSKELETAL / TRAUMA

- **Wounds**.

ONCOLOGY

- **Breast cancer** [Germany]; **cancer** [Italy, UK]; **stomach cancer** [Australia]; **tumors** [Guatemala].

PARASITES

- **Parasites** [Tanzania (internal)].

PEDIATRIC

- **Colic** [Dominican Republic].
- **Teething in children** [Houma (infused)].

PSYCHOSPIRITUAL

"*This and the former [Oxalis spp.] are under the influence of Venus.*"

- - Nicholas Culpepper

REPRODUCTIVE

"*The decoction of the leaves and stalks causeth abundance of milk in nurses, and their children to be well-coloured*" - - Nicholas Culpepper

"*Three spoonfuls of the juice taken, warmed in white wine, and some wine put thereto, causes women in travail to have so easy and speedy a delivery, that they may be able to walk presently after.*"

- - Nicholas Culpepper

- **"Caked breasts"** (leaves infused); **mastitis** [Ancient Greece, China].
- **Late menses** (infused); **uterine bleeding**, **irregular menses** [China, Bolivia].
- **Unwanted pregnancy** [New Zealand, Hoama (infused)].
- An herbalist in the 1200s recommended the addition of *Sonchus* to the diet in order **to "prolong the virility of gentlemen."**
- For **decreased lactation**.

RESPIRATORY

- **Asthma** (root).
- **Chest complaints** (root), **coughs** (root).
- **Coughing up blood** [China].

URINARY

"*Pliny saith, That it hath caused the gravel and stone to be voided by urine, and that the eating thereof helps a stinking breath.*"

- - Nicholas Culpepper

- **Gravel and stoppage of urine**; **urinary obstructions.**
- **Hematuria** [China].
- **Urinary stones** (infused) [Nicholas Culpepper].

VETERINARY

"W*hen fainting with the heat she (the rabbit) recruits her strength with this herb: or if a hare eat of this herb in the summer when he is mad, he shall become whole.*"

- - Author Unknown

- **A favorite food of rabbits and pigs**. Hence the names "sow thistle" and "hare's thistle." It was once said to cure rabbits of their "madness," and that predators could not attack a rabbit that rested under a hare's thistle.

OTHER MEDICINAL USES

- **"Cure for opium addiction"** [Pima]; **"morphinism"** [Iraq].
- **Snake bite** [China]; **scorpion bites** [New Zealand].
- **"Blood purifier"** [New Zealand]; **flux** (fluid discharge) [China].
- **Inflammation** [Nicholas Culpepper].
- **Rejuvenation**, **"low vitality"** [China].
- Used by Captain Cook for **scurvy** [New Zealand].

USE AS FOOD:

- Used as food throughout the ages. The ancients considered the leaves to be very wholesome and strengthening. It is eaten in such faraway places as Lapland, South Africa, and Indonesia. Grown for it's edible leaves by the Maoris of New Zealand. The Maori have a lower incidence of colorectal cancer than non-Maori New Zealanders, despite a higher intake of alcohol, saturated fat, red meat, and a higher incidence of obesity. It has been speculated that this is due to the presence of *Sonchus* leaves and *Nasturtium officinale* (watercress) in their diet. Both *Sonchus* and *Nasturtium* have been reported as cancer protective [Thomson 2002].
- The young leaves can be used in a salad or cooked green. The stems should be bruised and the latex washed out of them before cooking.
- The root is roasted as a coffee substitute.
- **NOTE**: **Because there is some question as to possible chronic toxicity, I cannot recommend using Sonchus as food until more information becomes available.**

OTHER USES: The sap has been used as "chewing gum" by the Maoris of New Zealand The sap contains 0.14% rubber, not enough for commercial use, but apparently enough to chew on.

CONSTITUENTS: Leaves high in Vitamin C (30-

60mg / 100g dry) and mineral salts. Protein, fat, carbohydrate, fiber, ash, calcium, phosphorus, iron, Vitamin A, thiamine, riboflavin, niacin. Also contains flavone glycoside compounds (quercetin-3-O-alpha-L-rhamnoside & kaempferol-3, 7-alpha-L-dirhamnoside).

POSSIBLE DRUG INTERACTIONS: Lithium toxicity may be exacerbated (in *Taraxacum* spp.) due to sodium depletion. (Speculative)

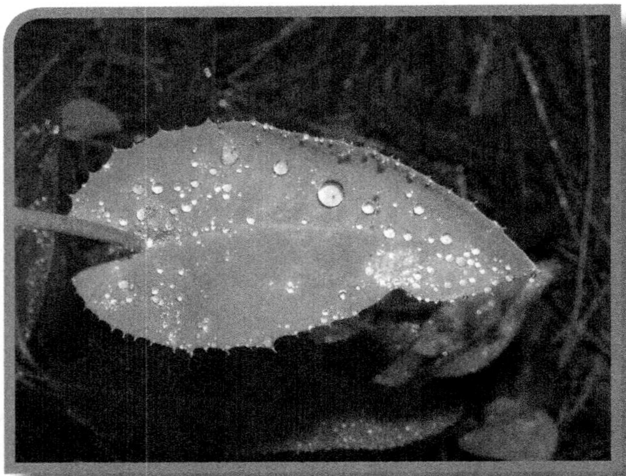

Sonchus oleraceus: Pualele leaf attachment

Pualele (Sow Thistle) Local Combinations

Hepatitis: Add *Bidens pilosa* (kīnehi / spanish needle), *Desmodium* spp. (pua pilipili), *Eclipta prostrata* (han lian cao).

Bronchitis: Add *Plantago major* (laukahi / plantain). With yellow / green phlegm: add *Musa* spp. (mai'a / banana) sap, *Waltheria indica* ('uhaloa) root cortex, *Tropaeolum majus* (pohe haole / nasturtium). With white / clear phlegm add *Curcuma longa* ('ōlena / Turmeric), *Zingiber officinale* ('awapuhi pākē / ginger).

Pualele (Sow Thistle) Cross-Cultural Combinations

Infectious hepatitis: Pualele is used with *Oxalis corniculata* ('ihi mākole / sorrel) and lean pork in China for infectious hepatitis and cirrhosis. This is not all that surprising considering that pualele is a close relative of the blesséd and cursed weed *Taraxacum officinale* (dandelion), another herb that is well known for treating liver disorders. The pork is another matter.

Unwanted pregnancy: With *Plantago major* [New Zealand].

Pain from "scalding urine": Young tops as food with oil and vinegar.

Post partum hemorrhage: With wild turnip [Pohatu].

Blood in the urine: Decocted and taken with wine.

Deafness: Topically with bitter almond oil and pomegranate skin [Nicholas Culpepper].

"Stuffing of the lungs": British traveler John Josselyn wrote in 1637 he had found several varieties in the gardens of the Pilgrims. When he came upon Native Americans who suffered from "stuffing of the lungs" he prepared a combination of European plants he had found in the New World. These included *Sonchus* spp, *Foeniculum vulgare* (xiao hui xiang), *Nepeta cataria* (catnip), and *Pimpinella anisum* (anise) [balanced formula!].

RANGE: Native to Europe. Found in Australia, Europe, Asia, Middle East, and North and South America.

HABITAT: *Sonchus* was part of the "Thistle Invasion" of North America three hundred years ago that involved as many as 120 different species. See *Notes 'n Quotes.* As all good asteraceaes are wont to do, *Sonchus* spp. spread quickly. It is known for its remarkable skill in adaptive radiation [Kim 1996]. In Hawai'i it lives upcountry on both wet and dry sides.

GATHERING: Please do. Flowers June through October in America. *Sonchus* can be differentiated from the common dandelion (*Taraxacum* spp.) in that the *Sonchus* stem will fork with leaves growing on the upper stem. In a true dandelion, the leaves only grow at the base of the stem, which never forks.

PROPAGATION & CULTIVATION: Please don't

RESEARCH: The leaves as a green are anti-oxidant [El 2004].

NOTES 'N QUOTES

"*The juice [of S. alpinus] is useful in deafness, either from accidental stoppage, gout or old age. Four spoonfuls of the juice of the leaves, two of salad oil, and one teaspoonful of salt, shake the whole well together and put some on cotton dipped in this composition into the ears and you may reasonably expect a good degree of recovery.*" Also: "*The juice boiled or thoroughly heated in a little oil of bitter almonds in the peel of a pomegranate, and dropped into the ears, is a sure remedy for deafness, singings, etc.*"

- - Nicholas Culpepper

[Please note: this is most likely "deafness" due to earwax.]

- It is recorded by Pliny (Caius Plinius Secundus, A.D. 23-79) that before Theseus encountered the bull of Marathon, he had a meal of sow thistles.
- According to the 16th century herbalist John Gerard, unscrupulous upholsterers filled mattresses and pillows with sow thistle down instead of goose down.
- *Sonchus* is a prime example of a "DYC" among botanists: a "Damned Yellow Compositae." They are so named because of the difficulty in differentiating species within the family. See *Habitat.*
- Traditionally used similar to dandelion.
- Like some mumbling old eccentric uncle, *Sonchus* has that familiar and raggedy appearance that is at once comforting and amusing. *Sonchus* is an old friend and I treat it as such. It is reasonably effective for bronchial infections with yellow phlegm; and if the phlegm has caused digestive disturbances, *Tropaoleum majus* (pohe haole) can be added. *Sonchus* also makes a good secondary herb in formulas for tonsilitis and sore throat. It is useful in small doses as a bitter tonic for the Spleen deficient patient with a sluggish liver.

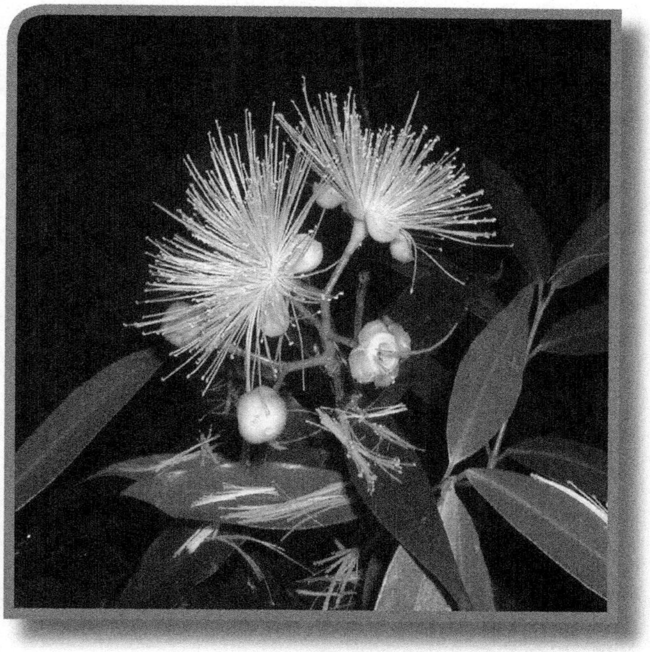

Syzygium jambos ('Ōhi'a Loke / Rose Apple)

PLANT NAME: *Syzygium jambos* (L.) Alston.

OTHER NAMES: *Eugenia jambos, E. vulgaris, Jambosa jambos, J. vulgaris*

Status: Tasty alien fruit. Bad pest.

Habitat: Shady and moist.

COMMON NAMES: **'Ōhi'a loke** ("rose 'ōhi'a") [Hawai'i]; **rose apple**, malabar plum, malay apple [English]; pu tao [China]; ahi'a popa'a [French Polynesia]; fekika papalangi [Tonga]; iouen wai, youenwai, apel en wai [Pohnpei]; jambosier, pommier rose [French]; kavika, kavika ni vavalangi, kavika ni india [Fiji]; pomme rose [Caribbean]; thulo jamun [Nepal]; pomarrosa [Spanish]; manzanito de rosa [Colombia]

NOMENCLATURE: Loke is the Hawaiian word for "rose."

FAMILY: Myrtaceae

CATEGORY: Stabilize and bind (fruit, root bark) ~

PROPERTIES: Undetermined. The fruit peel is said to be sweet, sour and hot.

PLANT PART USED: Bark, root bark, fruit, seeds

TOXICITY: The bark has very high tannin content, 77% in water extractions.

CAUTIONS AND CONTRAINDICATIONS: Caution in constipation.

ENERGETIC CAUTIONS: Caution with damp stagnation, heat stagnation or in exterior conditions ~.

PREPARATION OF MEDICINE: Bark infused or decocted.

DOSAGE: 5 - 10 grams of bark as single herb. 2 –4 fresh fruit.

STATUS IN HAWAI'I: A lovely tasty alien. High pest factor. Get rid of them all.

MERIDIAN AFFINITIES: Fruit peel: Spleen, lung.

WESTERN FUNCTIONS REPORTED: **Antimicrobial**; **astringent**; **antiseptic~**; **hemostatic**; **hypoglycemic**.

TRADITIONAL CHINESE ENERGETIC FUNCTIONS (~ = extrapolated):

Fruit, root bark

1) Astringes.
2) Cools the blood.

Fruit peel

1) Warms the stomach.
2) Strengthens the spleen.
3) Breaks blood stasis in deep ulcers and tumors.
4) Warms the lungs in lung deficient cold cough.

OTHER ENERGETIC FUNCTIONS: Benefits kapha and pitta.

'Ōhi'a Loke (Rose Apple) Cross-Cultural Medicinal Uses

CARDIOVASCULAR

- **High blood pressure** [Suriname (seeds)].
- **Bleeding** [India].

DIGESTIVE

- **Diarrhea**, **dysentery** [China (fruit, root bark), India (bark), Suriname]; **diarrhea with fever** [Suriname (leaves)]; **diarrhea with abdominal pain** [Suriname (fruit)].
- **Vomiting** [China (peel)].

ENDOCRINE

- **Diabetes** [Brazil, China (seeds), India, New Zealand, Suriname (seeds, leaves, bark)].

HEAD AND THROAT

- **Painful eyes** (leaves boiled).
- **Sore throat** [India].

HEPATIC

- **Liver problems** [Nepal (bark)].

INFECTION

- **Infectious diseases** [sub-Saharan Africa].

MUSCULOSKELETAL / TRAUMA

- **"Bleeding from knife wounds"** [China (fruit, root bark)].

RESPIRATORY

- **Wheezing and coughing**, **asthma** [India].

OTHER MEDICINAL USES

- **Hiccups** [China (fruit peel)].

'Ōhi'a Loke (Rose Apple) Common Medicinal Uses

- **Diarrhea**

USE AS FOOD: Rose apple tastes the way a rose smells. It is sweet and quite delicious. Can be eaten raw or made into preserves and jellies. Small amounts only as large amounts of tannins may be harmful, though the fruit contains much less than the bark.

OTHER USES: Bark is made into a brown dye. Used for erosion control, firewood, and as a windbreak. The distilled fruit has been made into "rosewater."

RANGE: Throughout Micronesia and Polynesia, Hawai'i, East Indies, & Malaya. Prehistoric introduction occurred through Southeast Asia, and more recently to Jamaica. First brought to Hawai'i from Rio de Janeiro in 1825 on the frigate "Blond."

HABITAT: Likes it shady and moist. Apparently gravity carries the seeds downhill and rats (& humans) carry them uphill. Supposedly it grows to 3500 feet on tropical islands and up to 6000 feet in Ecuador, but I've never seen it above 1200 feet or so.

GATHERING: By hand or with a fruit picker. Take care as the fruit bruises easily.

PROPAGATION & CULTIVATION: Don't. Creates monostands in Hawai'i, but it can also be a sub-canopy of other trees. Estimated rate of invasion is 3 feet per year. That's in all directions. In some places (South America, Pitcairn Island) rose apple as an invasive provides a safety zone for certain shade-tolerant native species, but not in Hawai'i. If cut it will re-sprout, so the roots must be removed. This is a gorgeous and psychopathic plant.

RESEARCH:
Water and acetone extractions are antimicrobial due to tannins. They are effective in vitro against numerous Staphylococci, and also against *Yersinia enterocolitica* [Djipa 2000].

NOTES 'N QUOTES

- Rose apple may be the legendary "gambu" or "jambu" tree of India that produced fruit of immortality. The seeds were said to produce gold and the fruit juice created the river Gambu. The Buddha is sometimes shown under a rose apple tree.
- The myrtaceae plant family often embodies extremes, and 'ōhi'a loke is no exception. The strong astringency of the bark is counterbalanced with the powerful and delicious sweetness of the fruit. It is usually an afterthought as a medicinal plant, but can be quite useful in an acute digestive disturbance. Given the alien impact of the plant, it is always a mixed blessing to come across a fruiting 'ōhi'a loke in the forest while gathering. The Chinese uses of the fruit peel are intriguing, and warrant further investigation.

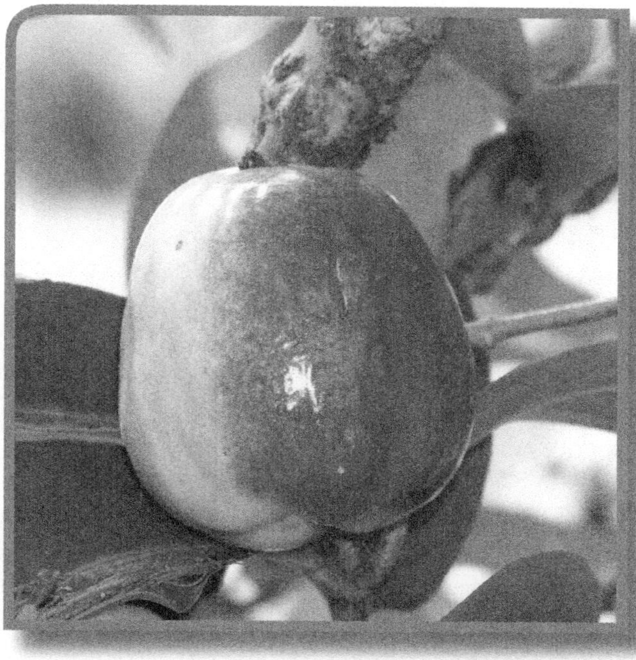

Syzygium malaccense ('Ōhi'a 'Ai / Mountain Apple)

PLANT NAME: *Syzygium malaccense* (L.) Merr. & Perry.

OTHER NAMES: *Eugenia malaccensis, Jambosa malaccensis.*

COMMON NAMES: **'Ōhi'a 'ai** [Hawai'i]; **hong hua qing tao**, ma liu jia qing tao [China]; **mountain apple** [English]; nonu fi'afi'a [Samoa] kafika ['Uvea, Futunu]; fekika kai [Tonga]; 'ahi'a [Tahiti]; kehika kehi'a [Marqueses]; pomerac [Suriname]; ka'ika [Cook Islands].

Status: Polynesian introduction. Minimal pest factor.

Habitat: Wet and shady. To 1800'.

NOMENCLATURE:

- *Syzygium* comes from the Greek "sys," which means "together" & "zygon" meaning "yoke"; a reference to the coherent petals in some species.
- In Hawaiian, "'ōhi'a 'ai" implies an 'ōhi'a tree that produces "'ai"(food).
- "Qing tao" is the Chinese name for some species of *Syzygium.* "Qing tao" means "clear peach." "Hong hua qing tao" means "red flowered *Syzygium*," a reference to the bright red flowers.

FAMILY: Myrtaceae.

CATEGORY: Stabilize and bind~.

PLANT PART USED: Bark, fruit, leaves, root.

CAUTIONS AND CONTRAINDICATIONS: Can cause stomach ache and vomiting in large doses.

PREPARATION OF MEDICINE: For sore throat the inner bark is scraped, or the whole bark can be decocted. The fruit can be eaten.

DOSAGE: A piece the size of the palm of one's hand was the traditional size of the bark used. I find that a piece one-half that size works just fine.

WESTERN FUNCTIONS REPORTED: **Abortifacient** (root bark); **diuretic** (root); **emetic**; **emmenagogue** (root bark); **febrifuge** (seed, fruit, or leaves decocted); **gastrointestinal aid**; **strengthener.**

'Ōhi'a 'Ai (Mountain Apple)
Common Medicinal Uses

- Sore throat (inner bark chewed)

'Ōhi'a Ai (Mountain Apple) Cross-Cultural Medicinal Uses

DERMATOLOGICAL

- **Eczema** [New Caledonia].
- **Itching**, **lice** [China (root)].
- **Skin lotion** (leaf juice)

DIGESTIVE

- **Bark for stomach ache** [Tonga].
- **Constipation** [Brazil].
- **Digestive tract disorders** [Hawai'i].
- **Dysentery** (root bark).
- In combination with other plants for **stomach pain and abdominal problems** [Tonga].

ENDOCRINE

- **Diabetes** [Brazil].

HEAD AND THROAT

"For sores about the mouth and the foul odor that comes from such sores, the 'Ōhi'a 'Ai is a good remedy."
- - *D.* M. Kaaiakamanu, 1922

- **Bad breath**, **mouth ulcers** [Hawai'i (bark juiced in combination or sap from petiole), Polynesia (bark and leaves)].
- **Mouth infections** (leaves and bark chewed or infused as mouthwash) [Samoa, Tonga]. Also for infants.
- **Thrush** [China (bark), New Caledonia (mouthwash)].
- **Sore throat** [Hawai'i (inner bark, old fruit), throughout Polynesia (bark and leaves)].
- **Tongue diseases** [China (leaves)]; **cracked tongue** [Malaya (leaf powder, topical)].
- **Headache** [Brazil].

INFECTION

- **Fever** [Cambodia (seed, fruit, or leaves decocted), New Caledonia].
- **Suppurating wounds** [New Caledonia].
- **Tuberculosis** [Hawai'i].

MUSCULOSKELETAL / TRAUMA

- **Cuts** [Hawai'i].

PARASITES

- **Lice** [China (root)].

PEDIATRIC

- **Thrush** [China (bark), Hawai'i, throughout Polynesia (bark and leaves), Spice Islands].
- **General debility in children** (bark juiced in combination) [Hawai'i].
- **Stomach weakness in children** (bark juiced in combination) [Hawai'i].

PSYCHOSPIRITUAL

- In old Tahiti, 'ōhi'a 'ai was used **for sacred ceremonies**.

REPRODUCTIVE

- **Vaginal infection** (bark decocted).
- **Venereal disease** [Hawai'i].
- Young reddish leaves and bark were used post partum or after miscarriage **to help clear the uterus and for cleansing** [Hawai'i]; with other herbs **for retained placenta** [Hawai'i]; **to cause a miscarriage** (infused).

RESPIRATORY

- **Cough** [Brazil, throughout Polynesia (bark and leaves)].
- **Phlegm in the lungs** [Brazil]; leaves "crushed and ingested" for **bronchitis** [Hawai'i]; the bark was chewed **to cause vomiting in cases of tenacious phlegm in the lungs** [Hawai'i].

URINARY

- **Edema** (root).

OTHER MEDICINAL USES

- **General debility** [Hawai'i].
- **To increase muscle mass** [Hawai'i (young buds, bark and leaves juiced)].

USE AS FOOD:

- Fruit is good fresh or chilled. Sometimes in Hawai'i it is dried or pickled. Eating too much fresh fruit can cause diarrhea.
- Fruit is sometimes cooked with cloves and served with cream as a dessert.
- In Puerto Rico mountain apple is made into red and white wines.
- Flowers in salads or in syrup. Very young shoots eaten raw or cooled as a green [Indonesia].

OTHER USES: Trunks used for posts, house rafters, ki'i (statues) carved from wood, poi boards, and bowls. Wood tends to warp [Hawai'i].
Kapa (clothing) was dyed using the root of 'ōhi'a 'ai [Hawai'i].

'Ōhi'a Ai (Mountain Apple) Local Combinations

Sore throat or the beginning of a respiratory infection: Inner bark chewed with *Musa* spp. (mai'a / banana) sap chaser.

'Ōhi'a Ai (Mountain Apple) Cross-Cultural Combinations

Please note some of the ingredients in the following combinations are toxic! Do not self-administer without the supervision of a licensed practitioner or an experienced Elder.

Deep cuts: Bark juiced with Pa'akai (Hawaiian salt) and used topically. "*The patient must exercise absolute self-control as the liquid buns its way into the flesh and nerves.*" - - Old Hawaiian Herbal

Mouth sores: The bark is juiced with *Psilotum triquetrum* (moa) & *Saccharum officinarum* (kō / sugarcane). Used as a mouthwash. Followed with *Bidens* spp. (native / ko'oko'olau) tea, poi, and fresh fish. [Old Hawai'i]

"Children afflicted with white coating of the tongue and having a tendency to become weak": With *Diospyros sandwicensis* (lama) fruit, leaves and buds. [Old Hawai'i]

General debility: The bark, buds and leaves. With *Aleurites moluccana* (kukui) flowers, onion bulbs, *Waltheria americana* ('uhaloa) aerial parts, and *Saccharum officinarum* (honua'ula / red sugarcane) (*Please Note*: There is a fourth ingredient in this old Hawaiian formula, but its identity is uncertain. The fourth ingredient is called hinahina kū kahakai. Hinahina kū kahakai is generally thought to be *Heliotropium anomalum*, but I have also heard *Artemisia australis* ('āhinahina) referred to as hinahina kū kahakai. That the ingredient might be *Artemesia australis* makes more sense from an herbalist's point of view. It could also be *Vitex rotundifolia* (pōhinahina / vitex). All three of these plants are found in coastal windward areas.) [Old Hawai'i].

Headache: 'Ōhi'a 'ai leaves topical with *Premna serratifolia* (aloalo) [Samoa].

Scrotal swelling: 'Ōhi'a 'ai leaves topical with *Eugenia corynocarpa* (young leaves), *Psychotria* spp. leaves, and oil [Samoa].

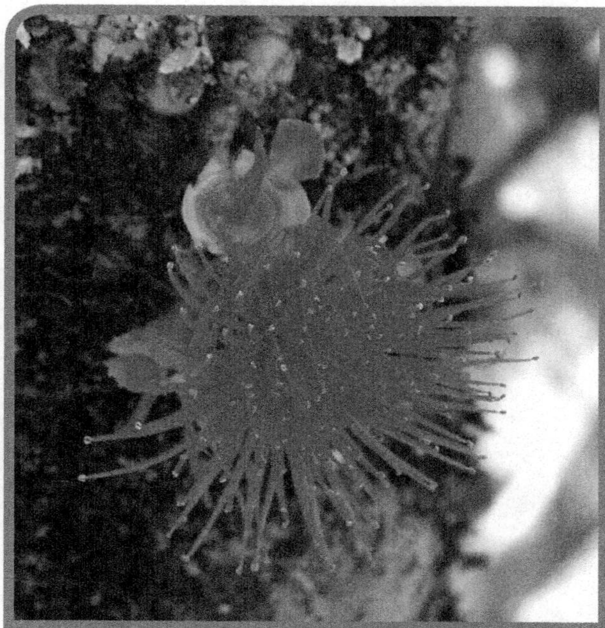

Syzygium malaccense: 'Ōhi'a 'Ai flower

RANGE: Native to India and Malaysia. Found in East Africa, Southeast Asia, and Polynesia. Cultivated in Central and South America. First brought from Tahiti to Jamaica by Captain Bligh in 1793. By 1839, 'ōhi'a 'ai was growing in a herbarium in Cambridge, Massachusetts, and by 1878 the fruit was growing in Bermuda.

HABITAT: Likes it wet 'n shady, up to 1800 feet. Can grow 50 – 60 feet.

GATHERING: Fruit picker... make it a long one. Inner bark is used fresh as needed. I've never heard of, nor seen it, stored for later use. 'Ōhi'a 'ai flowers in March / April & fruits in the summer. Sacred to Pele.

PROPAGATION & CULTIVATION: Propagate from fresh seed, germination in 2 – 4 weeks. Keep it moist. Cuttings and air layering sometimes work. Transplant cuttings 6 weeks after taking root. Transplant outdoors at 8 months. Bears fruit after 7 – 8 years. Can yield 50 - 200 lbs of fruit per tree.

RESEARCH:
Extracts inhibit *Staphylococcus aureus, Streptococcus pyogenes*, and three different fungi [Locher 1995].

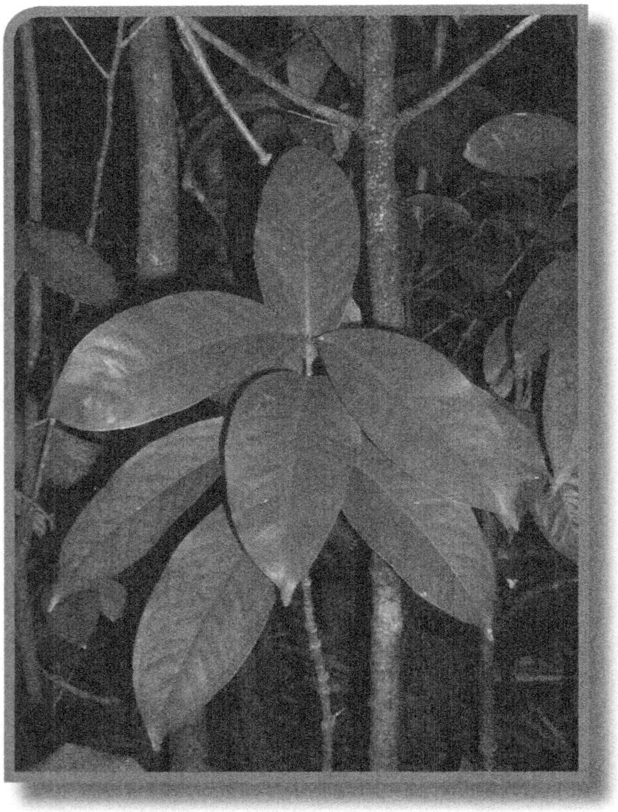

Syzygium malaccense: 'Ōhi'a 'Ai leaves.

NOTES 'N QUOTES

Hinaia'ele'ele ka malama, 'āluka ka pala a ka 'ōhi'a.
Hinaia'ele'ele is the month when
the mountain apples open everywhere.

"*... for it to rain while the sun shines, the old wise ones say that these showers are for strewing the petals of our mountain apples, preparation to the coming of the fruit - then another shower and the ripening of it. It is very poetical to us - the idea is continuity of life.*"
- - Queen Liliu'okalani, in a letter to a friend, 1901.

- There were many plants called "'ōhi'a" in old Hawai'i, and all of them were related. This plant, *Syzygium malaccense* ('ōhi'a 'ai) had another name: 'ōhi'a leo. 'Ōhi'a leo means "talking 'ōhi'a." The sister plant of *Syzygium moluccana* ('ōhi'a 'ai) was *Metrosideros polymorpha*, ('ōhi'a lehua). 'Ōhi'a lehua also had another name: 'Ōhi'a hāmau. 'Ōhi'a hāmau means "silent 'ōhi'a." This odd pairing of names was a reference to the fact that the Hawaiian bird catchers would often catch their prey among the bird's favorite food, 'ōhi'a hāmau, so it was best to be silent near those trees. But it was permissible to speak while close to 'ōhi'a leo.
- Featured in Fijian mythology.
- With the exception of a few native berries such as 'ōhelo (*Vaccinium reticulatum*), 'ōhelo kai (*Lycium sandwicese*), and 'ākala (*Rubus hawaiiensis*), the only edible fruit in pre-contact Hawai'i was 'ulu (breadfruit), mai'a (banana), niu (coconut), and 'ōhi'a 'ai (mountain apple).
- Considered sacred to (and possibly "kinolau" – manifestation of) Pele, the goddess of the volcano. 'Ōhi'a 'ai was made into ki'i (religious statues) by the ancient Hawaiians.
- Supposedly there is a seedless variety of 'ōhi'a 'ai with white flowers and white fruit called 'ōhi'a kea. I have never seen it.
- On more than one occasion, 'ōhi'a 'ai bark has turned a sore throat into a distant memory. But the bark, once tasted, will not be forgotten. The question then becomes: Which is less painful, the sore throat, or the taste of the bark?
- Speaking of memories... in spring, 'ōhi'a 'ai creates a brilliant carpet of red across the floor of the Hawaiian forest. This tree can transform a quiet walk into an unforgettable crimson memory.

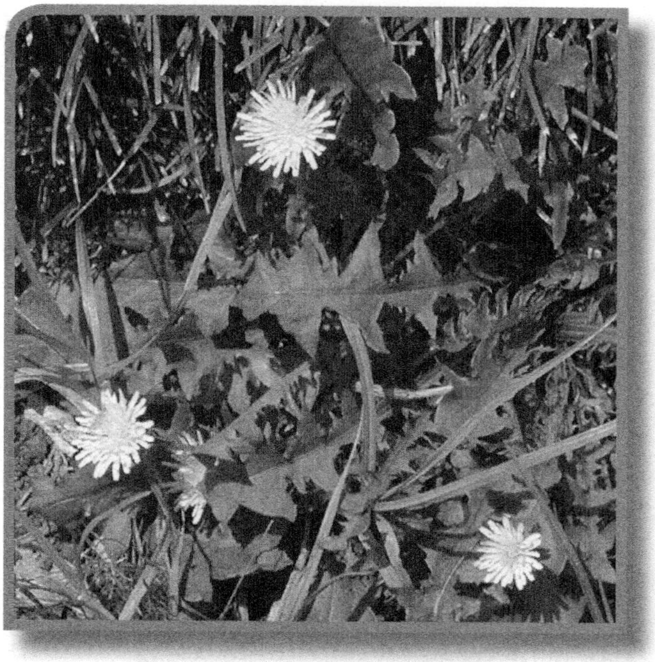

Taraxacum spp. (Laulele / Dandelion)

PLANT NAME: *Taraxacum* spp.

SYNONYMS OR SIMILARLY USED SPECIES: *T. officinale, T. albidum, T. coreanum, T. laevigatum, T. japonicum, T. mongolicum, T. magellanicum, T. platycarpum, Leontodon latiloba, Leontodon taraxacum.*

Status: Alien. Minimal pest factor.

Habitat: Where ever lawns are found.

COMMON NAMES: **Laulele**, lauhele [Hawai'i]; **pu gong ying** [China]; **dandelion** [English]; butterblume, lōwenzahn [Germany]; dent de lion, pissenlit [French]; dente de leone, soffione [Italy]; dente-de-leão [Portugese]; diente de león [Spanish]; doon-head clock [Scotland]; dughdapheni [Sanskrit]; hokoei [Japan]; mælkebøtte, løvetand [Denmark]; mniszek pospolity [Poland]; ogrāsmaskrosor, maskros [Sweden]; paardebloem [Netherland]; ugrasløvetann, løvetann [Norway]; voikukka [Finland].

PHARMACEUTICAL NAME: Herba Taraxaci.

NOMENCLATURE:
- The origins of the name "*Taraxacum*" are unclear. It is thought to possibly be from the Persian "tark hashgun" ("wild endive"), from the Persian "talkh chakok" ("bitter herb"), or from the Greek "taraxos" (disorder) and "akos" (remedy).
- "Dandelion" means "tooth of the lion," a reference to the serrated leaves.
- The French name "pissenlit" means "piss in the bed," alluding to dandelion's reputation as a diuretic.

FAMILY: Asteraceae (dandelion family).

CATEGORY: Clear heat and toxins.

PROPERTIES: Bitter, cold.

PLANT PART USED: All of it. Leaves will replace potassium loss through diuresis.

TOXICITY: The LD50 in mice is 59g / kg. [Bensky 1986]

CAUTIONS AND CONTRAINDICATIONS:
There is a single human case report of anaphylaxis after ingesting the pollens of *Taraxacum officinale* (dandelion), *Artemesia vulgaris* (mugwort), and *Salix alba* (willow) [Chivato 1996].
Caution with gall bladder problems, gastric ulcer, weak digestion, liver problems.

PREPARATION OF MEDICINE:
"*No part of the plant should be considered very potent after a year's storage.*"
- - Michael Moore
Decoction or tincture. Can also be used raw or juiced fresh.

DOSAGE: 10 - 15 grams dried herb in formulas. Up to 60 grams fresh as a single herb.

STATUS IN HAWAI'I: Alien. Pest factor is surprisingly minimal.

MERIDIAN AFFINITIES: Liver, stomach.

WESTERN FUNCTIONS REPORTED: **Aids digestion**; **alterative** [China, New Zealand, Turkey]; **analgesic** [Bella Coola, Iroquois, Papago]; **antibacterial** (juice topical, decocted internal); **antidiarrheal**; **anti-scorbutic**; **antiseptic for cystitis**; **aperient** [France, USA]; **astringent**; **bactericide**; **bitter tonic** [Potawatomi (root)]; **blood cleanser**; **blood medicine** [Cherokee, Iroquois]; **blood purifier**; **cathartic** [Mohegan]; **cholagogue** [China, Mexico, Turkey]; **clears the kidneys**; **depurative** [Native American, Spain, Turkey]; **dermatological aid**; **detoxicant** [China]; **diaphoretic** [India, Japan]; **diuretic** [Europe, India, Nepal, Turkey, USA]; **emetic** [Iroquois (roots infused)]; **eye medicine**; **febrifuge** [Japan]; **galactogogue**

[China]; **gastrointestinal aid** [Bella Coola]; **gland stimulating**; **gynecological aid**; **heals wounds** (juice topical); **hemolytic**; **hepatic** [India (root)]; **hypoglycaemic**; **intoxicant**; **kidney aid**; **lactogogue** [China, Japan]; **laxative** [Delaware, England, Iroquois, Mexico, Oklahoma, Turkey]; **love medicine**; **orthopedic aid**; **physic** [(leaves infused) Mohegan]; **promotes metabolism**; **pulmonary aid**; **regulates the stomach**; **sedative** [Cherokee]; **stimulant** (root) [India]; **stimulates the bile ducts**; **stimulates the digestive glands**; **stimulates the pancreas**; **stomachic** [China, Japan]; **strengthens the liver**; **tonic** [China, India, Japan, Mohegan, Nepal, Potawatomi, Shinnecock, USA, USSR]; **toothache remedy**; **urinary aid**; **urinary disinfectant**; **witchcraft medicine.**

TRADITIONAL CHINESE ENERGETIC FUNCTIONS (~ = extrapolated):

1) Clears heat and fire toxins.
2) Clears damp heat.
3) Breaks up congestion.
4) Strengthens the stomach.
5) Stimulates lactation.

OTHER ENERGETIC FUNCTIONS: Increases vata, reduces pitta and kapha.

Laulele (Dandelion)
Common Medicinal Uses

- As a diuretic
- Lung infections
- Liver disorders
- Poor digestion (as a bitter tonic)
- Skin disorders

Laulele (Dandelion) Cross-Cultural Medicinal Uses

BITES & STINGS

- **Bee sting**; **snake bite** [China].

COSMETIC

- Ligules (leaf appendages) are distilled in water and used topically **to "bleach" freckles**.

CARDIOVASCULAR

- **Anemia** (herb decocted) [Iroquois]; **blood medicine** [Algonquin (leaves eaten), Ojibwa (root), Rappahannock (root infused)]; **bleeding**; **poor circulation**.
- **Arteriosclerosis**; **hypertension and edema from cardiac weakness**; **heart problems** [USA]; **Used to ensure adequate potassium supply in cardiac disease** [Europe]; **chest pain** [Fox].

DERMATOLOGICAL

- **All eruptions on the surface of the body** [England]; **skin diseases** (root) [India, Mexico]; **inflammatory skin conditions.**
- **Acne**; **corns**; **liver spots** (herb infused in combination, topical) [Iroquois]; **moles**; **warts** (latex topical) [China, France, UK].
- **Dermatitis** [China]; **eczema** [England]; **psoriasis**.

DIGESTIVE

- **Atonic dyspepsia** [England]; **diseases of the stomach**; **dyspepsia** [China, Mexico, Rappahannock]; **impairment of the digestive functions**; **stomach pain** (root decocted) [Aleut (steamed leaves poulticed), Bella Coola, China]; **sluggish stomach**; **food sensitivities**; **loss of appetite** [Mexico]; **vitamin deficiency**; **weak digestion.**
- **Constipation**; **habitual constipation** [England].
- **Diarrhea**; **intestinal catarrh**; **intestinal diseases**; **intestinal inflammation**; **flatulence**.
- **Gastritis**; **gastro-intestinal disturbances**; **heartburn** (root infused) [Ojibwa].
- **Hemorrhoids**.

ENDOCRINE

- **Diabetes**, **glandular malfunctioning**, **hypoglycemia.**

HEAD AND THROAT

- **Conjunctivitis**; **dark circles and puffy eyes** (root infused in combination) [Iroquois]; **diseases of the eye**; **red**, **painful**, **and swollen eyes** [China (herb)].
- **Head pain**.
- **Mouth or pharynx inflammation**; **sore throats** [Aleut (steamed leaves poulticed); General]; **tooth decay** [Cherokee, China, Iroquois (flower stems chewed)].

HEPATIC

"*A diuretic for bile.*" - - James Snow

- **Cirrhosis**; **hepatic edema**; **hepatitis** (herb) [China, Mexico, Shaker]; **liver problems** [Colonial USA, Turkey]; **jaundice** [China, Iraq]; **liver enlargement**; **obstructions of the liver** [India (root)]; **sluggish liver function due to alcohol abuse or**

poor diet.
- **Gall bladder disorders**; **gallstones.**

INFECTION
- **Boils and abscesses** [Aleut (steamed leaves poulticed), China]; **sores caused by "bad blood"** (bark and roots decocted in combination) [Iroquois].
- **Fevers** [China].

LYMPHATIC
- **Enlarged spleen**, **malarial spleen** [Finland].
- **Scrofula** [England].

MUSCULOSKELETAL / TRAUMA
- **Arthritis**; **joint pain**; **orthopedic ailments**; **osteoarthritis**; **rheumatic diseases.**
- **Back pain** [Iroquois (root infused in combination)].
- **Bone fractures** [Tewa (poultice)]; **bruises** [USA]; **smashed testicles** [Iroquois (herb decocted, topical)]; **swelling** [China, Navajo (poultice)]; **swollen ankles**; **wounds** [China].
- **Gout**.
- **Swellings from bee stings**.

ONCOLOGY
- **Breast cancer** [Australia, China].
- **Cancer** [China, Germany, USA, Wales].
- **Esophageal cancer** [China].
- **Nose tumor** [China].
- **Skin cancers** (white sap topical).
- **Tumors** [USSR].

PSYCHOSPIRITUAL
"*It is under the dominion of Jupiter.*"
- - Nicholas Culpepper
- **Agitation** [Cherokee (herb infused)].
- **Anti-witch medicine** [Iroquois (root decocted, topical)].
- **Hypochondria**; **spring fatigue**; **mental atony**.
- **Love medicine** [Iroquois (root decocted, topical)].

REPRODUCTIVE
- **Lack of menstruation**; **menstrual cramps** [Kiowa (young leaves decocted), Papago (flowers infused)]; **premenstrual bloating**; **women's ailments**; **yeast infections**.
- **Firm, hard sores in the breasts** [China (herb)].
- **Inadequate milk supply** [China (herb decocted), (root infused in combination)].
- **Mastitis** [China (herb decocted)].
- **Speed delivery of baby** [Navajo (cold infusion)].
- **Uterine obstructions**.

RESPIRATORY
- **Bronchitis**; **inflamed mucous membranes with phlegm** [Iraq]; **swollen lungs and pain** [Iroquois (herb decocted in combination)].

URINARY
- **Chronic disorders of the kidney** (root) [India, Nepal].
- **Diseases of the bladder**; **urinary tract infection** [China (herb)].
- **Edema** (root) [England, India]; **kidney trouble and dropsy** [Iroquois (root infused in combination)].
- **Kidney stones and gravel** [England (root decocted)].

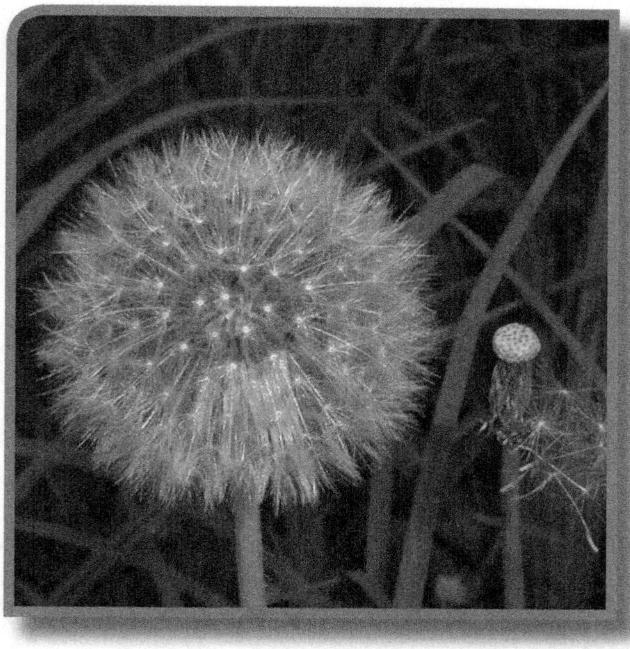

Taraxacum spp. (Laulele) seed heads

VETERINARY
"*Birds like the seeds, pigs devour the whole plant, goats eat the leaves, but sheep, cattle, and horses turn up their noses at this abundant weed.*"
- - James Duke
- **Said to increase lactation in cows. Rabbits like it as food.**

OTHER MEDICINAL USES
- **Allergies**.
- **Appendicitis** [China].
- **Chest pain when other remedies fail** (root infused) [Meskwaki].
- **General fatigue after illness or overwork**.
- **Hangover** [Europe].
- **Lipoma**.
- **Scurvy** [England].
- **Visceral diseases** (root) [India].

USE AS FOOD
"*... eat it with unleavened bread and bitter herbs...*"
- - Numbers 9.

"*You see here what virtues this common herb hath, and that is the reason the French and Dutch so often eat them in the Spring; and now if you look a little farther, you may see plainly without a pair of spectacles, that foreign physicians are not so selfish as ours are, but more communicative of the virtues of plants to people.*"
-- Nicholas Culpepper

- The leaves are universally eaten as greens or used as a potherb.
- The leaves are cooked with maple sap vinegar and sometimes combined with pork or deer meat [Menominee, Ojibwa, Potawatomi].
- Dandelion leaves are more nutritious than spinach and are a good source of vitamin C and pro-vitamin A. Leaves harvested in the spring are more bitter than those harvested in the fall. Bitter leaves can be blanched before eating if desired to reduce the bitterness.
- Dandelion sandwiches were eaten in Glencoe, Scotland to cure ulcers.
- The flowers can be dipped in batter and fried.
- The dried roots are used as a (poor) coffee substitute.
- Herbal Wine is made from fermented flowers and is used as a blood tonic.
- In Europe, dandelion wine and dandelion beer are both available.
- In England, an interesting medicinal brew is made from *Taraxacum officinale* (dandelion), *Urtica doica* (nettles), and *Rumex crispus* (yellow dock). Likely it's used for warm conditions.

OTHER USES:

- An evolutionary psychopath, dandelion releases ethylene gas, a hormone that causes nearby plant competitors to prematurely ripen and bear fruit. This stunts their growth. So if you place *Taraxacum* in a bag with unripe fruit it will speed the ripening process.
- Used as liquid plant food (leaf and root).
- Red dye is made from its roots and a yellow dye from its flowers [Native American].
- Hollow stems made into whistles [Hesquiat].
- Russian dandelion was cultivated during World War II to make a low quality rubber from the root.

CONSTITUENTS: High in vitamin C. More beta carotene than carrots.
Aesculin (leaf); ash; calcium salts (root); catortenoids (leaf); chicoric acid; chlorogenic acid; choline; chrysoeriol (leaf); cichoriin (leaf); coumarins (leaf); homotaraxasterol; hydroxycinnamic acid; inulin; iron; lecithin; levulin; luteolin (flower); luteolin 7-glucoside (flower); magnesium; manganese; monocaffeyltartaric acid; pectin; phenolic acids (root); phytosterols; potassium salts (whole plant); saponin; sesquiterpene lactones (taraxacin); silicon; sterols; sugar; tannins; taraxacerin; taraxacoside; taraxasterol; triterpenes; vitamins A, B, C, and D; zinc.

POSSIBLE DRUG INTERACTIONS: *T. mongolicum* enhances bioavailability of ciprofloxacin in rats [Zhu 1999].
Caution with pharmaceutical diuretics ~ (speculative).

Laulele (Dandelion) Local Combinations

Hepatitis and jaundice: Add *Plantago major* (laukahi / plantain) leaf, *Bidens pilosa* (kīnehi / spanish needle) herb.

Bladder infections: Add *Coix lacryma jobi* (pū'ohe'ohe / jobs tears) root, *Bidens pilosa* (kīnehi / spanish needle) herb, *Plantago major* (laukahi / plantain) seeds.

Skin disorders: Add *Oxalis* spp. ('ihi / sorrel), *Stellaria media* (chickweed).

Laulele (Dandelion) Cross-Cultural Combinations

Breast cancer: With *Smilax* spp. (sarsaparilla), *Trifolium pratense* (red clover), *Arcticum lappa* (burdock) [Christopher Hobbs].

Hemorrhoids: With *Plantago lanceolata* (long-leaved plantain), Polypody fern root, *Capsella bursa-pastoris* (shepherds purse), and *Rheum palmatum* (rhubarb) tincture internal. Celandine ointment is also administered topically [England].

Colitis: With *Hypericum perforatum* (st. johns wort), *Melissa officinalis* (lemon balm), *Calendula officinalis*, and *Foeniculum vulgare* (fennel) [Chakurski 1981].

"**Biliousness and dizziness**": With *Marrubium vulgare* (black horehound), *Acorus calamus* (sweet flag) rhizome, and "mountain flax" [England].

Arthritis: With *Apium graveolens* (celery) seed [Chris Hobbs].

Gall stones: With *Petroselinum crispum* (parsley) root, balm herb, *Zingiber officinale* ('awapuhi pākē / ginger), *Glycyrrhiza* spp. (licorice) root [England].

Jaundice in children: With *Zingiber officinale* ('awapuhi pākē / ginger), *Carum carvi* (caraway) seed, *Cinnamomum cassia* (cinnamon) bark, *Cassia* *senna* (senna) leaves [England].

Boils: *Taraxacum mongolicum* is sometimes combined with one or more of the following: *Forsythia suspensa* (lian qiao), *Chrysanthemum indicum* (ye ju hua), *Desmodium* spp. (jin qian cao), *Lonicera japonica* (jin yin hua / honeysuckle) flowers [China].

Urinary tract infection: With *Imperata cylindrica* (bai mao gen) and *Desmodium* spp. (jin qian cao) [China].

Lung abscess: With *Benincasa hispida* (dong gua ren) seeds and *Houttuynia cordata* (yu xing cao) [China].

Swollen lymph glands: With *Prunella vulgaris* (xia ku cao / self heal) [China].

Jaundice and hepatitis: Decocted with *Podophylum.*

Bad bruising: With dough as a poultice [Tewa].

RANGE: Everywhere in the Northern Hemisphere. Native to Greece. Introduced by European settlers to North America as food for bees.

GATHERING: Dig around it. Try to find areas unpolluted with chemicals. (Good luck...) 2 year-old cultivated roots are harvested in autumn.

PROPAGATION & CULTIVATION: Do not propagate in Hawai'i.

Propagation is by seed. Germinates in 14 days. Best cultivated in well-turned soil for ease of removal. Two-year-old roots are best, with non-forked taproot. If you don't cut the flower heads off before they go to seed your neighbors will hate you.

Dandelion is apomictic (reproduces non-sexually), so seeds are often clones of the parent.

RESEARCH:

- Immune modulating in mice with burns [Luo 1993].
- Constituents of *Taraxacum* spp. are immune potentiating and anticarcinogenic in mice [Jeong 1991; Takasaki (I) 1999; Takasaki (II) 1999]. However, effects on tumor necrosis factor and interleukin-1 are inconclusive [Kim 2000; Koo 2004]. Taraxinic acid, a constituent of *Taraxacum coreanum*, may inhibit human leukemia cells in vitro [Choi 2002].
- *Taraxacum mongolicum* is antimicrobial against *Bacillus dysenteriae, Corynebacterium diphtheriae,* ECHO virus, *Leptospira, Meningococci, Mycobacterium tuberculosis, Neisseria meningitidis, Pneumococci, Pseudomonas aeruginosa, Shigella* spp., *Staphylococcus aureus,* and *Streptococcus pneumoniae* [Bensky 1986] *Taraxacum mongolicum* is antiviral in vitro against type 1 *Herpes simplex* virus [Zhang 1990].
- A constituent of *Taraxacum platycarpum* has anti-allergic properties [Cheong 1998].
- Water extractions of dandelion flowers are antioxidant [Hu 2003].
- Extracts increase insulin secretion in vitro [Hussain 2004].
- A constituent of *Taraxacum platycarpum* is anticoagulant [Yun 2002].

First recorded use was in China in the 7th century, and in Arabian medical journals in the 10th century. In the West, the earliest reference found is by Hieronymus Bock in 1543. *Taraxacum* was established as a drug in Europe in the 16th Century.

NOTES 'N QUOTES

"*It is colde, but drieth more and doth withall clense and open by reason of the bitterness which it hath joined with it...*"- - John Gerard, 1597

- *Taraxacum officinale* (the name for the common dandelion) is not actually a single species but an aggregate of many different species.
- Because of its' high potassium content, dandelion replaces the potassium normally lost with herbs that promote urination.
- This and *Plantago* spp. (laukahi) are two of the most versatile plant medicines we have. Laulele is a great secondary herb for a multitude of conditions. Like laukahi, it does many things reasonably well.

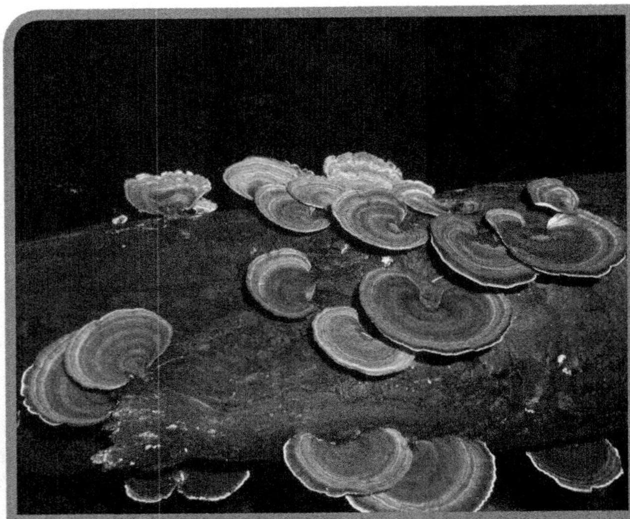

Trametes versicolor (Yun Zhi / Turkey Tails)

PLANT NAME: *Trametes versicolor.*

OTHER NAMES: *Boletus versicolor, Coriolus versicolor, Coriolus zonztus, Polyporus versicolor, Polystictus versicolor.*

COMMON NAMES: **Yun zhi** ("cloud mushroom") [China]; **turkey tails** [English]; kawaratake ("mushroom by the river") [Japan].

Status: Unknown. Low pest factor.

NOMENCLATURE: The word "*Trametes*" means skinny, and "*versicolor*" means multi-colored.

Habitat: Wet and shady

FAMILY: Polyporaceae.

CATEGORY: Tonify qi ~.

PROPERTIES: Sweet and slightly warm.

PLANT PART USED: Fruiting body

TOXICITY: Very safe. The reported oral LD5O of PSP is 10.0 gm / kg.

CAUTIONS AND CONTRAINDICATIONS: Not with gout.

PREPARATION OF MEDICINE: Dried, powdered and steeped, or taken in capsules. Long slow heating such as a crock-pot works well. Normal infusion or decoction will work though, as well as tincturing. The polysaccharides in yun zhi are bound to chitin in the fruiting body. Heat breaks down the chitin and releases the medicinal value.

DOSAGE: Powder in tea up to 60 g per day. Powder in capsules up to 5 grams per day. PSP dosage: 1 gram per day.

MERIDIAN AFFINITIES: Heart, Spleen.

WESTERN FUNCTIONS REPORTED: **Antibacterial**; **antimalarial**; **antimicrobial**; **antineoplastic**; **antioxidant**; **antitumor**; **antiviral**; **diuretic**; **immune enhancer**; **immunomodulating**; **mild tranquilizer**; **strengthens the physique**.

TRADITIONAL CHINESE ENERGETIC FUNCTIONS (~ = extrapolated):

1) Dispels damp.
2) Reduces phlegm.
3) Tonifies qi.
4) "Invigorates the spirit".
5) Stops cough.

Yun Zhi (Turkey Tails) Common Medicinal Uses

- Low energy
- Cancer
- Low Immune Function

Yun Zhi (Turkey Tails) Cross-Cultural Medicinal Uses

DERMATOLOGICAL

- **Impetigo**, **ring-worm** [Mexico].

DIGESTIVE

- **Digestive tract infection** [China].

HEPATIC

- **Hepatitis** (decocted) [China, Japan]; **chronic active hepatitis** [China].

INFECTION

- **Bacterial and viral infections** [China].

ONCOLOGY

- **Tumors** [China].
- **Adenosarcoma, carcinoma, fibrosarcoma, leukemia, mastocytoma, melanoma, plasmacytoma, sarcoma.**
- **Breast cancer.**
- **Lung cancer.**
- **Colon cancer.**

RESPIRATORY

- **Respiratory infections** (decocted) [China, Japan].

URINARY

- **Urinary tract infection** [China].

OTHER MEDICINAL USES

- **Immune weakness, fatigue** [China].

USE AS FOOD: Shelf fungi are technically not mushrooms and most are edible and nontoxic. *Trametes* is best used as a broth, as it is quite chewy.

CONSTITUENTS: Protein-bound polysaccharides (glucans), PSP (Polysaccharopeptide), PSK (Polysaccharide K), hydroxymethylquinoline, bioactive plant sterols (beta-sitosterol), provitamin D-2 (ergosterol).

POSSIBLE DRUG INTERACTIONS: PSK can increase survival time and potentiate numerous chemotherapeutic agents such as 5-fluorouracil, 6-mercaptopurine, cyclophosphamide, ftorafur, mitomycin C, and vincristine [Iino 1995, Mitomi 1992].

Yun Zhi (Turkey Tails) Local Combinations

Low immune function: Add *Morinda citrifolia* (noni), *Centella asiatica* (pohe kula / gotu kola) and *Auricularia auricula* (pepeiao).
Chronic bronchitis: Add *Usnea* spp. ('umi koa) and *Zingiber officinale* (ginger / 'awapuhi pākē).

RANGE: Asia, North America, and Europe.

HABITAT: Likes it wet and shady. Often seen growing on rotting *Aleurites moluccana* (kukui) logs in Hawai'i.

RESEARCH:

- PSK and chemotherapy increased survival rates in colonrectal cancer [Torisu 1990, Mitomi 1992], gastric cancer [Nakazato 1994], and leukemia [Nagao 1981] as compared to chemotherapy alone. Proper administration of PSK reduces the incidence of metastatic tumors in lab animals [Ebina 1989]. This may be through the modulation of immune response [Habelhah 1998(a), 1998(b); Matsunaga 1986; Oguchi 1986] and in conjunction with IL-2 [Sakamaki 1992]. It is directly mediated through the lymphatic system [Ebina 1989]. PSK decreases oxidative stress [Kobayashi 1994], boosts NK (natural killer) activity in rats [Kobayashi 1993] and induces interferon in mice at up to eight times the levels of controls [Li 1990].
- PSP (Polysaccharide-Peptide) has significantly extended five-year cancer survival and increased quality of life in double blind trials [Kidd 2000].
- Ethanol extracts of *Trametes* may reduce androgen sensitive prostate cancer cells and PSA levels [Hsieh 2001].
- PSK is anti fungal against *Candida albicans* in mice, probably through the boosting of immune function [Ohmura 2003].
- PSK boosts antiviral and antibacterial immunity in tumor bearing mice [Taniguchi 1984; Tsuru 1984(a), 1984(b)].
- *Trametes* spp. may be liver protective [Farghali 1998].
- Potent inhibitor of recombinant HIV-1 reverse transcriptase [Collins 1997].
- Analgesic in mice [Ng 1997].

NOTES 'N QUOTES

- In 1987, Japan spent 25% of its' national expenditure of anti cancer medication on PSK.
- *Trametes versicolor* is the most common species of the family Polyporaceae and one of the most beautiful medicines in the Hawaiian forest. I have seen huge kukui trees, like fallen warriors, reincarnating into hundreds of these marvelous fungi. Sometimes I am so impressed by their beauty that I am unwilling to harvest them and will search for more humble specimens. Dry and rubbery to the touch, they are a powerful addition to any herbal pharmacy.

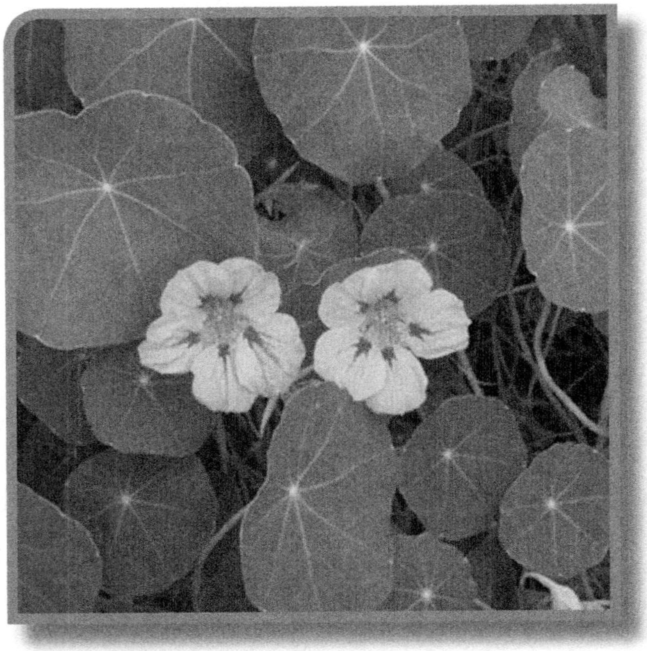

Tropaeolum majus (Pohe Haole / Nasturtium)

PLANT NAME: *Tropaeolum majus* L.

COMMON NAMES: **Pohe haole** [Hawai'i]; **nasturtium**, [USA]; han lian hua, jin lian hua, chin-lien-hua [China]; blomkarse, blomsterkarse [Norway]; blomsterkarse, landløber, tallerkensmækker, tropæolum [Denmark]; kapuzinerkresse [Germany]; masteruerzo, capuchina, pajarilla, pajarito [Bolivia]; nasturcja, nasturcja wieksza [Poland]; taxsawl, alpincu, thejsau yuyu, mallau [Aymara]; tijsaw thejsawi, chiri chiri [Quechua]; indian cress [England].

Status: Alien. Marginal pest factor.

Habitat: Sunny, built up areas.

NOMENCLATURE: The name *Tropaeolum* comes from the Greek tropaion, which means trophy. *Tropaeolum* is said to have sprouted from the spilled blood of a Trojan warrior. The round leaf was his shield and the flower was his helmet. The English common name "nasturtium" comes from "nasus tortus" (a twisted nose) and is given because of its pungent odor.

FAMILY: Tropaeolaceae.

CATEGORY: Clear heat and toxins ~.

PROPERTIES: Bitter, pungent. Cool.
PLANT PART USED: Aerial parts.

TOXICITY: Acute toxic effects in mice were observed at 200 mg / kg i.p. [Pintao 1995]

CAUTIONS AND CONTRAINDICATIONS: Sensitive stomachs may be irritated. Eating too much may cause vomiting. Not with GI ulcers or kidney disease. Not for infants or small children. Care should be taken in handling: may cause blisters.

PREPARATION OF MEDICINE: Leaves infused.

DOSAGE:

Internal

- 10-15 grams fresh in combination.
- As a single herb use 2 tsp. of fresh leaves in 1 cup boiling water. Steep 10-15 minutes. Take 2-3x a day.

Topical

- For athlete's foot, infuse 2 cups of leaves in 4 cups of boiling water for 15 minutes. Strain. Add 2 gallons of warm water. Soak feet for 2 weeks, 1 / 2 hour a day.
- For bacterial infections infuse 1 cup of leaves to 2 cups of boiling water.

MERIDIAN AFFINITIES: Lung, stomach, spleen ~.

WESTERN FUNCTIONS REPORTED: **Seeds are purgative. Antibacterial** (essential oil); **antibiotic** [Portugal, also essential oil); **anti-microbial**; **antimycotic** (essential oil); **antineoplastic**; **antisceptic**; **antiscorbutic** [Portugal]; **antispasmodic** [Portugal]; **antiviral** (essential oil); **aphrodisiac**; **bactericide**; **bacteriostatic**; **blood cleanser**; **clears phlegm**; **demulcent**; **depurative** [Turkey]; **digestive problems**; **diuretic** [Turkey]; **emmenagogue** [Haiti, Turkey]; **expectorant** [Turkey]; **fungicide**; **improving appetite**; **internal or external disinfectant**; **invigorates digestion**; **laxative** [Iraq, Turkey]; **promotes blood cells**; **promotes digestion**; **purgative**; **reduces mucus**; **rejuvenative**; **removes respiratory congestion**; **respiratory infections**; **rubifacient**; **seeds eliminate toxins through the bowels and kidneys**; **stimulant for hair growth** [Portugal]; **stimulates secretion of digestive enzymes**; **stimulates the appetite**; **tonic for weak digestion**; **urinary tract infections**; **very antimycotic** (topically); **virostatic**; **vulnerary**.

TRADITIONAL CHINESE ENERGETIC FUNCTIONS (~ = extrapolated):

1) Clears heat and toxins.
2) Cools blood and stops bleeding.

Pohe Haole (Nasturtium)
Common Medicinal Uses

- **Bronchitis with irritation, yellow phlegm**
- **Urinary infections**
- **Topical for bacterial and fungal infections**

Pohe Haole (Nasturtium) Cross-Cultural Medicinal Uses

COSMETIC
- **Hair rinse**.

DERMATOLOGICAL
- **Itching**, **skin fungi** (topically), **ringworm**, **tinia**, **fungus in fingernails** [Mexico].
- **Skin infections with "fierce toxins," sores** [China, General]; **skin wounds** [Peru]; used as an **antiseptic wash**.

DIGESTIVE
- **Low appetite**, **weak digestion**.

HEAD AND THROAT
- **Opthalmic conditions**; **opthalmologic infections** (internal). The Chinese use this topically for **red, swollen, and painful eyes**. (Do not try this at home!)
- In India, the leaves are used topically **to clean the gums**.
- **Chronic throat problems**; **thrush**.

INFECTION
- **Antiseptic wash** (leaves infused).
- **Any bacterial infection** (specific for lungs, leaves infused).
- **Candida**; **fungal infections** (infusion as foot bath).
- **Fever**.

LYMPHATIC
- **Scrofula** (lymph TB, juiced, internal)

MUSCULOSKELETAL / TRAUMA
- **Minor cuts and scratches** [Quechua (leaves poulticed)].
- **Wounds**; **wound healing**.

ONCOLOGY
- **Cancer** [Mexico].

PSYCHOSPIRITUAL
- **Stimulant** [Mexico].

REPRODUCTIVE
- **Infections of the female reproductive organs**.
- **Menstrual problems** [Quechua (leaves)]

RESPIRATORY
- **Bronchitis**, **chest plaster for coughs**, **influenza**, **influenzal pneumonia. Respiratory problems** [Mexico, Quechua (leaves)].
- **Coughs**, **common cold and the flu** [Quechua (leaves)].
- **Nasal and bronchial congestion** (leaves infused).

URINARY
- **Urogenital problems**, **urinary tract infections**, **stones.**

OTHER MEDICINAL USES
- **Inflammation**.
- **Scurvy** [Mexico, Spain, Turkey].

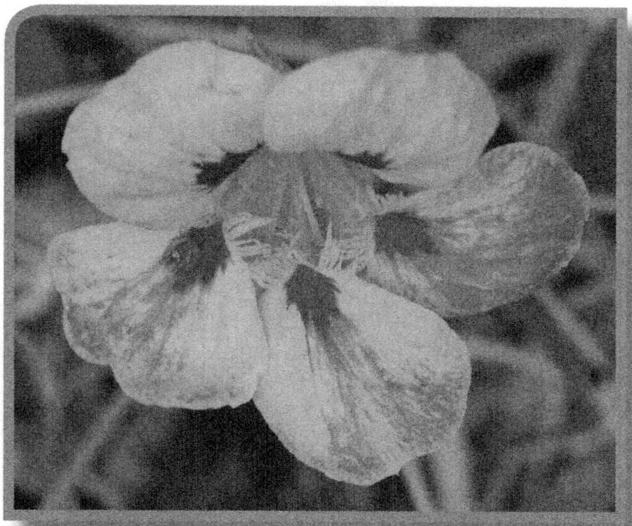

Tropaeolum majus: Pohe Haole flower

USE AS FOOD:
- The fresh flowers are used in salads as a garnish and "stimulant." The ground seeds were used as a pepper substitute during World War II. Young leaves can also be added to salads.
- Pickle flower buds in white wine vinegar, sugar, and salt for 3 weeks as a substitute for capers.
- Plants grown in the shade have a milder taste.

ESSENTIAL OIL: Contains mustard oil. Disinfectant.

CONSTITUENTS: Spilanthol, myrosin (an enzyme), oxalic acid, vitamin C (leaves), glucosinolates (a mustard-oil glycoside), glycotropeoline, iodine.

Pohe Haole (Nasturtium) Cross-Cultural Combinations

For thrush: With *Tabebuia impetiginosa* (pau d'arco).

RANGE: Hawai'i, North and South America, Europe

HABITAT: Native to Peru. Likes sunny built up areas.

GATHERING: Straight from the garden. Young plants are stronger. If gathering in large amounts use gloves.

RESEARCH:
- Extracts reduce blood clotting [de Medeiros 2000].
- *Tropaeolum tuberosum* is a related species with an edible tuber from in the Andes. It is reported to be an anti-aphrodisiac, either through the reduction of testosterone, or through its estrogenic activity. Animal studies have failed to confirm any effect on male fertility, only on libido [Johns 1982].
- In vitro cytotoxicity has been reported against ovarian carcinoma, human lung tumor, and leukemia [Pintao 1995].

NOTES 'N QUOTES

"*Shield-like Nasturtium, too, confusedly spread,*
with intermingling trefoil fills each bed-
once graceful youths, this last a Grecian swain,
The first an huntsman on the Trojan plain."
- - PAUL DE RAPIN (1661-1725)

- Indigenous to Peru. The original nasturtiums grown by the Quechua Indians had yellow flowers. The Conquistadors brought *Tropaeolum majus* to Spain from Peru in the sixteenth century. It reached herbalist John Gerard by the 1590s, and was brought to central Europe by Bewerning in 1684 as food and medicine.
- Nasturtiums were grown at Thomas Jefferson's home, Monticello, and in the royal gardens of France.
- On hot summer days the nasturtium flower can emit sparks. These may be caused by phosphoric acid.
- The nasturtium flower represents patriotism.
- The classification of nasturtium is one of those interesting examples of Chinese pragmatism. Although pohe haole tastes "warm," because it clinically clears heat, it is classified as "cool."

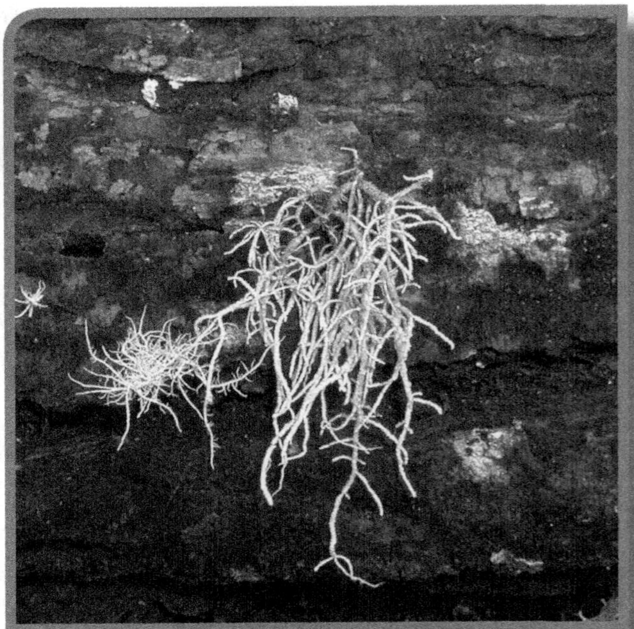

Usnea spp. ('Umi Koa)

PLANT NAME: *Usnea* spp.

SIMILARLY USED SPECIES: *U. barbata, U. ceratina, U. dasypoga, U. florida, U. hirta, U. filipendula, U. longissima*

COMMON NAMES: **'Umi koa** ("beard of koa"), limu 'o ke kuahiwi ("seaweed of the mountain") [Hawai'i]; **song lo** [China]; **old man's beard** [USA]; chan wiziye ("spirit of the north wind") [Lakota]; janggut tok adam ("adam's beard"), rumput angin ("air grass"), tahi angin ("excrement of air") [Malaysia].

Status: Unknown.

Habitat: Old growth trees in cool areas.

FAMILY: *Usneaceae.*

CATEGORY: Cool herbs that transform hot phlegm.

PROPERTIES: Bitter sweet neutral.

LICHEN PART USED: All of it

TOXICITY: None noted when using the whole lichen.
- Oral administration of hydro-alcoholic (tincture) extract has no mortality at 32g / kg. The acute LD50 for hydro-alcoholic extracts (tinctures) of *U. barbata* and *U. hirta* are as follows: *U. barbata* intraperitoneal: 22.53g (of lichen) / kg; *U. hirta* intraperitoneal: 21.02g (of lichen) / kg; *U. barbata* intravenous: 7.43g (of lichen) / kg; *U. hirta* intravenous: 4.52g (of lichen) / kg [Dobrescu 1993].
- Usnic acid in its pure extracted form at high dos-

es may be liver toxic to rats, [Ingolfsdottir 2002; Pramyothin 2004] causing damage from oxidative stress [Han 2004, Pramyothin 2004], although *Usnea* spp. also have antioxidant effects in mice.

CAUTIONS AND CONTRAINDICATIONS: Not in pregnancy. May cause contact dermatitis in topical use, discontinue if rash develops [Mitchell 1965; Goncalo 1987]. If used in autoimmune conditions, monitor immune status carefully.

PREPARATION OF MEDICINE: Because usnic acid is not water soluble, the tincture is preferred (1:3, 70% alcohol), or you can decoct. A crock pot works well. *Usnea* can also be made into a salve.

DOSAGE: 10 grams in combination, or powdered in a capsule. Tincture: 3-4 ml 3 times per day. For tuberculosis, tincture, 2-7 droppersful 3 times per day for 6 months. For acute bacterial infections, *Usnea* can be taken every 2 hours.
100 mg in capsules three times a day.

WESTERN FUNCTIONS REPORTED: **Antibacterial**; **antibiotic**; **antifungal**; **antiparasitic**; **antiseptic**; as **bitters**; **dermatological aid**; **eupeptic**; **general wound healer**.

TRADITIONAL CHINESE ENERGETIC FUNCTIONS (~ = extrapolated):

1) Opens the chest~, cleanses the lungs, transforms phlegm~.
2) Removes damp heat.
3) Invigorates blood~.
4) Clears heat and toxins.
5) Clears deficiency heat~, stops bleeding.

'Umi Koa (Usnea)
Common Medicinal Uses

- **Lung infections**
- **Bacterial infections**

'Umi Koa (Usnea) Cross-Cultural Medicinal Uses

COSMETIC

- **Baldness** [Ancient Rome].

DERMATOLOGICAL

- **Skin conditions** [Nitinaht].
- **Fungal infections**, **athlete's foot**, **ringworm** [Native American].

DIGESTIVE

- **Dysentery** [Native American].
- **Indigestion**; **poor digestion** [Italy].

HEAD AND THROAT

- **Headache** [China].
- **Sinus infections** [Native American].
- **Sore throat**.
- **Eye inflammation** [China].

IMMUNITY

- **Lupus** [Native American].

INFECTION

- Reportedly used over 3,000 years ago in ancient Egypt, Greece, and China to treat **infections**.
- **Abscesses**, **boils**, **carbuncles**, **bacterial infections** [China, Kiowa, Native American].
- ***Candida albicans.***
- **Leprosy** [Malaysia].

LYMPHATIC

- **Lymph tuberculosis** [China].

MUSCULOSKELETAL / TRAUMA

- **Bleeding from wounds** [China]; **wounds** [Soviet Union (*U. filipendula* powdered topical)].
- **Toxic snakebite** [China].

ONCOLOGY

- **Maligant tumors** [Chile].

PARASITES

- **Malaria** [China].

REPRODUCTIVE

- **Problems in the uterus** [Ancient Rome]; **abnormal uterine bleeding** [China]; **delayed menstruation** [Korea, Middle East].
- Diluted in a small amount of water for external application on the skin or for a vaginal douche. Douched for **trichomoniasis and yeast infections** [Native American]; **chlamydia**.
- **Vaginal discharge** [China].
- **Mastitis** [Native American].
- **Female sanitary napkins** [Nitinaht (*U. longissima*)].
- **Post partum as a potherb** (?) [Malaysia].

RESPIRATORY

- **Used to boost immunity in common cold, pleurisy, pneumonia, & tuberculosis.**
- **Common cold, flu** [China, Malaysia, Native American]; **cough** [Ancient Rome, China, Malaysia]. *Usnea* also contains mucilage, which can soothe an **irritated cough**.
- **Profuse phlegm, bronchitis** [Ancient Rome, Native American, China].
- **Pleurisy, pneumonia** [Native American].
- **Tuberculosis** [Native American].

URINARY

- **Urinary tract infections** [Native American].

OTHER MEDICINAL USES

- **Made into bandages** [Nitinaht].

OTHER USES: Made into bandages, diapers and sanitary napkins [Nitinaht tribe].

- Because of its ability to absorb heavy metals and pollutants, *Usnea* is used as a biomonitor to measure air pollution [Poblet 1997; Takani 2002], although its accuracy is in question [Carreras 2002]. It may only be valid for monitoring certain pollutants [Rossbach 1999]. It can also be used as a salt monitor [Figueira 2002].

'Umi Koa (Usnea) Local Combinations

Bronchitis: Add, *Musa* spp. (mai'a / banana) sap, *Waltheria americana* ('uhaloa) root cortex, and *Plantago* spp. (laukahi / plantain).

'Umi Koa (Usnea) Cross-Cultural Combinations

Bacterial infections: With *Lomatium.*

RANGE: Every continent except Australia.

GATHERING:

- *Usnea* is not actually a plant but a lichen, which is part algae and part fungus. A good way to identify this lichen is to pull it apart. Medicinal *Usnea* has a soft thread-like "core" and is always round.
- *Usnea* is becoming rare and should only be picked in genuine need. Only take what you will use! Take it from downed branches if possible. *Usnea* often grows on old-growth trees and it is imperative to not over-harvest. Avoid gathering *Usnea* from heavily polluted areas, as it might absorb heavy metals from the air. See *Other Uses* above.

RESEARCH:

Bacterial

- Most of the research points to usnic acid being an effective antibacterial against gram-positive bacteria; [Cocchietto 2002; Garcia, 1999], although one study showed it to be also antibacterial against gram-negative bacteria [Rowe 1989]. Its effect on gram-positive bacteria may be due to secondary metabolites of lichens [Lauterwein 1995]. Usnic acid may prevent bio-film colonization by *Staphylococcus aureus*, *Enterococcus faecalis*, and *Enterococcus faecium* on artificial implant devices [Francolini 2004].
- An usnic acid preparation can inhibit *Streptococcus mutans* in the oral cavity without altering the normal bacterial equilibrium of the mouth [Ghione 1988].

Viral

- Usnic acid inhibits Epstein-Barr virus activation [Yamamoto 1995] and is a potent inhibitor of mouse polyomavirus because of its ability to inhibit RNA transcription [Campanella 2002].
- Extracts of *Usnea complanta* are antiviral in vitro against *Herpes simplex* virus [Vijayan 2004].
- Usnic acid is used topically with zinc sulfate to prevent post-surgical recurrence of human Papilloma virus [Scirpa 1999].

Parasites

- Usnic acid is anti-parasitic against *Leishmania amazonensis* when applied intra-lesionally but not orally or subcutaneously in mice [Fournet 1997]. It has a strong effect against *Trichomonas vaginalis* in vitro [Wu 1995].

Cancer

- Some research points to *Usnea* spp. extracts being only mildly antineoplastic [Proska 1999], while others report stronger effects [Bezivin 2004; Campanella 2002]. Extracts of *U. fasciata* containing the polysaccharide raffinose inhibited close to 90% of sarcoma 180 and Ehrlich tumor cells [Periera 1994].

Fever, Pain & Inflammation

- Usnic acid is anti-inflammatory in lab animals for both acute and chronic conditions [Vijayakumar 2000]. It is analgesic and reduces induced fever in mice [Okuyama 1995].
- It is reportedly comparable to hydrocortisone and hemisuccinate phenylbutazone as an anti-inflammatory; noraminophenazone as an analgesic; and aminophenazone as an anti-pyretic [Dobrescu

1993].

- The compounds in *U. diffracta* responsible for its antipyretic and analgesic effects in mice appear to be diffractaic and usnic acids [Okuyama 1995].
- Usnic acid can function as a UVB light filter [Rancan 2002].

Antioxidant Functions

- Research results for *U. longissima* as an antioxidant range from mild [Bian 2002], to potent [Odabasoglu 2004]. Different species may have varying amounts of antioxidant potential [Caviglia 2001].

NOTES 'N QUOTES

- Used as medicine in Ancient Egypt, Rome, Greece, and China since before the time of Christ. The use of *Usnea* was documented in "The Formulary of Al-kindi", A.D. 850
- In Native American traditions *Usnea* represents the north and maintains the "lungs" of Planet Earth. In those traditions *Usnea* has a sacred primeval relationship with the trees, helping to protect them against infections.
- *Usnea* was historically used as a bitter tonic.
- One of our best plants for chronic respiratory problems. Because it does well as a tincture, it is often taken separately from the rest of an herbal formula.

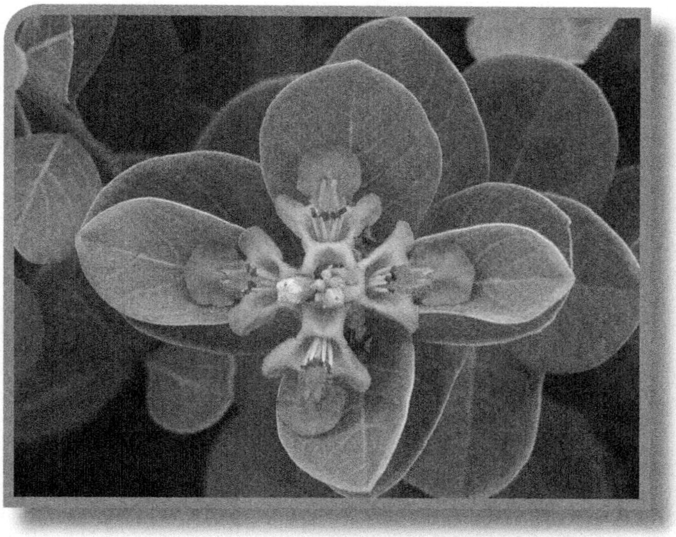

Vitex rotundifolia (Pōhinahina / Beach Vitex)

PLANT NAME: *Vitex rotundifolia* L. fil.

SIMILARLY USED SPECIES: *V. trifolia* L.

COMMON NAMES: **Pōhinahina**, kolokolo kahakai [Hawai'i]; **man jing zi**, man ching tzu [China]; **beach vitex** [English]; khon-thee so thale [Thailand]; lagundiang dagat [Philipines (Tagalog)]; lala tahi (*V. trifolia*) [Tonga]; mankeishi [Japan]; namulega ("mosquito") (*V. trifolia*) [Samoa]; rara (*V. trifolia*) [Cook Islands]; tawari [Aymara].

Status: Indigenous.

Habitat: Salty dry areas. To 30'.

NOMENCLATURE:
- *Vitex* comes from the Latin viere: to twist, referring to the twisting stems of some *Vitex* spp.
- Rotundifolia means, "round leaved."
- The Hawaiian name kolokolo kahakai means "beach creeper" and hinahina means "silver."
- Man jing means "trailing" in Chinese, and zi means "seed," the part used in Chinese medicine.

FAMILY: Verbenaceae (vervain family).

CATEGORY: Cool Acrid Release the Exterior.

PROPERTIES: Bitter, acrid, neutral to cold.

PLANT PART USED: Fruit and leaves.

CAUTIONS AND CONTRAINDICATIONS: Can cause respiratory irritation when trimmed as a hedge.

ENERGETIC CAUTIONS: Not with yin or blood deficiency. Traditionally not used with gypsum (shi gao) or *Aconitum carmichaeli* (wu tou).

PREPARATION OF MEDICINE: Decoct. Tincture the seeds [1:5, 65% alcohol].

DOSAGE: 3-15 grams.

STATUS IN HAWAI'I: Indigenous.

MERIDIAN AFFINITIES: Lung, urinary bladder, liver, stomach.

WESTERN FUNCTIONS REPORTED: **Alterative**; **analgesic**; **anhydrotic**; **anodyne** [India]; **antipyretic**; **antiseptic** [India (leaves)]; **bactericide**; **cephalic** (fruit); **demulcent**; **diaphoretic** [Samoa (*V. trifolia* bark and leaves)]; **diuretic** [India]; **emmenagogue** (fruit) [India]; **estrogenic**; **expectorant** [Thailand (leaf)]; **febrifuge** [India (powdered leaves)]; **insect repellant**; **nervine** (fruit); **sedative**; **stimulates pituitary gland function**; **tonic.**

TRADITIONAL CHINESE ENERGETIC FUNCTIONS (~ = extrapolated):

1) Disperses wind heat.
2) Cleanses the eyes and head.

Pōhinahina (Beach Vitex)
Common Medicinal Uses

- **PMS**
- **Eye inflammation**
- **Headache**
- **Back and joint pain**

Pōhinahina (Beach Vitex) Cross-Cultural Medicinal Uses

COSMETIC

- **Hair-tonic**.
- **Promotes the growth of the beard** [China (fruit)].

DERMATOLOGICAL

- **Itching** [Thailand (topical)].
- **Skin disease** [Thailand (topical)].
- **Puerperium**.

DIGESTIVE

- **Enterosis**.
- **Stomach ache** [Tonga (*V. trifolia*)].

HEAD AND THROAT

- **Brain disease** [Samoa (stems)].
- **Eye pain, redness and swelling, floaters** [China]; **tearing** [China]; **night blindness** [China].
- **Head congestion, heaviness** [China]; **migraine headache** [China]; **headache from "wind heat"** [China].
- **Toothache** [Futuna (*V. trifolia* infused)].

HEPATIC

- **Liver disease** [Thailand (root)].

INFECTION

- **Intermittent fever with scanty urine** [India (infused)].
- **Fever** (*V. trifolia*) [Malaya (root decocted), Samoa (bark, leaves)].

LYMPHATIC

- **Enlarged spleen** [India (infused)].

MUSCULOSKELETAL / TRAUMA

- **Arthritis** [Hawai'i]; **rheumatic conditions** [Bolivia, India (leaves topical)]; **cramping and numbness in the limbs** [China (fruit)].
- **Back pain** [Hawai'i]; **myalgia** [China (fruit)].
- **Sprains, contusions** [China (decocted or in wine, internal and topical), India (leaves topical)]; **fractures** [Fiji (leaves)]; **swelling** [Samoa (leaves)].
- **Swollen feet** [Hawai'i]; **burning sensation in the feet** ("quemaduras del pic o ignipedites") [Philippines (heated leaves topical)].

NEUROLOGICAL

- **Dizziness** [China].
- **Neuralgia** [China (fruit)].

ONCOLOGY

- **Breast cancer** [China (fruit)].
- **Cancer**.
- **Nose tumors**.

PEDIATRIC

- **Mouth infections in infants** [Tonga (*V. trifolia* leaves infused)].

PSYCHOSPIRITUAL

- **Nervous conditions** [Bolivia].

REPRODUCTIVE

- **Menopausal problems.**
- **PMS.**
- **Lack of menses.**
- **Post partum** [Cook Islands (*V. trifolia* as a bath), Malaya (root decocted, internal)].

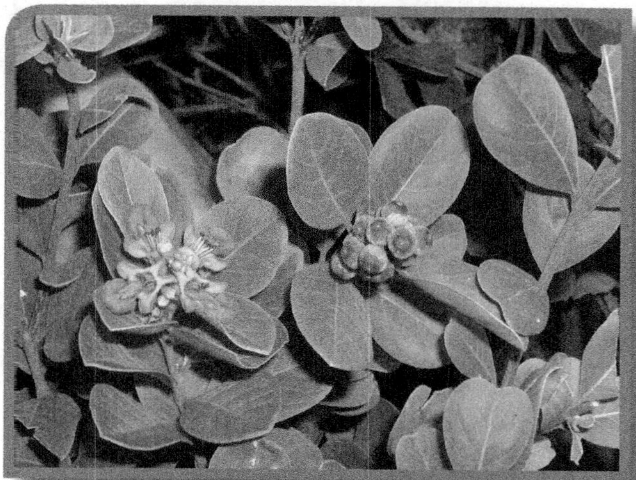

RESPIRATORY

- **Lung problems** [Samoa (*V. trifolia* bark & leaves)]; **breathlessness**.
- **Common cold, especially with eye pain or headache** [China (fruit)].
- **Cough; phlegm** [China (fruit)].
- **Tuberculosis** [Samoa (stems)].

OTHER MEDICINAL USES

- **"Ghost sickness"** [Tonga (*V. trifolia*)].
- **Beriberi** [India (as a bath)].
- **Inflammation.**
- **Sunstroke.**

OTHER USES: *V. trifolia* may function as an insect repellent. The Samoan name "namulega" means mosquito. In Malaysia the burned leaves are used to repel mosquitoes. Used as a sand binder.

CONSTITUENTS: Essential oils: l-d pinene, alpha-pinene, camphene, terpineol acetylester, diterpene alcohol. Alkaloid: Vitricine. Monoterpene glucoside: Agnuside. Flavonols: Vitexicarpin (castisin), camphene, casticin, vitamin A. Iridoid glycosides: Agnoside, aucbin. Flavonoids: Casticin, isovitexin, orientin.

Pōhinahina (Beach Vitex) Local Combinations

PMS: Add *Cyperus rotundus* (xiang fu / nutgrass).

Back pain with emotional agitation: Add *Siegesbeckia orientalis* (xi xian cao), *Cyperus rotundus* (xiang fu / nutgrass).

Back pain with insomnia: Add *Piper methysticum* ('awa / kava), *Mimosa pudica* (hilahila / sensitive plant).

Eye redness and pain: Add *Pandanus tectorius* (hala) and *Ficus microcarpa* (lao gong xu / banyan).

Pōhinahina (Beach Vitex) Cross-Cultural Combinations

"Qi deficient" dizziness, eye problems and ear ringing: With *Astragalus membranaceus* (huang qi) and *Panax ginseng* (ren shen / ginseng) [China].

Headache and body aches: With *Ledebouriella divaricata* (fang feng), *Ligusticum chuanxiong* (chuan xiong), and *Gentiana macrophylla* (qin jiao) [China (decocted)].

Headache and common cold: With *Angelica dahurica* (bai zhi), *Perilla frutescens* (zi su ye), *Chrysanthemum morifolium* (ju hua), and *Mentha arvensis* (bo he) [China (decocted)].

"Wind heat" dizziness and headache: With *Tribulus terrestris* (bai ji li), *Chrysanthemum morifolium* (ju hua), and *Cryptotympana atrata* (chan tui) [China (decocted)].

Sore eyes: With *Cassia tora* (jue ming zi), *Tribulus terrestris* (bai ji li), *Chrysanthemum morifolium* (ju hua), and *Equisetum debile* (mu zei) [China (decocted)].

"Consumption": Leaves with *Piper nigrum* (bi ba), *Curcuma longa* ('ōlena), *Allium sativum* (garlic) [Malaya].

RANGE: In coastal areas from India, China, and Japan through Australia and the Pacific Islands.

HABITAT: Does well in salty areas with little water. Up to 30' elevation. Sometimes used to bind soil.

PROPAGATION & CULTIVATION: By cuttings.

RESEARCH:

- Polymethoxyflavonoids, rotundifuran, and luteolin; all isolated from *V. rotundifolia*, inhibit proliferation of human leukemia [Ko 2000, 2001, 2002].
- Water extract inhibits plasma histamine [Shin 2000].
- Rotundial (a cyclopentene dialdehyde) is used as a mosquito repellant [Watanabe 1995].
- Numerous constituents of *V. rotundifolia* are antibacterial against methicillin-resistant *Staphylococcus aureus* [Kawazoe 2001].

- Flavonoids in *V. rotundifolia* inhibit T-lymphocyte proliferation but not B-lymphocyte proliferation in mice, suggesting a possible use in autoimmune disorders [You 1998].
- Extracts of *Vitex rotundifolia* are analgesic in mice [Okuyama 1998].
- Alcohol and hexane extractions of *Vitex trifolia* inhibit mast-cell activity and reduce histamine response [Ikawati 2001; Alam 2002].
- Ethanol and petroleum ether extracts of *Vitex trifolia* leaves moderately inhibit gram-negative & gram-positive bacteria [Hossain 2001].

NOTES 'N QUOTES

- There are 260 species in the genus *Vitex*.
- A good secondary herb for PMS, redness in the eyes or face, or rheumatic pain. It is easier to buy the Chinese seeds than to find the Hawaiian ones, but I will sometimes gather the leaves. Gathering can lead us to beautiful places, inside and out.

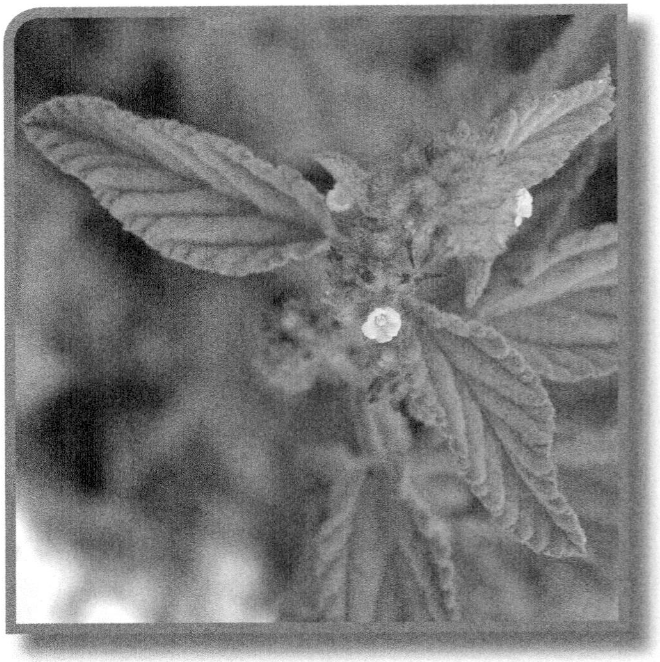

Waltheria indica ('Uhaloa)

PLANT NAME: *Waltheria indica* L.

OTHER NAMES OR **SIMILARLY USED SPECIES**: *W. americana; W. africana; W. angustifolia; W. arborescens; W. corchorifolia; W. detonsa; W. douradinha, W. elliptica; W. erioclada; W. guineensis; W. laevis; W. microphylla; W. ovata; W. pyrolifolia; W. wildii; W. viscosissim.*

Status: Indigenous.

Habitat: Dry disturbed areas, and on lava flows.

COMMON NAMES: **'Uhaloa**, **'uhuloa**, hi'aloa [Hawai'i]; buff coat [Virgin Islands]; guimauve [Martinique, Guadeloupe]; friega plato, hierba de soldado [Panama]; manrubio o tapacola [Mexico].

NOMENCLATURE: Named after A. F. Walther (1688-1746), a German educator.

FAMILY: Malvaceae (hibiscus family).

CATEGORY: Clear damp heat.~

PROPERTIES: Bitter, cool to cold, astringent ~.

PLANT PART USED: Whole plant. According to Hawaiian tradition, the yellow flowers are used for infants, the leaves and stems for young people, and the roots for adults. However, the whole plant is often used for adults.

CAUTIONS AND CONTRAINDICATIONS: Nasty Tastin'!
Not in pregnancy.

PREPARATION OF MEDICINE: Buds chewed and given to children. Whole plant or roots decocted. Root bark chewed for sore throat. Whole plant juiced fresh for asthma, or as a bitter tonic.

DOSAGE: 3-9 grams in decoction. For sore throat chew one thumbnail-sized piece of root cortex and swallow the juice.

STATUS IN HAWAI'I: Native plant. The rule of thumb when using non-threatened native Hawaiian plants is to give back to the 'Āina more than you take from her. Take only what you will use and use sparingly.

MERIDIAN AFFINITIES: Lung, liver, kidneys ~

WESTERN FUNCTIONS REPORTED: **Abortifacient** [Ghana, Gold Coast]; **anti diarrhea**; **depurative** [Mexico]; **emollient** [Haiti]; **purgative** [South Africa]; **sudorific** [Venezuela]; **prevents fever** [Ghana].

TRADITIONAL CHINESE ENERGETIC FUNCTIONS (~ = extrapolated):

1) Clears damp heat ~
2) Clears heat and poison ~
3) Cools the blood ~

'Uhaloa Common Medicinal Uses

- Sore throat
- Lung infections
- Asthma

'Uhaloa Cross-Cultural Medicinal Uses

COSMETIC

- **Eye shadow** [Ghana].

DERMATOLOGICAL

- **Eruption**, **skin problems** [Mexico]; **sores** [Gambia, Ghana].

DIGESTIVE

- **Diarrhea** [Ghana, Mexico].
- **Intestinal bleeding** [S. Africa].
- Juiced as a **bitter tonic** [Hawai'i].

HEAD AND THROAT

- **Sore throat**. The cortex (root bark) about the size of a thumbnail is chewed and the liquid swallowed [Hawai'i].
- **Eye baths** [Panama (root decoction)].
- The roots are used as a **chewstick** [Central America].

INFECTION

- **Fever** [Ghana, Guadelupe, Surinam].

MUSCULOSKELETAL / TRAUMA

- **Arthritis** [Hawai'i (internal)].
- **Wounds** [Mexico].

NEUROLOGICAL

- **Neuralgia** [Hawai'i (internal)].
- **Pain** [Hawai'i].
- **Vertigo**.

ONCOLOGY

- **Tumors** (*W. douradinha, W. viscosissima*) [Brazil].

PEDIATRIC

- In old Hawai'i the buds were chewed and given to infants as a **laxative**.
- **Children's diarrhea** [Panama (root decoction)].

PSYCHOSPIRITUAL

- In Nigeria, the leaves are used to treat **excess giddiness**. (If you've ever tasted 'uhaloa, you'll understand how it could stop giddiness.)

REPRODUCTIVE

- In Ghana, *Waltheria* is said **to cause abortion**
- **Sterility** [South Africa].
- In Mexico regularly drinking a decoction is supposed to impart **immunity to syphilis**.

RESPIRATORY

- In Hawaiian medicine 'uhaloa is used for **asthma** ("hānō"), and juiced in combination for **chronic asthma** and "**pulmonary complications.**"
- **Bloody sputum** [Panama].
- **Bronchial phlegm**, **mucous**, **chest congestion** [Hawai'i].
- **Common cold**, **cough** [Caribbean, Hawai'i, Panama, Togo]; **cough from vog** [Hawai'i].

URINARY

- **Urinary tract infections** [Caribbean].

VETERINARY

- **Open wounds and injuries in animals** [Africa].

OTHER MEDICINAL USES

- Whole plant in combination **for weight loss** [Hawai'i].
- **Fatigue**, **bitter tonic**; **in combination for debility** [Hawai'i]; **restorative** [South Africa].

OTHER USES: In Panama the leaves are used to wash dishes.

'Uhaloa Local Combinations

Sore throat: Add *Musa* spp. (mai'a / banana) sap and / or *Syzygium malaccense* ('ōhi'a 'ai / mountain apple) cortex.

Bronchial infections: Add *Musa* spp. (mai'a / banana) sap, *Hedyotis* spp. (bai hua she she cao), and / or *Phyllostachys nigra* (bamboo) shoots.

Asthma: Add *Desmodium* spp. (pua pilipili).

'Uhaloa Cross-Cultural Combinations

Please note that some of the ingredients in the following combinations are toxic! Do not self-administer without the supervision of a licensed practitioner or an experienced Elder.

Asthma: With *Solanum nigrum* (pōpolo), *Cheirodendron guadichaudii* ('ōlapa), *Acacia koa* (koa), *Saccharum officinarum* (kō / sugar cane), *Morinda citrifolia* (noni), *Sadleria cyantheoides* ('ama'u) [Old Hawai'i].

Asthma: With *Euphorbia* ('akoko) and *Saccharum officinarum* (kō / sugar cane) [Old Hawai'i].

Neuralgia: With *Piper methysticum* ('awa / kava) [Old Hawai'i].

Pain: With *Argemone glauca* (puakala) and *Psilotum complanatum* (moa) [old Hawai'i].

GATHERING: Easier to gather in lava cinders than in packed soils, you might have better luck on leeward sides. Some say 'uhaloa is the kinolau (physical manifestation) of Kamapua'a, while others consider it the kinolau of Kanaloa.

PROPAGATION & CULTIVATION: Propagate by seed.

RESEARCH: Inhibits HIV protease (branch, water extracted) [Miyashiro 1994].

NOTES

'Uhaloa is one of our best native plant medicines for sore throats and a good primary herb for bronchial or bacterial infections. It is somewhat astringent, so it needs to be properly combined to effectively deal with sticky phlegm in the lungs (pa'a).

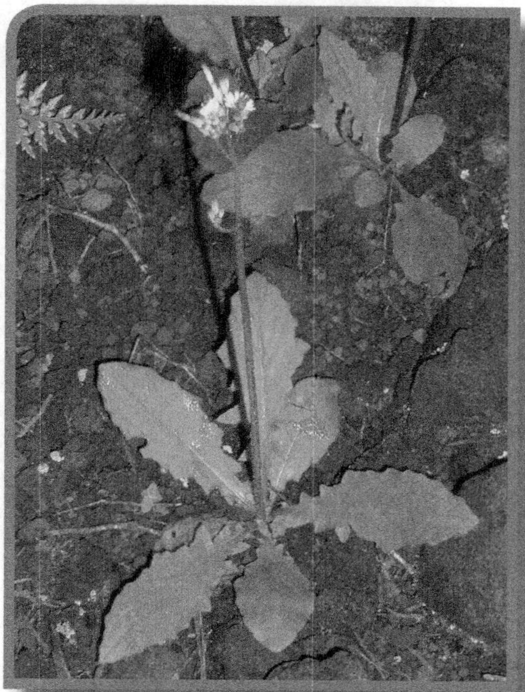

Youngia japonica (Hawksbeard)

PLANT NAME: *Youngia japonica* (L.) DC.

OTHER NAMES: *Chondrilla lyrata, Crepis japonica, Prenanthes japonica, Prenanthes lyrata, Prenanthes multiflora, Youngia lyrata, Youngia thunbergiana.*

COMMON NAMES: Oriental **hawksbeard**, asiatic hawksbeard [English].

NOMENCLATURE: *Youngia* is named after two British writers: Edward Young (1683-1765) and Thomas Young (1779-1829).

FAMILY: Asteraceae (daisy family).

CATEGORY: Clear heat and poison ~.

PROPERTIES: Sweet, bitter, cool.

PLANT PART USED: Whole plant.

ENERGETIC CAUTIONS: Caution with cold deficient Spleen / Stomach ~.

PREPARATION OF MEDICINE: Decocted. Mashed for topical use.

Status: Alien. Mild pest factor.

Habitat: Disturbed areas to 4000'.

DOSAGE: 10 - 30 grams in combination, 30 - 60 grams if used alone.

WESTERN FUNCTIONS REPORTED: **Antidote; anti-inflammatory; antitussive; diuretic; febrifuge.**

TRADITIONAL CHINESE ENERGETIC FUNCTIONS (~ = extrapolated):

1) Clears heat & reduces inflammation.
2) Drains dampness.

Hawksbeard Common Medicinal Uses

- Cold and flu
- Infections

Hawksbeard Cross-Cultural Medicinal Uses

BITES & STINGS

- **Snakebite**

HEAD AND THROAT

- **Conjuctivitis; tonsillitis; toothache** [China].

INFECTION

- **Boils.**

MUSCULOSKELETAL / TRAUMA

- **Rheumatic arthritis** [China].

REPRODUCTIVE

- **Mastitis** [China (decocted and mixed with wine)].

RESPIRATORY

- **Common cold** [China].

URINARY

- **Urinary tract infections, ascites** [China].

OTHER MEDICINAL USES

- **Calluses** (topical) [China].

USE AS FOOD: Leaves are edible.

Hawksbeard Local Combinations

Respiratory infections: Add *Vernonia cinerea* (yi chi xiang / ironweed) and *Prunella vulgaris* (xia ku cao / selfheal). **With sticky phlegm**: Add *Hibiscus tiliaceus* (hau), *Verbascum thapsus* (mullein), or *Malvastrum coromandelianum* (sai kui).

Hawksbeard Cross-Cultural Combinations

Sore throat: Juiced with vinegar topical [China].

RANGE: Native to Southeast Asia.

RESEARCH: Methanol extracts of *Youngia japonica* are antibacterial [Yang 1995].

NOTES

Although it is sometimes difficult to find enough to use in a a formula, it can be useful as a second level (back-up) herb in formulas for infections. Similar plants might include *Stachytarpheta, Vernonia, Emilia, Taraxacum,* and *Sonchus.* First level (primary) herbs might include *Bidens, Musa, Waltheria, Prunella, Hedyotis,* or *Usnea.*

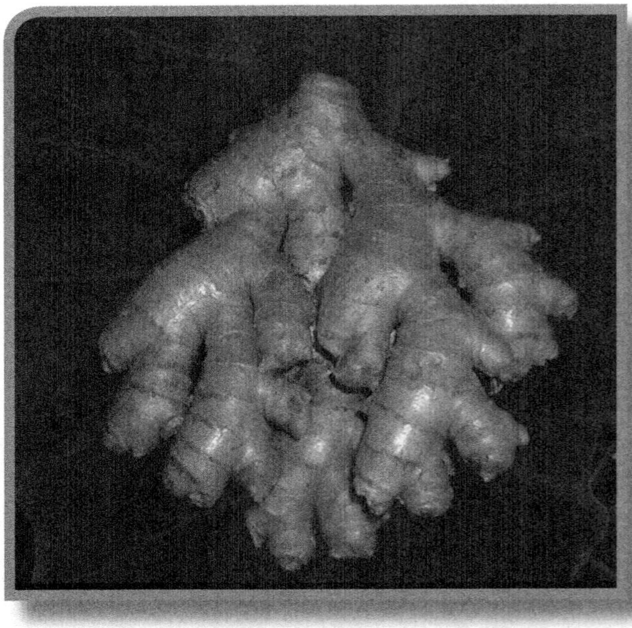

Zingiber officinale ('Awapuhi Pākē / Ginger)

PLANT NAME: *Zingiber officinale* Roscoe.

OTHER NAMES: *Amomum zingiber* L.

COMMON NAMES: **'Awapuhi pākē**, 'awapuhi 'ai [Hawai'i]; **ginger** [English]; **sheng jiang** (fresh), gan jiang (dry), jiang ye (leaves), jiang pi (cortex) [China]; aduwa, sutho [Nepal]; ardrakah (fresh) [Sanskrit]; fiu [Samoa]; gember [Nederland]; gemeiner ingber / ingwer [Germany]; gengibre / jengibre [Spain]; gingembre [France]; gingimbre [Caribbean]; imbir lekarski [Poland]; ingefær [Denmark & Norway]; jahe [Indonesia]; jengibre [Bolivia]; khing [Thailand]; saenggang [Korea]; sang geung [Canton]; shokyo [Japan]; shringara [Sanskrit]; sukku [India]; sunthi (dried) [Sanskrit]; sunthi (dry), nagara (dry), shingabera, ardakam, ardraka (fresh) [India]; ziggiberis, giggiberi [Greece]; zingiberis [Ancient Greek].

Status: Cultivated alien. No pest factor.

Habitat: Likes moisture and fertile soil.

NOMENCLATURE:

- 'Awapuhi is the Hawaiian name for ginger-like plants. Pākē means Chinese. 'Ai means food.
- 'Awapuhi pākē received the name "*Zingiber officinale*" from the British botanist William Roscoe in 1807. The name "ginger" comes from the Sanskrit "sringavera" meaning "horn body," a reference to the shape

of the rhizome. This became zingiberis in Greek and gingibar in Latin.

• The Chinese word for ginger is "jiang" and there are numerous characters that have the same pronunciation. Li Zi Shen, the great Chinese herbalist, used a different character (with the same pronunciation "jiang") than others of his day when referring to Ginger: One meaning "boundary" or "border." This may have implied ginger's function of expelling external pathogens, or it may have been a reference to ginger's status as an imported herb. Or maybe he just misspelled it.

FAMILY: Zingiberaceae. The family zingiberaceae claims more than1200 species in 53 genera. There are 85 species in the genus *Zingiber*.

CATEGORY: Fresh: Warm acrid release the exterior. Dried: Warm the interior.

PROPERTIES:

Fresh rhizome: Acrid warm (fresh rhizome).
Dried rhizome: Acrid hot (dried).
Sprouts: Acrid, neutral [China].

PLANT PART USED: Rhizome.

TOXICITY: Safe at therapeutic doses. The acute oral LD50 in rats of roasted ginger is 170 g / kg. Dry ginger is more than 250 g / kg [Wu 1990]. To put this into an inter-species perspective and extrapolating to humans, a 160 lb man would have to eat about 40 lbs of dried ginger all at once in order to do himself harm.

CAUTIONS AND CONTRAINDICATIONS:

• Caution with gastric ulcers or heartburn [Ody 1993].
• Can aggravate contact dermatitis [Futrell 1993].
• Some studies show a significant reduction in morning sickness when ginger is used [Keating 2002; Lien 2003; Niebyl 1992]. There is no evidence of teratogenic or embryotoxic effects in pregnant mice at doses of 1000 mg / kg [Weidner 2001]. I still try to avoid giving any herbs during pregnancy, although sometimes ginger may be called for with those who have severe morning sickness such as hyperemesis gravidarum. Many practitioners routinely will give up to 1 gram of ginger per day to pregnant women with nausea. If ginger is given during pregnancy, fresh is preferred over dried.

ENERGETIC CAUTIONS: Not with vomiting from stomach heat. Not with lung heat. Practically speaking, however, it can be easily balanced with other herbs. Traditionally not used with gua lou ren or tian hua fen (both are *Trichosanthes kirilowii*).

PREPARATION OF MEDICINE: Infused, decocted, fresh, powdered. Infused to cause a sweat. I almost always prefer fresh ginger to dried. Dried ginger has more "heating" qualities than fresh ginger. Tincture: Fresh 1:2 90% alcohol.

DOSAGE: 1-9g as food or in combination.
For motion sickness: 500 mg dried ginger every half hour, beginning one half hour before travel.

WESTERN FUNCTIONS REPORTED: **Adaptogenic**; **anodyne**; **anthelmintic**; **anti-inflammatory**; **antiallergenic**; **antibacterial**; **anticancer**; **anticarthartic**; **anti-coagulant**; **anticonvulsant**; **antidepressant**; **anti-diabetic**; **antifungal**; **anti-inflammatory**; **antimicrobial**; **antimutagenic**; **antioxidant**; **antirheumatic**; **antispasmodic**; **antithrombic**; **antitoxic**; **antitumor**; **antiulcer**; **antiviral**; **aphrodisiac**; **benefits digestion**; **carminative**; **cholinergic** (antagonizes adrenergic stimulation); **cleanses the throat and tongue**; **clears mucous from the lungs**; **cytoprotective**; **diaphoretic**; **diuretic**; **immune supportive**; **increases bile secretion**; **increases circulation**; **increases saliva**; **increases urination**; **inhibits prostaglandin biosynthesis**; **inhibits gastric secretions**; **inhibits gastric ulcers**; **kills germs topically**; **liver protective**; **lowers blood pressure**; **lowers fever**; **normalizes peristalsis**; **promotes digestion**; **promotes saliva**; **reddens the skin**; **reduces cough**; **reduces nausea and vomiting**; **reduces platelet aggregation**; **reduces serum cholesterol**; **reduces spasm**; **removes obstructions in the vessels**; **rubefacient**; **serotonergic enhancement**; **sialogogue**; **stimulant**; **stops pain**; **strengthens the heart**; **strengthens the intestines**; **strengthens the tissues**; **systemic stimulant**; **thermoregulatory**.

TRADITIONAL CHINESE ENERGETIC FUNCTIONS (~ = extrapolated):

Dried ginger

1) Warms the interior, expels cold, rebuilds the yang.
2) Promotes lactation.
3) Transforms phlegm.
4) Warms the lungs in chronic bronchitis.

Fresh ginger

1) Causes sweating, releases the exterior.
2) Expels cold, warms the middle burner.
3) Stops nausea.
4) Removes toxins.
5) Modifies the ying and wei qi. (For patients with exterior cold due to deficiency who sweat without improvement in their condition.)

Leaves

1) Invigorate blood

OTHER ENERGETIC FUNCTIONS: With honey, ginger relieves Kapha, with rock candy it relieves Pitta, and with rock salt it relieves Vata.

'Awapuhi Pākē (Ginger) Cross-Cultural Medicinal Uses

BITES & STINGS

- **Mosquito repellent** [Africa (rhizome internal)].

COSMETIC

- **Baldness** (paste topical) [China].

CARDIOVASCULAR

"*... promotes the circulation through the extreme vessels...*"

- - Robert Thorton, The Family Herbal (1814)

- **Anemia** [India].
- **Heart disease** [India]; **heart palpitations** [India]; **chest pain** [China].
- **Bleeding** (dried), **nosebleed** [China].
- **Poor circulation**, **cold hands and feet** [Eclectic, Europe, China, India]; **leg pain on exertion due to reduced circulation** ("intermittent claudication"); **phlebitis**.

> **'Awapuhi Pākē (Ginger)**
> **Common Medicinal Uses**
>
> - **A harmonizer in herb formulas**
> - **Joint or muscle pain**
> - **Nausea of any type**
> - **Bronchitis with white sputum**
> - **Impaired liver function**

DERMATOLOGICAL

- **Frostbite** [Europe, General].
- **To create softness and shine of the skin** [India].
- **Bleeding under the skin** [China (bruised leaves topical)].

DIGESTIVE

"*It is of an heating and digesting qualitie and is profitable for the stomacke*"

- - John Gerard, 1597

"*Dyspeptic patients from hard drinking, and those subject to flatulency and gout, have been known to receive considerable benefit by the use of ginger tea... it is to be advised in torbid and phlegmatic habits, where the stomach is subject to be loaded with slime, and the bowels distended with flatulency.*" -

- - Robert Thorton, The Family Herbal (1814)

- **Hunger** [India]; **loss of appetite** [Eclectic, France (on sugar lumps), India].
- **Indigestion**, **belching** [India]; **flatulence** [Eclectic, France (on sugar lumps), India]; **heartburn**; **borborygmus** [Eclectic]; **abdominal distention** [China]; **digestive stimulant** [China (bruised leaves, internal)].
- **Constipation** [China (dried), India].
- **Diarrhea**, **dysentery** [China, Eclectic, Europe, India (juice on the navel), Shakers]; **ulcerative colitis**.
- **Dried for vomiting with blood** [China]; **poisoning from bad meat or seafood** [China]; **mushroom poisoning**.
- **Stomach ache** [Philippines, Samoa]; **gastric and intestinal spasms** [Eclectic]; **to prevent abdominal pain** [Eclectic].
- **Nausea**: **motion sickness**, **seasickness**, **morning sickness**, **dizziness and vertigo**, **stomach flu**, **chemotherapy**. [Universal].

ENDOCRINE

- **Diabetes** [India].

HEAD AND THROAT

Used by Hippocrates and Dioscorides for digestion and "*against all darkness of the sight.*"

- **Eye disease**, **visual problems** [India, Medieval Europe]; **"opacity of the cornea"** [China (rhizome skin)].
- **Headache** [India (dried rhizome as paste topical)]; **migraines** [India]; **hypertensive headaches**.
- **Laryngitis** [India (infusion internal / paste on the throat)]; **toothache** [Medieval Europe, West Africa].
- **Inflammation of the inner ear** [India].

HEPATIC

- Specific for **liver inflammation** [India].

IMMUNITY

- **Allergies** [Nepal].

INFECTION

- **Fever** [France (on sugar lumps), India].

LYMPHATIC

- **Elephantiasis** [India].

MUSCULOSKELETAL / TRAUMA

- Gua sha is a Chinese "spoon massage" that is an

effective treatment for **muscle pain and spasm**. A hot ginger infusion topically can often increase its' effectiveness.

- **Muscle pain**; **stiff neck (compress topical)**; **low back pain** [China]; compress for **cramps**, **pain**, **and spasm** [India].
- **Osteoarthritis**, **rheumatism**, **chronic joint pain and tissue inflammation** (internal and topical) [India (specific), China, Europe. Nepal, West Africa; **rheumatoid arthritis**; **gout** [West Africa].

NEUROLOGICAL

- **Neurological diseases** [India].

PARASITES

- **Intestinal parasites** [Ancient Rome].
- **Parasites** [China (sprouts decocted)].
- **Cholera** [Eclectic, India].

PEDIATRIC

- **Cool the surface in children's diseases** [Eclectic].
- **Colic** [India].

PSYCHOSPIRITUAL

- Ginger is used in India **to increase memory**, **intelligence**, **courage**, **determination and mental clarity**.
- **Depression**.
- **Insomnia** [Medieval Europe].
- **Reported to be hallucinogenic** in large doses [Lewis 1977]. Doubtful.

REPRODUCTIVE

In Senegal, a woman who wanted to arouse a man would wear a belt with ginger in it.

"[Ginger is]... *provoking to venerie and lust*"
- - John Gerard, 16th century

"*Eat ginger and you will love and be loved in your youth.*"
- - from a Medieval medical university in Salermo, Italy

- **Aphrodisiac** [Africa, Middle East].
- **Contraception** [New Guinea (dried root eaten)].
- **Morning sickness**; **pathological vomiting in pregnancy** (hyperemesis gravidarum).
- **Painful menstruation** [China, Eclectic, Medieval Europe]; **scanty menses** [Medieval Europe]; **clots in the menses.**
- Ginger is given to mothers 30 days post partum as a **diaphoretic "cleanse"** [Indonesia].
- **"Perverted lochia"** [China (dried)].

RESPIRATORY

"*For a long sweat use ginger, for a short sweat use cayenne, and for a very short sweat use prickly ash.*"- - James Snow

- **Common cold and flu**, **fever** [China, Eclectic, Hawaii, India, Jamaica, Medieval Europe, Nepal].
- **Asthma**, **wheezing** [China, India]; **respiratory difficulties** [Samoa, West Africa].
- **Lung congestion with phlegm**; **bronchitis with copious white phlegm**; **cough** [China, India].
- **Pertussis** [India (fresh root)].

Due to its familiarity, ginger is often underrated as a medicinal plant. While it has not naturalized in Hawai'i, (or anywhere else, for that matter), I have included it here because it is so commonly used, particularly in Chinese and Hawaiian medicine. It is a powerful and safe remedy for many conditions.

URINARY

- **Incontinence** [India].
- **Painful urination** [India]; **urinary difficulties** [China (dried)]; **kidney problems** [Europe].
- **Ascites** [India].

OTHER MEDICINAL USES

"*... a corrective of many medecines... taketh away their malice*"
- - Henry Barham, 1794

- **Snakebite** [Medieval Europe].
- **Fatigue**.
- **Thirst** [India].
- **Hiccough**.
- **Wasting of the flesh** [China (sprouts decocted)].
- Used in approximately half of all Chinese herb formulas, ginger is **used as a "harmonizer" to soften the harsh effects of other herbs**. It is **used to "detoxify" toxic herbs** such as Aconite or *Pinellia* [China].

USE AS FOOD: One of the best. In the Koran ginger is one of the foods served in Paradise.

"*While most ginger is imported, the best this writer has ever sampled was organic ginger grown on a limited scale in Hawaii.*" - - Steven Foster

- Ginger ale.
- More than 4000 years ago the Ancient Greeks cov-

ered ginger in bread to help them digest food, thus creating the first "gingerbread." Ginger was brought to Greece by Alexander the Great.
- Chinese sailors ate ginger to prevent scurvy.
- The gingerbread *man* was made popular by Queen Elizabeth I.
- Ginger can be used as a meat tenderizer.

ESSENTIAL OIL: The essential oil is composed of more than 200 different ingredients. Reported functions include: Increases circulation, boosts immunity, aphrodisiac, relieves exhaustion, treats lethargy and depression.

CONSTITUENTS:
- Volatile oils (bisabolene, borneol, camphene, cineol, citral, citronellol, geranial, limonene, linalool, phellandrene, zingiberene, zingiberol).
- The aromatic principles are bisabolene & zingiberene.
- The pungent principles are gingerols & shogaols which are anti-nausea. Gingerols turn into shogaols when exposed to heat and air.
- Other ingredients: Calcium, capsaicin, curcumin, high in iron and calcium, limonene, linoleic acid, magnesium, phosphorus, potassium, riboflavin, vitamin B6, vitamin C, zingibain,
- Ginger has proteases (GP-I and GP-II) that are similar to digestive aids bromelain in pineapple, and papain in papayas [Choi 2000].

POSSIBLE DRUG INTERACTIONS:
- May potentiate platelet aggregation inhibitors [Krueth 2004]. Potential potentiation of warfarin (speculative) [Heck 2000].
- Can prevent vomiting when taken prior to cyclophosphamide [Brinker 2001].
- May increase absorption of oral drugs (empirical) [Brinker 2001].

'Awapuhi Pākē (Ginger) Local Combinations

Common cold ("wind cold"): Add *Cymbopogon refractus* (wāpine / lemongrass).

Impaired liver function: Add *Bidens pilosa* (kīnehi / spanish needle), *Curcuma longa* ('ōlena / Turmeric), *Desmodium* spp. (pua pilipili), *Eclipta prostrata* (han lian cao).

Bronchitis with white sputum: Add *Capsicum* spp. (nīoi / cayenne), *Coronopus didymus* (laukāne / swinecress).

'Awapuhi Pākē (Ginger) Cross-Cultural Combinations

Poor circulation, vessel problems
- With *Centella asiatica* (pohe kula / gotu kola).
- With *Ginkgo biloba*, *Cinnamomum cassia* (cinnamon), and / or *Rosmarinus officinalis* (rosemary).

Motion sickness, hiccups and vomiting
- With orange juice. Or with *Bambusa breviflora* (bamboo / zhu ru) shavings [China].
- With *Marrubium nigrum* (black horehound) and *Matricaria camomilla* (chamomile).
- With *Pinellia ternata* (ban xia) rhizome [China].

Common cold
- With *Zizyphus jujuba* (da zao) fruit [China (infused)].
- With *Amomum cardamomum* (cardamom), *Crocus sativus* (saffron), *Eugenia caryophyllata* (clove), and *Myristica fragrens* (nutmeg) [India].

Indigestion
- With *Zizyphus jujuba* (da zao) fruit [China (infused)].
- With *Amomum cardamomum* (cardamom), *Crocus sativus* (saffron), *Eugenia caryophyllata* (clove), and *Myristica fragrens* (nutmeg) [India].
- With rock salt and lemon juice [India].
- With *Cornus florida* (dogwood) and *Hydrastis canadensis* (golden seal).

Asthma
- With *Amomum cardamomum* (cardamom), *Crocus sativus* (saffron), *Eugenia caryophyllata* (clove), and *Myristica fragrens* (nutmeg) [India].
- With *Allium sativum* (garlic) juice and honey [19th century India].

Bronchitis with copious phlegm: With *Pinellia ternata* (ban xia) rhizome [China].

Cough, headaches, and after a stroke: With *Bambusa breviflora* (bamboo / zhu li) sap. [China]

Headache or toothache: Topical mashed with *Aloe vera* gel [India].

Earaches or dandruff: Grated ginger with olive oil for topical.

Backaches: With *Piper methysticum* ('awa / kava).

Chronic joint pain in the elderly: With *Curcuma longa* ('ōlena / Turmeric).

Acute bacillary dysentery: With brown sugar [China].

Amoebas: With *Berberis aristata*, *Boerhavia diffusa* (alena / huang xi xin), *Terminalia chebula* (he zi), and *Tinospora cordifolia* [India] (Cure rate with this formula for liver amoebas in hamsters was reported to be 73%. Immune response was also stimulated) [Sohni 1996].

RANGE: Tropics and sub-tropics throughout the world.

HABITAT: Native to Southeast Asia. Likes moisture and fertile soil.

GATHERING: In your garden or at the market. *Zingiber officinale* has not naturalized in Hawai'i, although in a pinch local *Hedychium* rhizomes can be used.

PROPAGATION & CULTIVATION: Commercial ginger doesn't flower, thus bears no fruit. Propagated by rhizome. Best propagated with large starts and in mounds. Harvest after it dies back and hardens off, unless you want to make pickled ginger. Do not propagate in the same soil two years in a row; it should be rotated with another crop.
Expect 20-25,000 lbs an acre, although my herb-nerd friend Mike Moriarty has seen yields of 60,000 lbs an acre.

Before the first potato was ever eaten in Ireland, ginger was a common spice in Europe. Ginger was served to the Knights of the Round Table in Camelot. Medieval Europeans were so smitten with ginger that some claimed it had come from the Garden of Eden. In the 1300s in Britain, the price for one pound of ginger root was one sheep. Francisco de Mendoca introduced Ginger to the New World, and by the 1600s the Spanish had created ginger plantations in Jamaica.

RESEARCH:

Antimicrobial

- Reduces swelling and fever in rats [Mascolo 1989].
- Some sesquiterpenes are antirhinoviral in vitro [Denyer]. Constituents inhibit Epstein-Barr virus in vitro [Vimala 1999]. Ethanol extract inhibits both gram-positive and gram-negative bacteria [Mascolo 1989]. The essential oil is antimicrobial [Martins 2001].
- A methanol extract of dried ginger inhibited 19 strains of *Helicobacter pylori* in vitro [Mahady 2003].

Cardiovascular

- Effect on blood pressure is inconclusive. Ginger lowers cholesterol in lab animals through interruption of biosynthesis [Fuhrman 2000] and reduces atherosclerotic lesions, possibly through antioxidant effects [Liu 2003]. Gingerol is cardiotonic in lab animals [Kobayashi 1988].
- There are conflicting data regarding ginger's effect on production of thromboxane and platelet aggregation [Janssen 1996; Thomson 2002; Koo 2001; Srivastava 1986]. The effect on platelet aggregation may be dose dependent. In one study 4 grams per day for 3 months did not affect platelet aggregation but one single dose of 10 grams did [Bordia 1997].

Digestion

- Ginger constituents inhibit gastric ulcers in lab animals [Yamahara 1988 & 1992;Yoshikawa 1994], including gastric damage by chemicals, NSAIDs and stress [al-Yahya 1989].
- More effective than conventional medicines for post-operative nausea [Pongrojpaw 2003]. Also effective for motion sickness [Lien 2003; Schmid 1994], although there are some conflicting data [Stewart 1991]. Other effective uses include nausea [Fischer-Rasmussen 1991], nausea from chemotherapy [Meyer 1995], and hyperemesis gravidarum [Fischer-Rasmussen 1991]. Please note caveats in *Cautions and Contraindications.*
- (6)-shogaol firms the intestinal muscles in guinea pigs [Hashimoto 2002].
- One gram of ginger in humans may reduce " hyperglycemia-evoked gastric dysrhythmias" through the blockage of prostaglandin production [Gonlachanvit 2003]. Reduces prostaglandin production in rats at therapeutic doses [Thomson 2002]. See *Inflammation* below.

Inflammation

- Ginger constituents inhibit arachadonic acid metabolism and prostaglandin synthesis. This may account for some of its anti-inflammatory properties. One constituent specifically, (6)-Shogaol, (found in semi-dry, but rarely fresh ginger), appears to interfere with the arachadonic / inflammatory cascade. It inhibits cyclo-oxygenases and prevents specific prostaglandin release in rabbits [Suekawa 1986] and rats [Mascolo 1989] Ginger may be a stronger inhibitor of prostaglandin synthesis than indomethacin [Flynn 1986; Guh 1995; Kiuchi 1992; Srivastava 1984]. It can be used for either rheumatoid or osteoarthritis [Altman 2001].
- Ginger extract is antiinflammatory on osteoarthrotic sow cartilage in vitro [Shen 2003].

Oncology

- Ginger has antimutagenic, anticarcinogenic, and chemoprotective properties due to its antioxidant and anti-inflammatory activities [Surh 2002]. Ginger oil is antioxidant in vitro [Lu 2003; Patro 2002].

Constituents such as [6]-gingerol and [6]-paradol show direct anti-tumor activity, blocking tumor production [Bode 2001; Surh 1998]. [6]-gingerol and [6]-paradol may also be cytotoxic / cytostatic against human promyelocytic leukemia cells (HL-60) [Lee 1998]. Ethanol extracts can prevent and inhibit live skin tumors in mice [Katiyar 1996], possibly through the improvement of immune function [Liu 2002]. Some of these anti-tumor and anti-inflammatory constituents have a structure similar to those found in vanilla [Surh 1999].

- Ginger inhibits COX-2 enxyme activity [Tjendraputra 2001]. Zerumbone (a ginger constituent) reduces inflammatory bowel conditions and colon cancer in mice (possibly through COX-2 inhibition) [Murakami 2003, 2004]. It may suppress free radical generation and cancer cell proliferation [Murakami 2002].

Other research

- Water extraction may be androgenic in rats [Kamtchouing 2002]. Sperm motility increased in animals given ginger for 3 months [Qureshi 1989].
- Intraperitoneal injection in mice reduces radiation sickness and mortality from exposure to gamma radiation [Jagetia 2003].
- Ginger juice is anticholinergic and antihistiminic [Qian 1992].
- Gingerols increase bile secretion [Yamahara 1985].
- Ethanol extract lowers blood glucose in rabbits [Mascolo 1989].
- Extracts kill *Schistosoma mansoni* parasites in vitro but not in vivo [Sanderson 2002].

Pythagoras used ginger for digestion, Roman doctors used it during military marches, and it was employed by King Henry VIII to protect against plague.

NOTES 'N QUOTES

"*... it doth corroborate the natural heate*"
- - Henry Barham (1794)

- First recorded use: Shen Nong's Ben Cao, 3000 B.C. Confucius wrote about ginger in the 5th century B.C., and the 13th century Welch herbal "Physicians of Myddvai," included ginger as one of its' 175 plants.
- The Romans taxed ginger in the second century A.D, as did the French in the 13th.
- Large ginger rhizomes are called "hands."
- During the 1990s, over 4000 metric tons of ginger were imported into the USA annually.
- Indian ginger consumption is estimated to be 8-10 grams per person per day and India has more than 45 different varieties of ginger. It is called "vishwabhesaj " or "universal medicine" in the oldest Ayurvedic text, the Charaka Samhita. Ginger, garlic, and onion are called the "Trinity Roots" in Ayurveda.
- Ginger reduces inflammation by eliminating free radicals, and reportedly has ingredients that are better antioxidants than vitamin C.

Hawaiian Plants Listed by Condition

PLEASE NOTE: SOME OF THE FOLLOWING PLANTS ARE TOXIC.
THIS LIST IS FOR INFORMATIONAL PURPOSES ONLY.
(Not all of these plants have been featured in this book. In addition, some at-risk native medicinal plants have been omitted. This list is not exhaustive.)

BITES & STINGS

Ageratum conyzoides (maile hohono) herb (centipedes)
Aloe vera (aloi / lu hui) gel
Carica papaya (mīkana / papaya) sap
Hibiscus rosa-sinensis (aloalo / red hibiscus) bud
Plantago lanceolata (laukahi / plantain) herb
Plantago major (laukahi / plantain) herb
Portulaca oleracea ('ākulikuli / purslane) herb as food
Scaveola spp. (naupaka) berries
Solanum americanum (pōpolo) leaf, topical

COSMETIC

Balding
Adiantum spp. ('iwa'iwa / maidenhair) herb
Polygonum multiflorum (he shou wu) root

Grey Hair
Eclipta prostrata (han lian cao)
Polygonum multiflorum (he shou wu) root

Sagging Breasts
Nicotiana tabacum (paka / tobacco) herb topical

CARDIOVASCULAR

Bleeding
Amaranthus spp. (pakai)
Capsella rubella (shepherd's purse) herb
Erigeron canadensis (fleabane) oil

High Blood Pressure
Cymbopogon citratus (wāpine / lemongrass) herb

Varicose Veins
Capsella rubella (shepherd's purse) herb
Centella asiatica (pohe kula / gotu kola) herb

DERMATOLOGICAL

Broussonetia papyrifera (wauke) leaves
Cannabis sativa (pakalōlō / huo ma ren) seeds
Momordica charantia (bitter melon / ka'ukama) herb
Stellaria media (chickweed) herb
Trifolium pratense (red clover) herb
Sophora chrysophylla (māmane) root cortex
Xanthium sibiricum (cang er zi) herb

Ringworm (Tinea / "Haole Rot")
Ageratum conyzoides (maile hohono) herb topical
Musa paradisica (mai'a / banana) sap topical

DIGESTIVE

Constipation
Aleurites moluccana (kukui) roasted nut
Aloe vera (aloi / lu hui) gel, sap
Musa paradisica (mai'a / banana) ripe fruit
Pipturus spp. (māmaki) fruit

Diarrhea
Psidium guajava (kuava / guava)
Musa paradisica (mai'a / banana) unripe fruit

Dysentery
Melastoma candidum (puna rose) root

GI Bleeding
Capsella rubella (shepherd's purse) herb
Erigeron canadensis (fleabane) herb / oil

Poor Digestion
Bidens pilosa (kīnehi / spanish needle) herb
Brassica nigra (mākeke / mustard) seeds
Capsicum frutescens (nīoi / cayenne) fruit
Carica papaya (mīkana / papaya) green fruit
Coix lachryma jobi (pū'ohe'ohe / jobs tears) leaves
Curcuma longa ('ōlena / tumeric / jiang huang) rhizome
Pandanus tectorius (hala) fruit
Pipturus spp. (māmaki) leaves, fruit
Pluchea indica (plukia) herb
Taraxacum officinale (laulele / dandelion) leaf eaten before meals

ENDOCRINE

Diabetes (NIDDM - Type II)
Annona muricata (soursop) leaf
Bauhinia forficate (cameltoe) leaf
Bixa orellana ('alae'a / anatto) leaf
Cecropia obtusifolia (guarumo) leaf
Cocos nucifera (niu / coconut) water
Momordica charantia (bitter melon / ka'ukama) herb
Opuntia spp. (pānini / prickly pear) leaf pad
Plantago major (laukahi / plantain) herb

Thyroid Imbalances
Seaweed (limu)

HEAD AND THROAT

Headache ('Aki)
Caffea arabica (kōpe / coffee) kernal
Piper methysticum ('awa / kava kava) root
Styphelia tameiameiae (pūkiawe) branch tips

Sore throat
Adiantum spp. ('iwa'iwa / maidenhair) herb
Commelina spp. (honohono / wandering jew) herb
Eriobotrya japonica (loquat / pi pa ye) leaf, fruit
Hedyotis corymbosa (shui [?] cao) herb
Musa paradisica (mai'a / banana) root, sap
Syzygium malaccense ('ōhi'a 'ai / mountain apple) bark or root
Verbena littoralis (ha'uoi) herb
Waltheria indica ('uhaloa) herb

Thrush
Aleurites moluccana (kukui) herb
Pipturus spp. (māmaki)

HEPATIC

Acute hepatitis
Bidens pilosa (kīnehi / spanish needle) herb
Boerhavia spp. (alena)
Cecropia obtusifolia (guarumo) leaf
Lonicera japonica (honeysuckle / jin yin hua / honekakala) flower
Musa paradisica (mai'a / banana) root, sap
Prunella vulgaris (xia ku cao) flower spike
Sonchus oleraceus (pualele / sow thistle) herb
Taraxacum officinale (laulele / dandelion) herb

Chronic hepatitis
Adiantum spp. ('iwa'iwa / maidenhair) herb
Annona muricata (soursop) leaf
Bidens pilosa (kīnehi / spanish needle) herb
Boerhavia spp. (alena)
Cecropia obtusifolia (guarumo) leaf
Curcuma longa ('ōlena / tumeric) rhizome
Desmodium spp. (puapilipili) leaves
Eclipta prostrata (han lian cao) herb
Pipturus spp. (māmaki) leaf
Verbena littoralis (ha'oui) herb
Zingiber officinale ('awapuhi pākē / ginger) fresh rhizome

IMMUNITY

Lowered immunity
Auricularia cornea (pepeiao)
Centella asiatica (pohe kula / gotu kola) herb
Morinda citrifolia (noni) fruit
Trametes versicolor (yun zi / turkey tail) herb

INFECTION

General Bacterial Infections
Bidens pilosa (kīnehi / xian feng cao) herb
Citrus limon (lemon kāne)
Musa paradisica (mai'a / banana) root, sap
Phylostachys nigra (shoot)
Plantago major (laukahi / plantain) herb
Portulaca oleracea ('ākulikuli / purslane) herb
Prunella vulgaris (xia ku cao) flower spike
Sonchus oleraceus (pualele / sow thistle) herb
Taraxacum officinale (laulele / dandelion) herb
Usnea spp. ('umi koa) lichen
Vernonia cinerea (yi chi xiang / little ironweed) herb
Youngia japonica (asia hawksbeard) herb

Fever
Commelina spp. (honohono / wandering jew) herb
Prunella vulgaris (xia ku cao) flower spike
Rumex acetosella (sheep sorrel) herb

MUSCULOSKELETAL / TRAUMA

Burns
Aloe vera (aloi / lu hui) gel, sap
Cibotium spp. (hapu'u)
Musa paradisica (mai'a / banana) root, sap

Bruises / Contusions
Boerhavia spp. (alena)
Cecropia obtusifolia (guarumo) leaf
Centella asiatica (pohe kula / gotu kola) herb
Ipomoea indica (koali / morning glory) stems as

poultice
Morinda citrifolia (noni) fruit
Pa'akai (Hawaiian salt)
Ricinus communis (koli / castor)
Verbena littoralis (ha'uoi)

Gout
Bidens pilosa (kīnehi / spanish needle) herb
Capsella rubella (shepherd's purse) herb
Vaccinium spp. ('ōhelo) fruit

Osteoarthritis / Joint Pain / Low Back Pain
Desmodium spp. (puapilipili) leaves
Morinda citrifolia (noni) fruit
Piper methysticum ('awa / kava kava)
Ricinus communis (koli / castor)
Siegesbeckia orientalis (xi xian cao) herb
Xanthium sibiricum (cang er zi) herb

ONCOLOGY

Cancer
Annona muricata (soursop) leaf
Auricularia cornea (pepeiao)
Carica papaya (mīkana / papaya) seeds
Curcuma longa ('ōlena / tumeric) rhizome
Hedyotis corymbosa (shui [?] cao) herb
Momordica charantia (peria / ka'ukama) herb (for prostate)
Morinda citrifolia (noni) fruit
Trametes versicolor (yun zi / turkey tail) fungus

PARASITES

Areca catechu (da fu pi)
Carica papaya (mīkana / papaya) seeds

PEDIATRIC

Osteomeles anthyllidifolia ('ūlei)
Stachytarpheta spp. (ōwīwī)

Thrush
Aleurites moluccana (kukui) herb
Pipturus spp. (māmaki)

Heart Problems
Drymaria cordata (pilipili) herb

Colic
Pluchea indica (plukia) herb

PSYCHOSPIRITUAL

Depression
Annona muricata (soursop) leaf
Morinda citrifolia (noni) fruit
Pandanus tectorius (hala) fruit
Sida rhombifolia (huang hua mu) herb & root

Insomnia/ Irritability
Annona muricata (soursop) leaf
Bidens pilosa (kīnehi / spanish needle) herb
Melaleuca quinquenervia (bai ding / paperbark) bark
Mimosa pudica (hilahila)
Oxalis corniculata ('ihi / sorrel)
Oxalis martianna ('ihi / sorrel)
Pandanus tectorius (hala) fruit
Passilora incarnata (passionflower) herb
Piper methysticum ('awa / kava kava)
Pipturus spp. (māmaki) leaf
Verbena littoralis (ha'uoi) herb

Stress
Cyperus rotundus (xiang fu / nutgrass)
Morinda citrifolia (noni) fruit
Oxalis corniculata ('ihi / sorrel)
Oxalis martianna ('ihi / sorrel)
Piper methysticum ('awa / kava kava)
Pipturus spp. (māmaki) leaf
Passilora incarnata (passionflower) herb
Verbena littoralis (ha'uoi)

REPRODUCTIVE

Birth Control (not recommended)
Carica papaya (mīkana / papaya) seeds
Hibiscus rosa-sinensis (aloalo) flower

Impotence
Centella asiatica (pohe kula / gotu kola) herb
Pandanus tectorius (hala) pollen
Tribulus terrestris (bai ji li) thorns

Infertility
Broussonetia papyrifera (wauke) fruit (not in Hawai'i)
Morus alba (sang shen zi / mulberry) fruit

Menstrual Pain
Adiantum spp. ('iwa'iwa maidenhair) herb
Piper methysticum ('awa / kava kava) root
Zingiber officinale ('awapuhi pākē / ginger) fresh

rhizome

Menopause
Oenothera biennis (evening primrose)
Trifolium pratense (red clover) herb
Vitex rotundifolia (pōhinahina / beach vitex) seeds

Labor
Capsella rubella (shepherd's purse) herb
Rubus rubifolius (thimbleberry) leaf

Threatened Miscarriage
Cordyline suffruticosa (lā'ī) herb

PMS
Cyperus rotundus (xiang fu / nutgrass) rhizome
Pipturus spp. (māmaki)

RESPIRATORY

Cold / Flu
Adiantum spp. ('iwa'iwa / maidenhair) herb
Cecropia obtusifolia (guarumo) leaf
Cymbopogon citratus (wāpine / lemongrass) herb
Desmodium spp. (puapilipili) leaves (sinus)
Pandanus tectorius (hala) aerial root
Melaleuca quinquenervia (paperbark) flower
Musa paradisica (mai'a / banana) root, sap
Sambucus mexicana (elder) flower
Vernonia cinerea (yi chi xiang / little ironweed) herb
Waltheria indica ('uhaloa) herb
Youngia japonica (asia hawksbeard) herb
Zingiber officinale ('awapuhi pākē / ginger) fresh rhizome

Cough ('Ako'ako)
Cecropia obtusifolia (guarumo) leaf
Eriobotrya japonica (loquat / pi pa ye) leaf, fruit
Hibiscus rosa-sinensis (aloalo)
Marrubium vulgare (horehound)
Musa paradisica (mai'a / banana) root, sap
Psidium guajava (guava) leaf
Waltheria indica ('uhaloa) herb

Bronchitis
Adiantum spp. ('iwa'iwa / maidenhair) herb
Bidens pilosa (kīnehi / spanish needle) herb
Capsicum frutescens (nīoi / cayenne) fruit
Cecropia obtusifolia (guarumo) leaf
Cordyline suffruticosa (lā'ī / ti) herb
Coronopus didymus (lau kāne / swinecress) herb
Desmodium spp. (puapilipili) leaves
Hedyotis corymbosa (shui [?] cao) herb
Hibiscus rosa-sinensis (aloalo)
Marrubium vulgare (horehound)
Plantago lanceolata (laukahi / plantain) herb
Plantago major (laukahi / plantain) herb
Solanum americanum (pōpolo) leaf, fruit
Sonchus oleraceus (pualele / sow thistle) herb
Taraxacum officinale (laulele / dandelion) herb
Verbascum thapsus (mullein) herb
Zingiber officinale ('awapuhi pākē / ginger) fresh rhizome

URINARY

Urinary Tract Infections
Bauhinia forficate (cameltoe) leaf
Bidens pilosa (kīnehi / spanish needle) herb
Bixa orellana ('alae'a / anatto) leaf
Boerhavia spp. (alena) herb
Capsella rubella (shepherd's purse) herb
Cecropia obtusifolia (guarumo) leaf
Hedyotis corymbosa (shui [?] cao) herb
Taraxacum officinale (laulele / dandelion) herb
Waltheria indica ('uhaloa) herb

Urinary Stones
Mimosa pudica (hilahila / sensitive grass)
Rumex acetosella (sheep sorrel) herb
Triumfetta rhomboidea
Stellaria media (chickweed) herb

VETERINARY

Fleas
Indigofera suffruticosa ('inikō)

Injuries
Aloe vera (aloi / lu hui) leaf topical

OTHER MEDICINAL USES

Cold Hands and Feet
Capsicum frutescens (nīoi / cayenne) fruit
Foeniculum vulgare (xiao hui xiang / fennel) fruit
Zingiber officinale ('awapuhi pākē / ginger) fresh rhizome

Fatigue and Low Energy

Auricularia cornea (pepeiao)
Caffea arabica (kōpe / coffee)
Centella asiatica (pohe kula / gotu kola) herb
Coix lachryma jobi (pū'ohe'ohe / jobs tears)
Pandanus tectorius (hala) fruit
Syzygium jambos ('ōhi'a 'loke / rose apple) skin
Trametes versicolor (yun zi / turkey tail) fungus

Hangover
Pandanus tectorius (hala) fruit

Inflammatory Conditions
Bacopa monnieri ('ae'ae / brahmi) herb
Bidens pilosa (kīnehi / spanish needle) herb
Cecropia obtusifolia (guarumo) leaf
Centella asiatica (pohe kula / gotu kola) herb
Curcuma longa ('ōlena / tumeric) rhizome
Desmodium spp. (puapilipili) leaves
Rumex acetosella (sheep sorrel) herb
Zingiber officinale ('awapuhi pākē / ginger) fresh rhizome

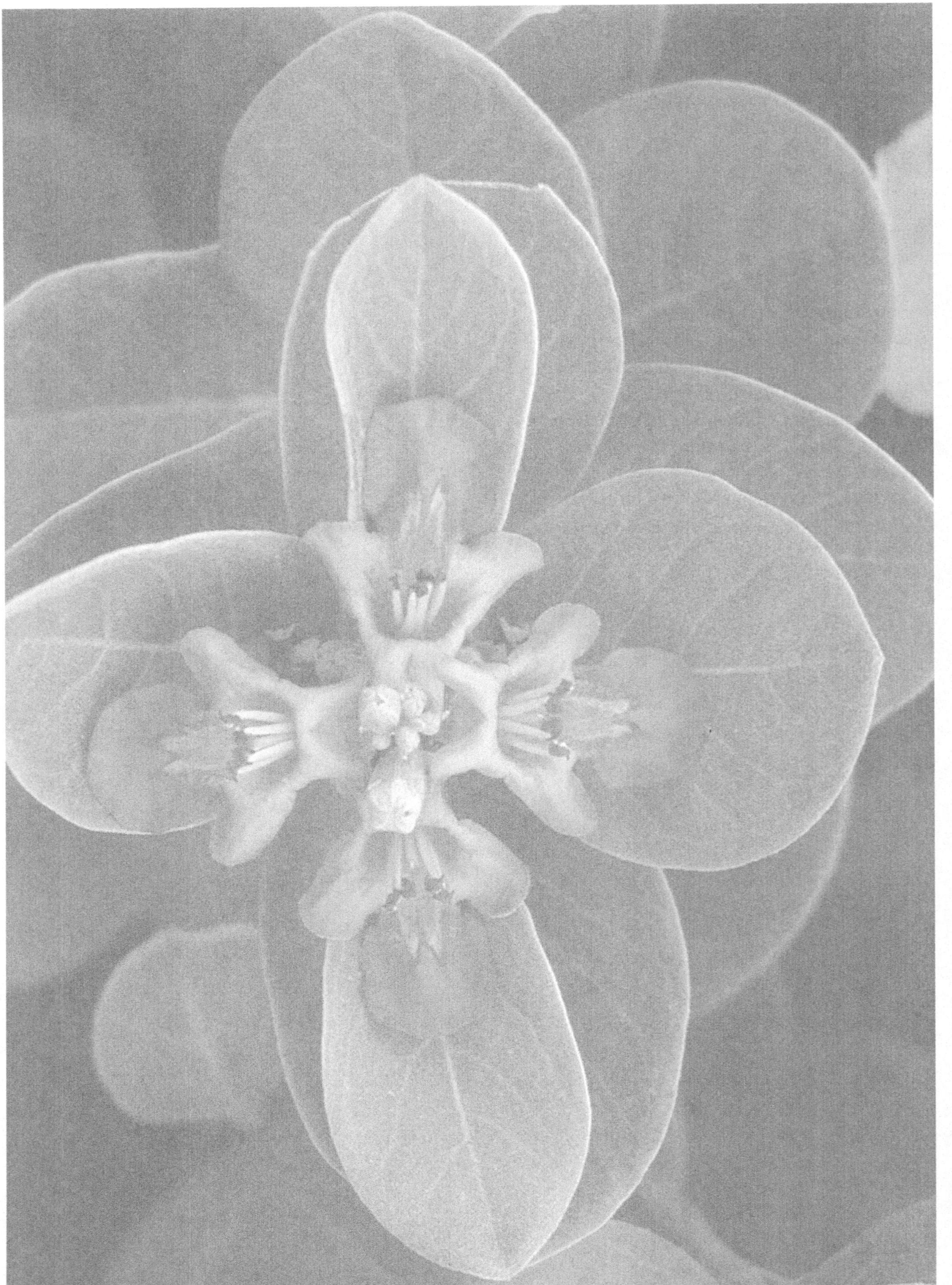

Hawaiian Plants in Traditional Chinese Medicine Categories

PLEASE NOTE: SOME OF THE FOLLOWING PLANTS ARE TOXIC.
USE ONLY UNDER PROFESSIONAL SUPERVISION.
(Some at-risk native medicinal plants have been omitted)

Warm, Acrid Herbs that Release the Exterior
Cymbopogon citratus (wāpine) herb
Melaleuca quinquenervia (bai ding / paperbark) flower ~
Perilla frutescens (zi su ye) leaf
Zingiber officinale ('awapuhi pākē / ginger) fresh rhizome

Cool, Acrid Herbs that Release the Exterior
Ficus microcarpa (banyan) aerial roots
Kyllinga spp. (kili'o'opu) herb
Morus alba (sang ye) leaf
Pandanus tectorius (hala) aerial root
Pueraria lobata (ge gen) root
Sambucus mexicana (elder) flower ~
Vitex rotundifolia (pōhinahina / man jing zi) seeds

Herbs that Drain Fire
Commelina spp. (honohono / ya zhi cao) herb
Prunella vulgaris (xia ku cao) flower spike

Herbs that Cool the Blood
Broussonetia papyrifera (wauke) fruit
Centella asiatica (pohe kula / gotu kola) herb
Cordyline suffruticosa (lā'ī) herb

Herbs that Clear Damp Heat
Sida rhombifolia
Sophora chrysophylla (māmane) ~
Waltheria indica ('uhaloa) herb ~

Herbs that Clear Heat and Poison
Ageratum conyzoides (maile hohono) herb
Bidens pilosa (kīnehi / xian feng cao) herb
Desmodium spp. (puapilipili) leaves
Hedyotis spp. (bai hua she she cao) herb
Lonicera japonica (jin yin hua / honekakala) flower
Musa paradisica (mai'a / banana) root, sap
Portulaca oleracea ('ākulikuli) herb
Selaginella doederleinii (shi shang bai) herb
Solanum nigrum (pōpolo) leaf, fruit
Sonchus oleraceus (pualele) herb
Taraxacum officinale (laulele / dandelion) herb
Trifolium pratense (red clover) herb
Vernonia cinerea (yi chi xiang / little ironweed) herb
Youngia japonica (asia hawksbeard) herb

Herbs that Clear and Relieve Summer heat
Dolichos lablab (bai bian dou) seed

Purgatives
Aleurites moluccana (kukui) herb ~
Aloe vera (aloi / lu hui) gel, sap

Moist Laxatives
Cannabis sativa (pakalōlō / huo ma ren)

Herbs that Drain Dampness
Coix lachryma jobi (pū'ohe'ohe / jobs tears) kernals, root
Dioscorea hypoglauca (bei xie) tuber
Juncus effusus (deng xin cao) herb
Malva verticillata (dong gua zi) seed
Plantago lanceolata (laukahi / che qian cao) herb
Plantago major (lau kahi / che qian cao) herb

Herbs that Dispel Wind-Dampness
Morus alba (sang zhi) branch
Piper methysticum ('awa / kava kava) ~
Siegesbeckia orientalis (xi xian cao) herb
Xanthium sibiricum (cang er zi) herb

Herbs that Cool and Transform Phlegm-heat
Adiantum spp. ('iwa'iwa) herb
Usnea spp. ('umi koa) lichen ~

Warm Herbs that Transform Phlegm-cold
Brassica alba (mākeke / bai jie zi) herb
Coronopus didymus (lau kane) herb ~

Herbs that Relieve Coughing and Wheezing
Eriobotrya japonica (loquat / pi pa ye) leaf, fruit
Morus alba (sang bai pi) root cortex
Perilla frutescens (zi su zi) seeds
Verbascum thapsus (mullein) herb ~

Aromatic Herbs that Transform Dampness

Pluchea indica (plukia) herb

Herbs that Relieve Food Stagnation

Carica papaya (mīkana) fruit ~

Herbs that Regulate the Qi

Areca catechu (da fu pi)
Citrus retuculata (chen pi)
Cyperus rotundus (xiang fu)
Pipturus spp. (mamaki) ~
Santalum spp. (sandalwood)

Herbs that Stop Bleeding

Amaranthus spp. (pakai) ~
Artemisia vulgaris (mugwort / ai ye) herb
Capsella rubella (shepherd's purse) herb
Cirsium vulgare (thistle) herb
Erigeron canadensis (fleabane) herb ~

Herbs that Invigorate the Blood

Boerhavia spp. (alena)
Curcuma longa ('ōlena / tumeric / jiang huang) rhizome, tuber
Leonurus sibiricus (yi mu cao / motherwort) herb
Melastoma candidum (puna rose) root
Selaginella doederleinii (shi shang bai) herb

Herbs that Warm the Interior and Expel Cold

Capsicum frutescens (nīoi) fruit
Foeniculum vulgare (xiao hui xiang) fruit
Zingiber officinale ('awapuhi pākē / ginger) dried rhizome

Herbs that Tonify the Qi

Auricularia spp. (pepeiao)
Coix lachryma jobi (pū'ohe'ohe / jobs tears) leaf
Morinda citrifolia (noni) fruit ~
Trametes versicolor (yun zi / turkey tail) herb
Pandanus tectorius (hala) fruit

Herbs that Tonify the Blood

Polygonum multiflorum (he shou wu) root
Colocasia esculenta (kalo / taro) prepared root ~

Herbs that Tonify the Yang

Pandanus tectorius (hala) pollen ~

Herbs that Tonify the Yin

Alternathera sessilis (han lian cao)
Dendrobium nobile (shi hu)
Eclipta prostrata (han lian cao)
Ophiopogon japonicus (mai men dong)

Herbs that Stabilize and Bind

Psidium cattleianum (waiwi / strawberry guava) ~
Psidium guajava (kuava / guava) ~
Rubus rubifolius (thimbleberry) ~
Syzygium cumini (java plum) ~
Syzygium jambos ('ōhi'a 'loke) ~
Syzygium malaccense ('ōhi'a 'ai) ~

Herbs that Nourish the Heart and Calm the Spirit

Oxalis corniculata ('ihi mākole, 'ihi `ai)
Oxalis martianna ('ihi pehu)
Melaleuca quinquenervia (bai ding/paperbark) bark ~
Mimosa pudica (hilahila) ~

Aromatic Substances that Open the Orifices

Caffea arabica (kōpe / coffee) ~

Herbs that Extinguish Wind and Stop Tremors

Tribulus terrestris (bai ji li)

Herbs for Parasites

Chenopodium ambrosiodes ('aweoweo) herb

Herbs for External Application

Ricinus communis (koli) ~

Hawaiian Herbs Not Yet Categorized

Anagallis arvensis (jian feng hong / scarlet pimpernel) herb
Argemone glauca (puakala) herb
Argemone mexicana (mexican poppy) herb
Bacopa monnieri (brahmi) herb
Cannabis sativa (pakalōlō)
Capparis sandiwchiana (maiapilo) flower
Chamaecrista nictitans (laukī)
Casuarina equisetifolia (ironwood / paina) herb
Chenopodium ambrosiodes ('aweoweo) herb
Cirsium vulgare (bull thistle)
Clerodendrum philippinum (pīkake hohono)
Clidemia hirta (koster's curse)
Cocos nucifera (niu / coconut)
Colocasia esculenta (taro / kalo)
Cuscuta sanwichiana (kauna'oa)
Dicranopteris spp.

Drymaria cordata ('ihi) herb
Elephantopus mollis herb
Eucalyptus spp. (nuhōlani / palepiwa) leaves
Fragaria chiloensis (strawberry) herb
Galinsoga parviflora
Geranium cunneatum(hinahina)
Geranium homeanum
Glycine wightii
Gossypium tormentosum (ma'o) root cortex
Heliotropium anomalum (hinahina) herb
Heteropogon contortus (pili grass)
Hibiscus rosa-sinensis (aloalo)
Hibiscus tiliaceus (hau)
Hypericum perforatum (st johns wort) herb
Impatiens spp. seeds
Indigofera suffruticosa ('inikō)
Ipomoea batatas ('uala)
Ipomoea cairica (koali 'ai)
Ipomoea indica (koali) stems
Ipomoea pes-caprae (pōhuehue) stems
Jaquemontia ovalifolia (pā'ūohi'iaka)
Justicia betonica herb
Lablab purpureus (pāpapa / bai bian dou) seed
Lantana camara (lākana) herb
Leonotis nepetifolia herb
Leonurus sibiricus (motherwort / yi mu cao)
Lepidium bidentatum ('anaunau)
Lepidium virginicum (maca) herb
Lespedeza cuneata
Leucana leucocephala (haole koa)
Litchi chinensis seed
Lycium sandwicense ('ōhelo kai) fruit
Lycopodium cernuum (wāwae'iole) herb
Malva parviflora
Malvastrum coromandelianum
Marrubium vulgare (horehound)
Medicago lupulina
Melia azedarach
Melilotus alba
Metrosideros polymorpha
Microsorium scolopendria
Mirabilis jalapa herb
Momordica charantia (peria / ka'ukama) herb
Monstera deliciousa fruit
Nasturtium officinale (watercress) herb
Nephrolepis spp. (kupukupu)
Nicotiana glauca (tree tabacco)
Nicotiana tabacum (paka / tobacco) herb
Ocimum basilicum (basil)
Oenothera biennis (evening primrose)
Opuntia spp. (pānini)
Osteomeles anthyllidifolia
Passilora edulis (passionflower) herb
Passiflora foetida
Peperomia spp. ('ala'alawainui) herb
Persea americana (avocado)
Petasites japonicus
Phlebodium spp.
Phylostachys nigra
Phymatosorus scolopendria
Physalis peruviana (poha) fruit
Phytolacca spp. (pōpolo kū mai)
Plumbago zeylanica ('ilie'e) herb
Plumeria spp.
Polygala paniculata
Portulaca oleracea ('ākulikuli) herb
Psilotum nudum (moa) herb
Raphanus sativus
Rumex acetosella (sheep sorrel) herb
Rumex crispus (curley dock) herb
Rumex gigantus (pāwale)
Saccharum officinarum (kō) herb
Sambucus mexicana (mexican elder)
Schefflera octophylla
Selaginella doederleinii (shi shang bai) herb
Sesuvium portulacastrum
Sida fallax ('ilima)
Stachytarpheta spp. (ōwīwī)
Stellaria media (chickweed) herb
Terminalia catappa (kamani haole)
Thespesia populnea (milo)
Tremella fuciformis
Trifolium repens (white clover)
Triumfetta rhomboidea
Tropaeolum majus (nasturtium)
Vaccinium spp. ('ōhelo)
Verbena littoralis (ha'uoi)
Veronica perigrina
Wedelia spp.
Wikstroemia spp. ('ākia)
Zingiber zerumbet ('awapuhi kuahiwi)

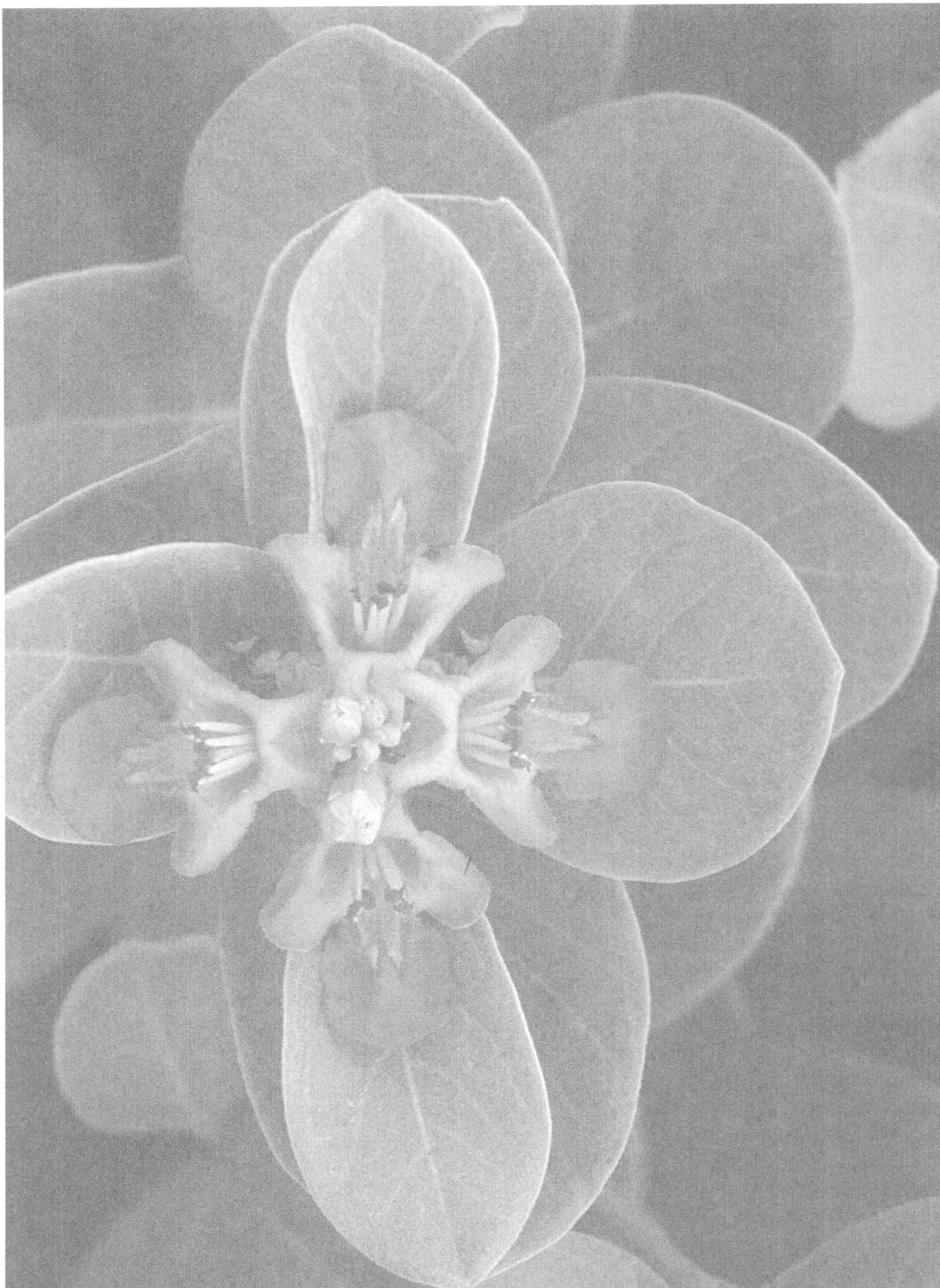

Cultural differences between Chinese and Hawaiian herbal medicine

Chinese and Hawaiian medicines often have diametrically opposed methods of plant preparation due to the significant differences between the cultures. Because this is a cross-cultural and somewhat schizophrenic tome, that dichotomy is reflected herein.

Hawaiian medicine is seated in a tradition of using fresh plant materials, gathered for one person at a time, and usually in combinations of less-than six ingredients. Flowers and leaves are used more commonly than roots, and the materials are usually used raw or boiled for only a short period of time. Materials are often gathered from nearby one's home, or for a more serious condition, gathered by a family practitioner from Wao Akua (an upland forest).

China has been an urban culture for thousands of years, with vast numbers of people packed into very small areas. The gathering of fresh herbal medicines was impractical in such a setting, so the Chinese learned how to dry and store their plant materials for future use. Because of volatile oils and other plant constituents, roots were discovered to have a longer ”shelf life” than flowers or leaves. As a result, Chinese herbal medicine has more roots in its pharmacy than does Hawaiian medicine. A typical Chinese herbal pharmacy has 300-400 different plant medicines on hand at any one time, around half of which are roots. These are gathered, prepared, and transported from across China. Herbs in a Chinese pharmacy are stored in drawers to facilitate easy access, but when dealing with this many herbs, identification can be a problem. Dried leaves often just look like dried leaves, dried roots often just look like dried roots, and the whole mess could easily be something that you just raked up out of your yard. So how can practitioners tell these herbs apart when preparing herb formulas? Being the innovators that they are, the Chinese came up with a system of dried plant identification that allows one to identify each herb almost from across the room. Each herb is cut in a specific way and to a specific length, making it instantly recognizable. This preparation is somewhat standardized across China. As an example, the result is that the prepared root *Paeonia alba* (bai shao) in Beijing will look identical to *Paeonia alba* (bak chut) in Guangzhou.

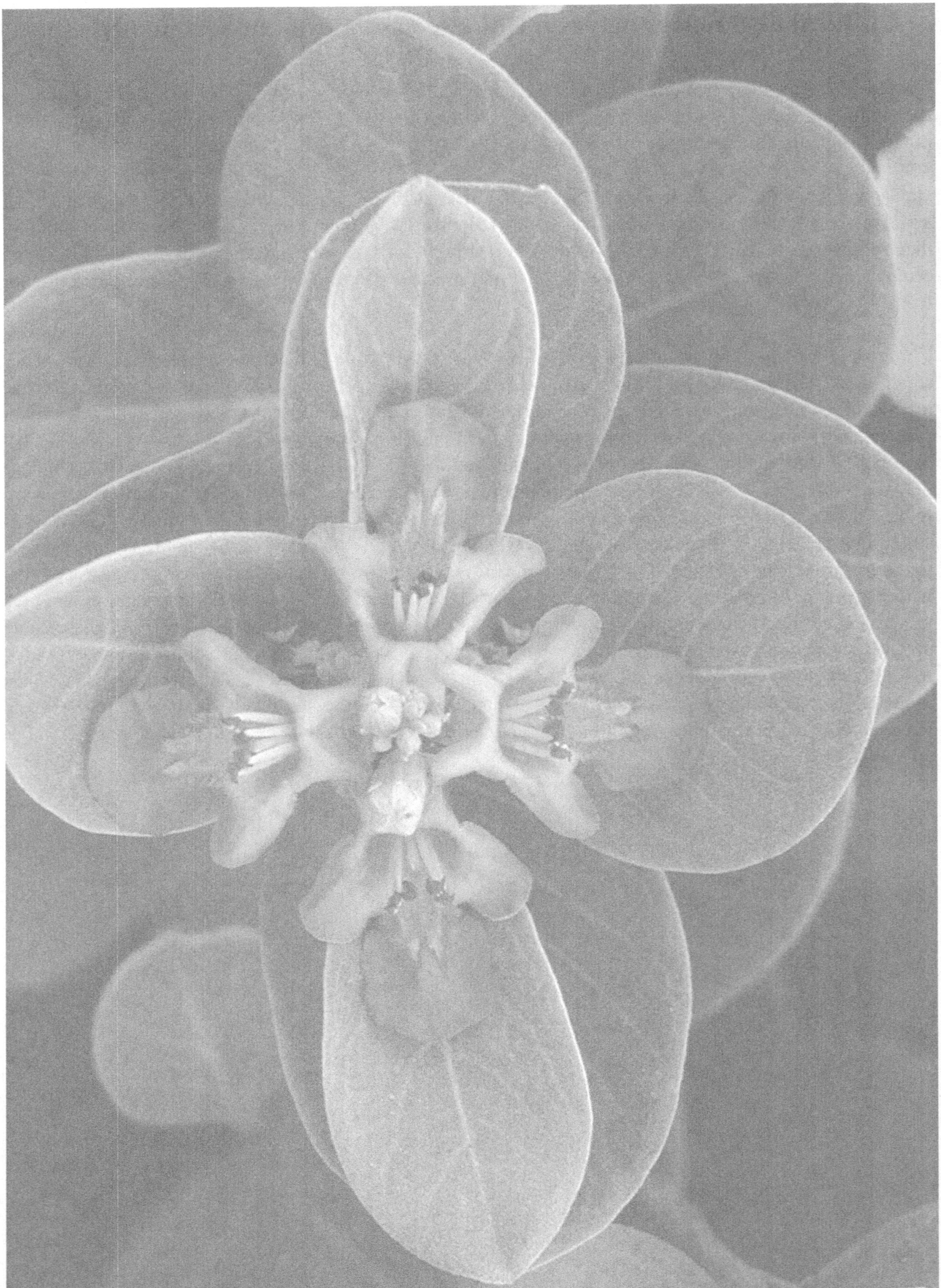

Definitions Of Medical Terms

Abortifacient: Can cause miscarriage.
Adjuvant: Seasoner for medicines.
Adenopathy: Enlargement of the lymph glands.
Aftosa: Hoof and Mouth disease.
Ague: Malarial fever.
Alexipharmic: An antidote for poison.
Alexiteric: A remedy.
Alterative: A plant that corrects and enhances bodily functions slowly over time.
Amebicide: Kills amoebas.
Amenorrhea: A lack of menses.
Amygdalitis: Inflammation of the amygdala, a cerebellar tonsil.
Analgesic: Reduces pain.
Anodyne: Reduces pain.
Anthlemintic: Expels worms.
Antiamoebic: Stops the growth of, or destroys, amoebas.
Antianaphylactic: A substance that reduces the effects of anaphylaxis.
Antiacariasis: Removes roundworms.
Antiasthmatic: A substance that reduces the effects of asthma.
Antibacterial: Stops the growth of, or destroys, bacteria
Antibilious: Reduces bile secretion.
Antibiotic: Stops the growth of, or destroys, bacteria
Anticatarrhal: Reduces inflammation of mucous membranes.
Anticarcinogenic: Reduces or prevents cancer.
Anticoagulant: Prevents or slows the clotting of blood.
Anticonvulsive: Reduces convulsions.
Antidote: An herb that counteracts a poison.
Antidysenteric: Prevents or reduces the severity of dysentery.
Antiemetic: Reduces vomiting.
Antifibrinolytic: Prevents the destruction of fibrin, a necessary component of a blood clot. Increases clotting.
Antihemorrhagic: Reduces bleeding.
Antileukopenic: Prevents white blood cell reduction.
Antineoplastic: Prevents or inhibits the formation of tumors.
Antihyperglycemic: An herb that prevents blood sugar swings.
Anti-implantation: Prevents the implantation of a fertilized egg.
Antimicrobial: Kills viruses or bacteria.
Antinociceptive: A substance that stops pain.
Antioxidant: Aids in the elimination of free radicals.
Antiplogistic: Reduces inflammation.
Antipruritic: Reduces itching.
Antipyretic: Lowers fever.
Antirheumatic: An herb that reduces inflammation and joint pain.
Antiscorbutic: Rich in vitamin C.
Antiseptic: Kills germs topically.
Antispasmodic: Reduces muscle spasms.
Antispermatogenic: Prevents the creation of sperm.
Antitussive: Supresses cough.
Anti-viral: Kills or prevents the reproduction of viruses.
Anxiolytic: Reduces anxiety.
Aperient: Gently laxative.
Aphrodisiac: Increases libido.
Astringent: Causes tissue constriction and reduces the flow of secretions.
Bactericide: Kills bacteria.
Balsamic: Soothing.
Beri-beri: Deficiency of thiamine (vitamin B1).
Bitter tonic: Increases digestive function using a bitter tasting herb.
Blenorrhagia: Urinary abscess.
Blepharitis: Inflammation of the eyelid.
Bradycardic: Slows heartbeat.
Bronchiodilator: Opens the breathing passages in the lungs.
Buboes: Lymph swelling
Calculi: Urinary stones.
Calmative: A sedative, hypnotic, or tranquilizer.
Cardiotonic: Improves heart function.
Cicatrix: New scar tissue over a wound.
Cicatrizant; An agent that promotes the healing of a wound
Cachexia: The loss of body mass associated with patients with advanced diseases.
Calculi: Stones, such as kidney stones.
Candidicide: Kills Candida albicans.
Cardiotonic: Strengthens heart function.

Carminative: Reduces intestinal gas.
Catamenial: Menstrual.
Catamenial seizures: Seizures associated with the menstrual cycle.
Cataplasm: Poultice.
Catarrh: Mucous membrane inflammation.
Cathartic: A strong laxative.
Cephalic: Treats diseases of the upper body and head.
Cholagogue: Increases the flow of bile.
Choleretic: Increases bile production.
Chyluria: Lymphatic fluid in the urine causing a milky white color.
Cicatrizant: Promotes healing of wounds or sores.
Climacteric: Menopause.
CNS depressant: Depresses the central nervous system.
Coagulant: Increases platelet aggregation.
Consumption: A disease that causes wasting of the body. Usually pulmonary tuberculosis.
Contraceptive: Prevents conception.
Collyrium: Cosmetic eye shadow.
Conjunctivitis: An inflammation of the conjunctiva of the eye.
Cositiveness: Bowel cramping.
Counterirritant: an herb that produces an irritation or heating sensation on the skin, increasing circulation and speeding the healing process.
Cynanche: Throat diseases.
Cyanogenetic: May produce cyanide.
Cyanogenic: Materials that can create hydrocyanic acid and cause cyanide poisoning.
Debridment: The cleaning of a wound.
Decoagulant: Reduces blood coagulation.
Decongestant: Removes respiratory mucous and phlegm.
Demulcent: Soothes internal membranes.
Dentifrice: Cleans the teeth.
Deobstruent: Removes urinary stones.
Depilatory: Removes hair.
Depurative: Expels waste and impurities from the blood or tissue.
Dermatological: Benefits the skin.
Detergent: Cleans out wounds.
Dermatosis: Any skin disease.
Diaphoretic: Causes sweating.
Discutient: Resolves tumors or inflammation.
Diuretic: Increases the flow of urine.
Dysentery: An intestinal infection.
Dysmenorrhea: Painful menstruation.
Dysuria: Painful urination.
Ecbolic: A substance that stimulates uterine contractions
Ecthyma: A bacterial skin infection similar to impetigo, but deeper.
Embryotoxic: Damaging to a fetus.
Emetic: Causes vomiting.
Emollient: Soothes external membranes.
Emmenagogue: Stimulates menstruation
Enuresis: Involuntary urine discharge.
Erysipelas: Skin disease caused by blood infection
Escharotic: Caustic to the skin, causing sloughing.
Estrogenic: Increases estrogen.
Eupeptic: Improves digestion.
Excitant: Stimulant.
Excrescence: A skin growth
Expectorant: Promotes the discharge of lung mucous.
Febrifuge: Lowers fever.
Filariasis: Infection by nematodes.
Flux: A bodily discharge of fluid.
Fumigant: A substance that is vaporized in order to kill pests.
Fungicide: Kills fungi.
Fungistatic: Stops the proliferation of fungi.
Gastritis: Inflammation of the stomach.
Galactogogue: Promotes the flow of breast milk.
Gingivosis: Any disorder of the gums.
Gravel: Urinary stones.
Hepatic: Relating to the liver.
Hepatitis: Inflammation of the liver.
Hepatoprotective: Prevents liver damage.
Hepatotonic: Improves liver function.
Hepatosis: Any disorder of the liver.
Hematochezia: Blood in the stools
Hematuria: Blood in the urine
Hemicrania: Migraine headache
Hemolytic: Increases the breakdown of red blood cells.
Hemorrhage: Uncontrolled bleeding.
Hemostatic: Stops bleeding.
Hydrocele: Fluid buildup in the scrotum.
Hypocholesterolemic: Lowers cholesterol.
Hypolipemic: Lowers blood lipids.
Hypotensive: Lowers blood pressure
Immunomodulatory: Stabilizes immune function.
Insecticidal: Kills insects.
Icteric hepatitis: Jaundice.

Intoxicant: Enhances reality.
Lactafuge: Reduces the flow of breast milk.
Lactogenic: Stimulates the production of breast milk.
Lactagogue: Promotes the flow of breast milk.
Larvicide: Kills insect larvae.
Laxative: Promotes mild evacuation of the bowels.
Leishmaniais: A parasitic disease spread by sand flies.
Leukoderma (vitiligo): A reduction of melanin in patchy areas of the skin, resulting in a mottled appearance.
Leucorrhea: Vaginal discharge.
Lipid lowering: Lowers fat levels in the blood.
Litholytic: Eliminates stones.
Lithontripic: Eliminates stones.
Lumbago: Lumbosacral (low back) pain.
Marasmus: Wasting of the flesh. It may be caused by malnutrition or by intestinal disorders.
Masticatory: Increases salivation.
Mastitis: An inflammation of the breast, usually bacterial in origin.
Melena: Tarry stools.
Menoxenia: Any abnormality of menstruation.
Menorrhagia: Excessive menstrual bleeding
Menorrhalgia: Painful menstruation.
Metritis: Inflammation of the uterus
Metrorrhagia: Bleeding between menses, spotting.
Mitogenic: Affects cell division.
Mucilaginous: A gelatinous and slippery herb that soothes and cools inflamed tissue and mucous membranes.
Mycosis: A fungal infection.
Myorelaxant: A muscle relaxant.
Narcotic: Stops pain by sedating the central nervous system.
Nephritis: Degeneration of the kidneys
Nervine: Relaxes nervous excitement.
Neuralgia: Nerve pain.
Neuroblastoma: A tumor of the adrenal medulla occurring in children.
Odontalogic: Temporarily reduces toothache
Oliguria: Decreased urination
Onychosis: Any disease of the nails
Ophthalmic: Benefits the eyes.
Ophthalmia: Inflammation of the conjunctiva of the eye.
Orexigenic: Increases appetite.
Orthopedic aid: Benefits musculoskeletal disorders.
Oxytocic: Accelerates childbirth.
Oxyuris: Intestinal worms.
Parturition: Childbirth.
Parulis: Inflammation of the gums
Pectoral: Benefits respiratory diseases.
Pediculicide: Kills body lice.
Philter: A potion.
Phthisis: Any disease that causes the body to waste away; tuberculosis
Pneumonitis: Respiratory allergies
Pock: pus filled lump on the skin
Polyuria: Excessive urination.
Post-partum: After childbirth.
Poultice: Herbs applied topically.
Prostaglandigenic: Increases prostaglandins.
Pruritis: Itching
Psoriasis: A chronic skin disease characterized by redness, itching and white scales.
Puerperium: Following childbirth
Puerperal: Relating to childbirth, as puerperal fever.
Purgative: Causes a drastic evacuation of the bowels.
Pyelitis: Inflammation of the kidney pelvis.
Pyoderma: Pus-containing skin conditions, (such as impetigo), caused by bacteria.
Quinsy: Streptococcal tonsillitis.
Ranula: A cyst on the floor of the mouth caused by a blocked salivary gland.
Restorative: An herb that restores health and strengthens the body.
Retinitis: Inflammation of the retina of the eye.
Rhagades: (pronounced "raggedies") Whistle lines around the lips.
Refrigerant: Cools the body.
Rejuvenative: Restores healthy function.
Rubefacient: An herb that reddens the skin.
Sapraemia: Blood poisoning from eating putrid food.
Sapremia: Blood poisoning from eating putrid food.
Scirrhus: A hard tumor.
Secretagogue: Increases secretions.
Secretolytic: Increases secretions.
Sedative: Reduces excitement, irritation, or stress.
Serotonergic enhancement: Increases serotonin.
Sialogogue: Increases saliva.

Sinapism: A plaster, often of Mustard seeds
Splenitis: Inflammation of the spleen.
Splenomegaly: Enlargement of the spleen.
Sterilant: Kills soil organisms.
Sternutatory: Causing sneezing.
Stimulant: Excites physiological processes and increases physiological activity.
Stomachic: Benefits digestion.
Strangury: Painful and dribbling urination from kidney stones, scars, or interstitial cystitis.
Styptic: An astringent herb that stops bleeding locally.
Sudorific: Increases sweating.
Suppurative: Helps expel pus.
Teratogenic: Causes birth defects.
Teratologic: Causes birth defects.
Thermogenic: Increases metabolism and the burning of stored fat.
Tic-douloureux: Trigeminal neuralgia
Tonic: An herb that maintains, restores, or increases health.
Tracheorelaxant: Relaxes the trachea.
Vaginitis: Vaginal inflammation.
Vasodialatory: Relaxes blood vessels.
Venereal: Treats venereal disease.
Vermifuge: Expels worms.
Vesicant: Causes blistering.
Vicarious menstruation: Discharge of blood from a non-genital source during a time that a menstrual period is normally expected.
Vulnerary: Speeds the healing of tissue.
Whitlow: A lesion of the finger. Whitlow may be viral or melanoma.
Yaws: an infectious disease caused by Treponema pertenue resulting in skin eruptions and ulcers.

BIBLIOGRAPHY BY PLANT

Adiantum spp. References

Bresciani 2003; Palmer 2003; Wagner 1999.

http: / / ars-genome.cornell.edu
http: / / www.ijp-online.com / archives / 1985 / 017 / 01 / r0073-0076le.pdf
http: / / www.ncbi.nlm.nih.gov / entrez / query.fcgi?db=PubMed
http: / / www.rain-tree.com / avenca.htm
http: / / www.swsbm.com / AJP / AJP_1883_No_1.pdf.

Aleurites moluccana References

Abbott 1992; Baldwin 1979; Degener 1945; Gibbons 2000; Gross; Gutmanis 1987; Handy 1934; Hargreaves 1964; Kaaiakamanu1922; Kepler 1990; Krauss 2001; Krauss; Lapulapu; Lamoureaux 1976; Locher 1995; Merlin 1999; Pedrosa 2002; Walker, Bill 1978; Whistler1992; World Health Organization 1998.

http: / / www.hort.purdue.edu / newcrop / duke_energy / Aleurites_moluccana.html
http: / / www.ncbi.nlm.nih.gov:80 / entrez / query.fcgi?CMD=Display&DB=PubMed

Aloe spp. References

Arvigo 2001; Bensy 1986; Beppu 2003; Brinker 2001; Chen 2004; Chithra 1998; Choi 2001; Corsi 1998; Davis 1989(a); Davis 1989(b); Davis 1989(c); Duansak 2003; Furukawa 2002; Ghannam1986; Lee CK 1997; Lee 2000(a); Lee KH 2000(b); Leonard 2003; Lewis 1977; Lim 2003; Macias 2004; Malterud 1993; Mindell 1992, 2000; Norikura 2002; Okyar 2001; Pecere 2000; Qiu 2000; Saada 2003; Shamaan 1998; Shimpo 2000; Shimpo 2002; Somboonwong 2000; Strehlow 1988; Vazquez 1996; Visuthikosol 1995; Womble 1988; World Health Organization; 1998; Yagi 2002.

http: / / chili.rt66.com / hrbmoore / ManualsMM / HerbRep3.txt
http: / / metalab.unc.edu / herbmed / eclectic / kings / aloe.html
http: / / newsbureau.upmc.com / Medsurg3 / FinkShockStudy2004.htm
http: / / www.medscape.com / server-java / MedLineApp? / member-search / getdoc.cgi?ord=6&searchid=1&have_local_holdings_file=0&local_journals_only=0
http: / / www.ncbi.nlm.nih.gov:80 / entrez / query.fcgi?CMD=Display&DB=PubMed
http: / / www.wholehealthmd.com / refshelf / substances_view / 1,1525,10001,00.html#Dosage_Information

Amaranthus spp. References

Berger 2003; Chaturvedi 1993; Chevallier 1996; Cribb 1986; De Lucca 1992; Elpel 2000; Haselwood 1983; Larsen 2003; Klimczak 2002; Moerman 1986; Neal 1965; Oladosu 1979; Schamber 1985.

http: / / bicn.com / wei / resources / nerp / wrs / ch3.htm
http: / / www.borneofocus.com / vaic / R&D / article1.htm
http: / / www.borneofocus.com / vaic / R&D / article18.htm
http: / / www.dweckdata.com / Published / Indian.htm
http: / / www.ethnobotany.com / seeds / Seed_a-e.html
http: / / www.floridaplants.com / Med / nausea.htm
http: / / www.google.com / search?q=cache:BOixxY1zZFg:www.fao.org / WAICENT / FAOINFO / AGRICULT / AGP / AGPS / Pgrfa / pdf / tanzania.pdf+Amaranthus+spinosus+medicine&hl=en
http: / / www.ibiblio.org / pfaf / cgi-bin / arr_html?Amaranthus+spinosus
http: / / www.mssrf.org.sg / 9-Table2-12.htm
http: / / www.mssrf.org / fris9809 / fris1014.html
http: / / www.mssrf.org / fris9809 / planti13.html
http: / / www.mssrf.org / fris9809 / planti52.html
http: / / www.natureproducts.net / Ecology / Biodiversity%20Products / biodiversity_products.html
http: / / www.pfaf.org
http: / / www.purr.demon.co.uk / Food / RelatedPlantList.html
http: / / www.rbgkew.org.uk / peopleplants / regions / africa / aen1 / review.htm
http: / / www.scs.leeds.ac.uk / pfaf / relations / weeds.html
http: / / www.soton.ac.uk / ~icuc / tambib / tam-u-e2.htm

Artocarpus communis References

Abbott 1992; Ahuna 1978; Degener 1945; Gibbons 2000; Higgs 1993; Kaaiakamanu 1922; Koshihara 1988; Krauss; Neal 1965; Wiart 2002; Whistler 1992; Whistler 1996; World Health Organization 1998.

http: / / ars-genome.cornell.edu:80 / cgi-bin / WebAce / webace?db=ethnobotdb&grep=artocarpus&longgrep=1
http: / / newcrop.hort.purdue.edu / newcrop / morton / breadfruit.html#Description
http: / / www.batcon.org / discover / ffecon4.html
http: / / www.bootlegbooks.com / Reference / Webster / data / 702.html
http: / / www.borneofocus.com / vaic / R&D / article41.htm
http: / / www.borneofocus.com / vaic / R&D / article42.htm
http: / / www.botgard.ucla.edu / html / botanytextbooks / economicbotany / Artocarpus / index.html
http: / / www.hawaii.edu / sciref / paccrops.html
http: / / www.hawaii-nation.org / canoe / ulu.html
http: / / www.k12.hi.us / ~kapunaha / TOJr.files / LiveLifeLiveLong / medicine%20files / hawaiian / hawaiian%20.htm
http: / / www.k12.hi.us / ~kapunaha / ulu.html
http: / / www.koaseeds.com / RWB / woodlist.html
http: / / www.ncbi.nlm.nih.gov:80 / entrez / query.fcgi?CMD=Text&DB=PubMed
http: / / www.purr.demon.co.uk / Food / RelatedPlantList.html
http: / / www.rrz.uni-hamburg.de / biologie / b_online / ibc99 / dr-duke / m.html
http: / / www.umd.umich.edu / cgi-bin / herb /
http: / / www.webhealthplus.com / alternativemedicine / currenttrends / anti.asp
http: / / www.wilderness-survival.net / plants-1.php

Auricularia spp. References

Agarwal 1982; Babineau 1994; Hobbs 1995; Jordon 2003; Misaki 1981; Wasser 1999; Yuan 1998.

http: / / www.gmushrooms.com / HEALTH.HTM

Bidens spp. References

Brandao 1997; Chin 1995; Chin 1996; Dimo 1999; Geissberger 1991; Hsu 1986; Hudson 1986; Jāger 1996; Li 1989; Matsunaga 1990; Mirvish 1979; Pereira 1999; Rabe 1997; Wang 1999; Wat 1979; Wat 1980.

http: / / bodd.cf.ac.uk / BotDermFolder / BotDermC / COMP.html
http: / / clinical.caregroup.org / altmed / interactions / Herb_Groups / Hyperglycemic-H.htm
http: / / hawaiianherbalteas.com / kookoolau.html
http: / / pppis.fao.org / GPPIS.exe$ShowHost?Host=517
http: / / spas.about.com / library / bllucayabush.htm
http: / / stuartxchange.com / OtherHerbals.html

http: / / uts.cc.utexas.edu / ~bramblet / ant301 / sixc.html
http: / / www.abc.net.au / gardening / stories / s237448.htm
http: / / www.abc.net.au / gardening / stories / s56380.htm
http: / / www.agricta.org / Spore / spore94 / spore94_brief.html
http: / / www.ann.com.au / herbs / Monographs / bidens.htm
http: / / www.ars-grin.gov / duke / dictionary / tico / b.html
http: / / www.brazil-brasil.com / cvrjul97.htm
http: / / www.britannia.com / panorama / seedbank.html
http: / / www.chs-connection.org / departments / science / rainforestplants / mikee / hola.htm
http: / / www.ethnobotany.com / seeds / Seed_a-e.html
http: / / www.fao.org / docrep / T9450E / t9450e0t.htm
http: / / www.fao.org / docrep / X5325e / x5325e07.htm
http: / / www.geocities.com / HotSprings / 5670 / natanon2.html
http: / / www.hepatitis-c.de / hyperic.htm
http: / / www.herbtrade.com / b.htm
http: / / www.ibiblio.org / pfaf / cgi-bin / arr_html?Bidens+pilosa
http: / / www.icomm.ca / survival / plants.don / plantnfo.htm
http: / / www.ilanet.net.au / clients / willoughby / bushnews.htm
http: / / www.itmonline.org / arts / bidens.htm
http: / / www.leafforlife.com / PAGES / HONORABL.HTM#aa460
http: / / www.mssrf.org / Fris9809 / planti64.html
http: / / www.nyu.edu / projects / summermst99 / groupprojects / rainforest / med.html
http: / / www.rain-tree.com / picaopreto.htm
http: / / www.rbgkew.org.uk / peopleplants / regions / africa / aen1 / review.htm
http: / / www.reyals.scarlet.nl / Bidens-AB.txt
http: / / www.sertek.com.tw / temp / bmtcg / english / knowlodge / production.htm
http: / / www.swsbm.com / Constituents / Bidens_pilosa.txt
http: / / www.thieme.de / plantamedica / 01_00 / planta82.html
http: / / www.unh.edu / herbarium / Poisonous / plantdict.html
http: / / www.uz.ac.zw / medicine / pharmacy / pubs / 1990.html
http: / / www-aes.tamu.edu / mary / brmrape / Br-iwwb.htm

Boerhavia spp. References

Bajracharya 1979; Bista 1997(a); Bista 1997(b); Chandan 1991; Cribb 1986; De Lucca 1992; Elpel 2000; Hiruma-Lima 2000; Honychurch 1986; Johnston 1997; Mehrotra 2002; Merlin 1999; Moerman 1986; Neal, 1965; Rawat 1997; Singh 1991; Sivarajan 1994; Sohni 1996; Taylor 1998; Wagner 1999; Whistler 1995; Whistler 1996; Wrench 1999; Xie 1996; Xu 1993; Zhong 1993.

http: / / 216.239.57.104 / search?q=cache:mNCpXQmiTrgJ:www.nybg.org / bsci / staf / KhanBalickAyurvedaArticle.pdf+Boerhavia+medicine&hl=en&ie=UTF-8
http: / / 216.239.57.104 / search?q=cache:udpFlT-cM1QJ:www.infinityfoundation.com / mandala / t_es / Himalayan_Materia_Medica_Table.pdf+Boerhavia+medicine&hl=en&ie=UTF-8
http: / / ayurveda-foryou.com / treat / liver.html
http: / / botanical.com / botanical / mgmh / i / ipecac07.html
http: / / botanical.com / botanical / mgmh / i / ipecac07.html
http: / / bush-tucker.tripod.com / html / textonly.html#Urpa
http: / / flora.huh.harvard.edu / china / mss / volume05 / Nyctaginaceae-US_edited.htm
http: / / herb.umd.umich.edu / herb / search.pl
http: / / medind.nic.in / imvw / imvw1886.html
http: / / translate.google.com / translate?hl=en&sl=es&u=http: / / www.niam.com / corp-web / mediplnt.htm&prev= / search%3Fq%3DBoerhavia%2Bmedicine%26start%3D10%26hl%3Den%26lr%3D%26ie%3DUTF-8%26sa%3DN
http: / / www.aromaherbshow.org / Article7.html
http: / / www.ars-grin.gov / cgi-bin / duke / ethnobot.pl
http: / / www.ayurvedahc.com / research.htm
http: / / www.ayurvedainsrilanka.com / Tumers%20and%20ulcers%20article.htm
http: / / www.calflora.net / botanicalnames / pageC-D.html
http: / / www.comp.leeds.ac.uk / cgi-bin / pfaf / arr_html?Boerhavia+diffusa
http: / / www.elephantcare.org / disquest.htm
http: / / www.geocities.com / judyseden / noni-pharmacy.html
http: / / www.healthwell.com / hnbreakthroughs / apr98 / vasantlad.cfm?path=hw
http: / / www.herbalfields.com / ayurveda.html
http: / / www.hinduonnet.com / folio / fo0010 / 00100140.htm
http: / / www.holistic-online.com / Herbal-Med / _Herbs / h178.htm
http: / / www.ibiblio.org / pfaf / cgi-bin / arr_html?Boerhavia+diffusa
http: / / www.ibiblio.org / pfaf / cgi-bin / arr_html?Boerhavia+diffusa&CAN=LATIND
http: / / www.inasp.info / ajol / journals / sajb / vol68no3abs.html
http: / / www.indiaoz.com.au / health / ayurveda / h_r / herbs_Punarnava.shtml
http: / / www.indmedplants-kr.org / Boerhavia_diffusa.htm
http: / / www.k12.hi.us / ~waianaeh / HawaiianStudies / natplants.html
http: / / www.ncbi.nlm.nih.gov:80 / entrez / query.fcgi?CMD=Display&DB=PubMed
http: / / www.niam.com / corp-web / mediplnt.htm
http: / / www.niam.com / corp-web / TradUses.html#boer
http: / / www.oneearthherbs.com / VanishingPlants.htm
http: / / www.pjbs.org / ansinet / ojbs / journal / 2001 / toc1(1).htm
http: / / www.rain-tree.com / ervatostao.htm
http: / / www.telmedpak.com / agricultures.asp?a=medplantpak&b=med_plant3a
http: / / www.vedahealth.com / html / abs.html

Broussonetia papyrifera References

Cheng 2001; Hsu 1986; Li 1976; Li 1994; Maui Community College database

http: / / apdl.kcc.hawaii.edu / ~ahupuaa / botany / fiber / wauke.htm
http: / / campus.ksbe.edu / middle / yellow / students / 1084208 / plant / default.html
http: / / hua.huh.harvard.edu / china / mss / volume05 / Moraceae-CAS_coauthoring.htm
http: / / www.awagami.or.jp / english / grossary.html
http: / / www.garynull.com / Documents / Continuum / AntibioticAlternatives.htm
http: / / www.huntington.org / BotanicalDiv / Timeline_org.html
http: / / www.ibiblio.org / pfaf / cgi-bin / arr_html?Broussonetia+papyrifera
http: / / www.jlhudsonseeds.net / SeedlistAp-B.htm
http: / / www.labyrinth.net.au / ~saul / history / garden.html
http: / / www.ncbi.nlm.nih.gov:80 / entrez / query.fcgi?CMD=Display&DB=PubMed
http: / / www.nps.gov / plants / alien / fact / brpa1.htm
http: / / www.pfaf.org
http: / / www.treeguide.com / nn / Species.asp?SpeciesID=188&Region=NorthAmerican
http: / / www.umd.umich.edu / cgi-bin / herb /

Capsella rubella References

Bliss 1973;Brown 1989; Commonwealth; Duke1985; El-Abyad 1990; Foster 2000; Gruenwald 1998; Heinerman 1996; Hoffman 1988; Hsu 1986; Hutchens 1983; Kuroda 1975; Kuroda 1976; Li 1976; Lust 2001;Mabey 1988;Miller1988; Moerman 1986; Moore 1989; Moore 1993; Mowrey 1986; Ody 1993; Peterson 1999; Shipochliev 1981; Thomson 1983, USDA-NRCS.

http: / / BoDD.cf.ac.uk / BotDermFolder / BotDermC / CRUC.html
http: / / chili.rt66.com / hrbmoore / ManualsMM / HerbMedContra1.txt
http: / / health.yahoo.com / health / Alternative_Medicine / Herbal_Remedies_Tree / Herbal_Remedies / shepherd_s_purse /
http://plants.usda.gov
http: / / thriveonline.oxygen.com / medical / library / herbs / ame0158.html
http: / / vitalvillage.net / nmc / nmc-pages / shepherdspurse.htm
http: / / www.backcountryrangers.com / edibles / plants_soloframe.html?CAPSELLA.html
http: / / www.bibliomania.com / 2 / 1 / 66 / 113 / frameset.html
http: / / www.botanical.com / botanical / mgmh / s / shephe47.html
http: / / www.central.edu / biology / botany / wild / plantsS.html
http: / / www.drgenie.com / Naturaopathic / S / Shepherd's%20 Purse.htm
http: / / www.healthy.net / asp / templates / article.asp?PageType=article&ID=1183
http: / / www.herbweb.com / herbage / A94.htm
http: / / www.holisticonline.com / Herbal-Med / _Herbs / h290.htm
http: / / www.ibiblio.org / herbmed / eclectic / kings / capsella.html
http: / / www.ibiblio.org / pfaf / cgi-bin / arr_html?Capsella+bursa%2dpastoris
http: / / www.naturalhealthnotebook.com / Herbs / Latin_Herbs / Genus-C / Capsella_bursa-pastoris.htm
http: / / www.ncbi.nlm.nih.gov:80 / entrez / query.fcgi?CMD=Display&DB=PubMed
http: / / www.odont.aau.dk / LibHerb2 / Pn0044.HTM
http: / / www.purplesage.org.uk / profiles / shepherdspurse.htm
http: / / www.reyals.scarlet.nl / Capsella-AB.txt
http: / / www.scotweb.co.uk / kitchen / wild / plants.html#shepherdspurse
http: / / www.scs.leeds.ac.uk / cgi-bin / pfaf / arr_html?Capsella+bursa%2dpastoris
http: / / www.umd.umich.edu / cgi-bin / herb /

Capsicum spp. References

Agrawal 1985; Agrawal 1986; Akagi 1998; Andoh 1986; Bernstein 1986; Biggs1990; Bista 1997(a); Bista 1997(b); Bliss 1973; Bouraoui 1988; Brinker 2001; Carper 1988; Castleman 1991; De Lucca 1992; Farnsworth 1975; Frawley 1988; Gruenwald 1998; Han 2001; Heinerman 1996; Henderson 1999; Hobbs 1998; Holzer 1989; Honychurch 1986; Hussain 1994; Jang 1991; Jones 1997; Kang 1995; Kato 2003; Kawada 1986; Kawada 1988; Kim 1997; Kim 1998; Kim 2003; Kim 2004; Kim J1985; Kogure 2002; Kowalchik 1987; Lejeune 2003; Li Ninghan 1976; Li Ninghan1994; Lopez-Carrillo 1994; Lu 1990; Lundberg 1983(a); Mabey 1988; McIntyre 1996; Miller 1983; Mindell 2000; Modly 1986; Moerman 1986; Monsereenusorn 1983; Monsereenusorn 1985; Moore; Mowrey 1986; Notani 1987; Ody 1993; Oh 2003; Page 1998; Park 1997; Park 2004; Pitchford 1993; Ramakrishna 2003; Readers Digest Editors 1986; Reilly 2003; Richeux 1999; Richeux 2000; Rosa 2002; Sicuteri 1990; Singh 2001; Stander 2001; Surh 1995(a); Surh 1995(b); Surh 1995(c); Surh 1996; Surh 1998; Surh 2000; Szolcsanyi 1998; Tolan 2004; Tsuchiya 2001; Vogel 1970; Watanabe 1987; Watanabe 1988(a); Whistler 1992(b); Whistler 1992(c); Whistler 1996; Yeoh 1995;

http: / / BoDD.cf.ac.uk / BotDermFolder / BotDermS / SOLA.html
http: / / www.ars-grin.gov / duke / dictionary / tico / c.html
http: / / www.botanical.com / botanical / mgmh / c / cayenn40.html
http: / / www.cfsan.fda.gov / ~djw / pltx.cgi?QUERY=Capsicum
http: / / www.dittmar.dusnet.de / english / suche-e.php?term=capsicum
http: / / www.fiery-foods.com / dave / bushmedicine.html
http: / / www.herbs2000.com / herbs / herbs_cayenne.htm
http: / / www.herbweb.com / herbage / A95.htm
http: / / www.holisticonline.com / Herbal-Med / _Herbs / h43.htm
http: / / www.ibiblio.org / herbmed / eclectic / kings / capsicum.html
http: / / www.medicinescomplete.com / mc / herbals / current / noframes / hrb0027.htm
http: / / www.mothernature.com / asp / category_list.asp?category=60
http: / / www.naturalproducts.org / inpr / mono_html / capsi_html / capsi_botan1.html
http: / / www.ncbi.nlm.nih.gov:80 / entrez / query.fcgi?CMD=Display&DB=PubMed
http: / / www.odont.aau.dk / LibHerb2 / Pn0357.HTM
http: / / www.swsbm.com / Constituents / Capsicum_frutescens.txt
http: / / taninos.tripod.com / capsaicin.htm
http: / / www.umd.umich.edu / cgi-bin / herb /
http: / / www.wrc.net / phyto / Cayenne.html

Carica papaya References

Blanco 1998; Chen 1981; Chevallier 1996; Duke1984; Emeruwa 1982; Eno 2000; Giordani1996; Gruenwald 1998; Hewitt 2000; Kermanshai 2001; Krauss; Lohiya 1994; Lohiya 1999; Lohiya 2000; Moerman 1986; Osato 1993; Quinones 1999; Starley 1999; Udoh 1999; Whistler 1992; Whistler 1992; World Health Organization 1998.

http: / / stuartxchange.com / Lists2.html
http: / / www.ansci.cornell.edu / plants / medicinal / papaya.html
http: / / www.ars-grin.gov / duke / dictionary / tico / c.html
http: / / www.ars-grin.gov / duke / syllabus / module14.htm
http: / / www.botanical.com / temp / mgmh-no-products / p / papaw-02.html
http: / / www.goinggreen.net / alternative / azherbs.htm
http: / / www.herbmed.org / herbs / Morinda_Noni.htm
http: / / www.herbweb.com / herbage / A98.htm
http: / / www.hort.purdue.edu / newcrop / duke_energy / Carica_papaya.html
http: / / www.ibiblio.org / herbmed / eclectic / kings / carica.html
http: / / www.indiangyan.com / books / healthbooks / food_that_heal / papaya.shtml
http: / / www.ncbi.nlm.nih.gov:80 / entrez / query.fcgi?CMD=Text&DBΔPubMed
http: / / www.parentspitara.com / health / alternate / online.asp?unit=10
http: / / www.philippineherbs.com / philippineherbindex.htm#P
http: / / www.purr.demon.co.uk / Food / RelatedPlantList.html
http: / / www.siu.edu / ~ebl / leaflets / papaya.htm
http: / / www.sunfood.net / papaya-wonderfruit.html
http: / / www.tlahui.com / medic / medic7 / papaya.htm
http: / / www.umd.umich.edu / cgi-bin / herb /
http: / / www.unh.edu / herbarium / Poisonous / plantdict.html

Centella asiatica References

Arpaia 1990; Babu 1995; Belcaro 1990; Bonte 1994; Bonte 1995; Bosse 1979; Brinkhaus 2000; Cesarone 2001(a); Cesarone 2001(b); Cesarone 2001(c); Chatterjee 1992; Cheng 2000; Cheng 2004; Chevallier 1996; Gupta 2003; Incandela 2001(a); Incandela 2001(b); Incandela 2001(c); Lee 2000; Li 1976; Li 1994; Maquart 1990; Medda 1995; Michael Moore's plant tincture brochure; Pukui 1986; Sairam 2001; Shukla 1999; Suguna 1996; Sunilkumar 1998; Translation of A Barefoot Doctor's Manual 1977; Veerendra 2003; Wagner 1999; Widgerow 2000; World Health Organization 1998; Zheng 1989.

http: / / 128.242.211.97 / healthnotes / Herb / Gotu_Kola.cfm
http: / / BoDD.cf.ac.uk / BotDermFolder / BotDermU / UMBE.

html
http: / / chili.rt66.com / hrbmoore / ManualsMM / HerbMedContra1.txt
http: / / herbsforhealth.about.com / library / weekly / aa121297.htm
http: / / herbwalk.com / remedy / herb_Gotu_Kola_103.html
http: / / members.aol.com / _ht_a / godshaer / herbal-bc.htm
http: / / thriveonline.oxygen.com / medical / library / herbs / ame0087.html
http: / / www.altnature.com / Library / gotukola.htm
http: / / www.ann.com.au / herbs / Monographs / centella.htm
http: / / www.apr.ch / ingred.htm
http: / / www.ayurveda.com / materiamedica / Centella%20asiatica--Gotu%20Kola.htm
http: / / www.dweckdata.com / Plant_month.htm
http: / / www.floridata.com / ref / C / cent_asi.cfm
http: / / www.healthwell.com / healthnotes / Herb / Gotu_Kola.cfm
http: / / www.herbmed.org / herbs / centella.htm
http: / / www.herbs2stopsmoking.com / herbdesc / 2gotukol.htm
http: / / www.herbweb.com / herbage / A109.htm
http: / / www.holisticonline.com / Herbal-Med / _Herbs / h18.htm
http: / / www.ibiblio.org / pfaf / cgi-bin / arr_html?Centella+asiatica
http: / / www.intelihealth.com / IH / ihtIH / WSIHW000 / 8513 / 28326.html
http: / / www.ion.com.au / ~iridology / Centella.html
http: / / www.linnea-worldwide.com / products / centella.html
http: / / www.mssrf.org / Fris9809 / Fris1065.html
http: / / www.naturalhealthnotebook.com / Herbs / Latin_Herbs / Genus-C / Centella_asiatica.htm
http: / / www.niam.com / corp-web / centella.htm
http: / / www.nybg.org / gardens / medicine.html
http: / / www.pharm.usyd.edu.au / hmrec / research.htm
http: / / www.phytotherapies.org / monograph_detail.cfm?id=62
http: / / www.quipo.it / abcfiori / curiosit.html#CENTELLA ASIATICA
http: / / www.rxvitamins.com / pets / posttech.asp
http: / / www.searsphytochem.com / product / centella.htm
http: / / www.swsbm.com / Constituents / Centella_asiatica.txt
http: / / www.thehimalayadrugco.com / h-centel.htm
http: / / www.time.com / time / reports / heroes / plant.html
http: / / www.uspharmacist.com / NewLook / DisplayArticle.cfm?item_num=696
http: / / www.viable-herbal.com / herbdesc1 / 1centell.htm
http: / / www.zestrsa.co.za / products / applecider.htm

Chamaesyce hirta References

Chevallier 1996; Huxley 1992; Johnson 1999; Lanhers 1990; Lanhers 1991; Li 1976; Matthews 1994; Pukui 1986; Sivarajan 1994; Tona 1999(a); Tona 1999(b); Tona 2000; Translation of A Barefoot Doctor's Manual 1977; Vijaya 1995; Wagner 1999.

http: / / bodd.cf.ac.uk / BotDermFolder / BotDermE / EUPH.html
http: / / hometown.aol.com / godshaer / herbal-def.htm
http: / / pc4.sisc.ucl.ac.be / prelude / getahun.html
http: / / pub1.ezboard.com / ftheausnaturopathicnetworkherbalmedicine.showMessage?topicID=4.topic
http: / / stuartxchange.com / OtherHerbals.html
http: / / thriveonline.oxygen.com / medical / library / herbs / ame0067.html
http: / / www.ann.com.au / herbs / Monographs / euphorbi.htm
http: / / www.ars-grin.gov / duke / dictionary / tico / e.html
http: / / www.ars-grin.gov / duke / syllabus / module9.htm
http: / / www.borneofocus.com / vaic / R&D / article1.htm
http: / / www.botanical.com / botanical / mgmh / s / spurge84.html
http: / / www.bri.net.au / medicine.html
http: / / www.cpreec.org / edu / medi-pln.htm
http: / / www.fao.org / docrep / T9450E / t9450e04.htm
http: / / www.fao.org / docrep / T9450E / t9450e0t.htm
http: / / www.hc-sc.gc.ca / hpb-dgps / therapeut / zfiles / english / policy / issued / herbnmi_e.html
http: / / www.healthandage.com / html / res / com / ConsConditions / Bronchitiscc.html
http: / / www.healthy.net / asp / templates / article.asp?PageType=Article&ID=783
http: / / www.herbmed.org / herbs / Morinda_Noni.htm
http: / / www.ibiblio.org / herbmed / eclectic / kings / euphorbia-pilu.html
http: / / www.ibiblio.org / pfaf / cgi-bin / arr_html?Euphorbia+hirta
http: / / www.indiangyan.com / books / therapybooks / Herbs_That_Heal / euphorbia.shtml
http: / / www.motherearthherbs.com / tincture.html
http: / / www.mssrf.org / fris9809 / planti28.html
http: / / www.mssrf.org / Fris9809 / planti48.html
http: / / www.mydr.com.au / default.asp?article=2708
http: / / www.nalusda.gov / afsic / AFSIC_pubs / qb93-02.htm
http: / / www.ncbi.nlm.nih.gov:80 / entrez / query.fcgi?CMD=Text&DB=PubMed
http: / / www.phytotherapies.org / monograph_detail.cfm?id=95
http: / / www.sonic.net / melissk / planta-e.html#e
http: / / www.swosu.edu / ~longs / phcl / alteinfl.htm
http: / / www.umkit.com / therapeutic.htm
http: / / www.vshiva.net / biodiversity / pirate.htm
http: / / www.vshiva.net / naturefacts / euphorb.html

Coix lachryma-jobi References

Andoh 1986; Bensy 1986; Bliss 1973; Chang 2003; Chen 2004; Gomita 1981; Hsu 1986; Hung 2003; Li 1976; Lu 1994; Moerman 1986; Otsuka 1988; Park 1988; Roman 1992; Seo 2000.

http: / / www.ars-grin.gov / cgi-bin / duke / ethnobot.pl
http: / / www.ars-grin.gov / duke / dictionary / tico / c.html
http: / / www.dittmar.dusnet.de / english / suche-e.php?term=Coix
http: / / www.holisticonline.com / Herbal-Med / _Herbs / h376.htm
http: / / www.ibiblio.org / pfaf / cgi-bin / arr_html?Coix+lacryma%2djobi
http: / / www.medscape.com / server-java / MedLineApp?MedscapeSURI=getdoc&multi=yes&op=none&searchid=1&sformat=medlars&eformat=quickdoc&vformat=citation&tformat=pc&totalselected=200&navcheckboxes=0&beginnumber=1&endnumber=9&ord=6&ord=7&x=18&y=18
http: / / www.ncbi.nlm.nih.gov:80 / entrez / query.fcgi?CMD=Display&DB=pubmed http: / / www.umd.umich.edu / cgi-bin / herb /

Commelina diffusa References

Bista 1997(a); Bliss 1973; Duke; Foster 2000; Haselwood 1983; Honychurch 1986; Huang 1993; Li 1976; Moerman 1986; Montagna; Naone; Neal 1965; Peterson 1999; Tang 1994; Translation of A Barefoot Doctor's Manual 1977; Wagner 1999; Whistler 1996; World Health Organization 1998.

http: / / 2bnthewild.com / plants / H65.htm
http: / / ars-genome.cornell.edu:80 / cgi-bin / WebAce / webace?db=mpnadb&class=Specific_use&object=Commelina%20dianthifolia%3a%20Navaho-Ramah%20Veterinary%20aid
http: / / www.africam.com / Articles / FieldGuide / FlowerGuide / YellowFlowers / yellowflowersindex.html
http: / / www.ars-grin.gov / cgi-bin / duke / ethnobot.pl
http: / / www.ars-grin.gov / duke / dictionary / tico / c.html
http: / / www.cgriffith.net / servlets / SearchBases
http: / / www.didgeridoo-australia.com / bushmedicine.htm
http: / / www.enwei.com.cn / english / enwei_home_doctor / product / single_herb / Ya%20zhi%20cao.htm

http: / / www.fau.edu / divdept / science / envsci / ethno-list.html
http: / / www.gse.buffalo.edu / FAS / Johnston / Sexlife_and_Folklore_of_D6B.htm
http: / / www.huis.hiroshima-u.ac.jp / ~nomura / T / tsuyuku.html
http: / / www.ibiblio.org / pfaf / cgi-bin / arr_html?Commelina+communis
http: / / www.medscape.com
http: / / www.montana.com / manu / paper.html
http: / / www.mssrf.org / fris9809 / planti23.html
http: / / www.ncbi.nlm.nih.gov:80 / entrez / query.fcgi?CMDΔText&DBΔPubMed
http: / / www.rrz.uni-hamburg.de / biologie / b_online / ibc99 / dr-duke / s.html
http: / / www.umd.umich.edu / cgi-bin / herb /
http: / / www.vetwork.org.uk / pune12.htm

Cordyline fruticosa References

Abbott 1992; Cambie 2003; Gutmanis 1987; Kaaiakamanu 1922; Kawai'ae 1980; Leonard 1992-2004; Ooi 1993; Whistler 1992(a); Whistler 1992(b); Whistler 1996; World Health Organization 1998.

http: / / bodd.cf.ac.uk / BotDermFolder / BotDermA / AGAV.html
http: / / hoolokahi.vizip.com / laau.html
http: / / library.kcc.hawaii.edu / ~soma / krauss / ki.html
http: / / uneli.unitec.ac.nz / our_auckland / greylynn / Forest%20Trees.htm
http: / / www.abc.net.au / ra / carvingout / issues / tjibaou.htm
http: / / www.aircav.com / survival / appb / asappb45.html
http: / / www.ars-grin.gov / cgi-bin / duke / ethnobot.pl
http: / / www.borneofocus.com / vaic / R&D / article41.htm
http: / / www.ccc.govt.nz / Streamside / PLANTS / Cordaust.html
http: / / www.cic-valencia.org.ve / gardens.htm
http: / / www.dittmar.dusnet.de / english / suche-e.php?term=cordyline
http: / / www.fao.org / ag / AGA / AGAP / FRG / afris / Data / 379.HTM
http: / / www.floweressences.com / Essences / Aloha.html
http: / / www.geocities.com / RainForest / 7109 / flax.htm
http: / / www.hawaii.edu / nhcoe / newsletter.html
http: / / www.ibiblio.org / herbmed / database / plant-names-c-e.html
http: / / www.k12.hi.us / ~kapunaha / ti.html
http: / / www.ktropicals.com / flowers / foliage.shtml
http: / / www.oak-tree.org / eden-seeds.html
http: / / www.rbgkew.org.uk / peopleplants / pdf / wp3e.pdf
http: / / www.rbgkew.org.uk / peopleplants / wp / wp3 / conservation.htm
http: / / www.terralingua.org / TLPublications / DiscussionPapers / DiscPaper9.html
http: / / www.textfiles.com / food / seeds42.txt
http: / / www.umd.umich.edu / cgi-bin / herb /
http: / / www-nceph.anu.edu.au / htc / pdfs / Hughes1.pdf

Curcuma longa References

Aggarwal 2003; Ahuna 1978; Ambegaokar 2003; Antony 1999; Barthelemy 1998; Calabrese 2003; Chainani-Wu 2003; Charles 1992; Chen 1999; Cheng 2001; Ciolino 1998; Cleghorn 1990; Dikshit 1995; Egan 2004; Elattar 2000; Ferreira 1992; Frautschy 2001; Fujisawa 2004; Gross; Hussain 1992; Hussain 1994; Ikezaki 2001; Kaaiakamanu 1922; Kandarkar 1998; Kawamori 1999; Kuttan 1985; Lans 1998; Life Extension Magazine December 2004; Lim 2001; Liontas 2004; Mahady 2002; Miquel 2002; Ono 2003; Ono 2004(a); Ono 2004(b); Polasa 1992; Qureshi 1992; Rafatullah 1990; Rajakrishnan 1999; Ramirez-Tortosa 1999; Reddy 1994; Sakagami 2000; Selvam 1995; Sidhu 1998; Spingarn 1998; Srivastava 1995; Sui 1993; Ushida 2000; Zava 1998.
http: / / acprx.pharmacy.arizona.edu / about / turmeric.html
http: / / BoDD.cf.ac.uk / BotDermFolder / BotDermZ / ZING.html
http: / / getnoni.com /
http: / / hawaiianherbalteas.com / olena.html
http: / / lists.ibiblio.org / mailman / listinfo / herbalhall
http: / / neuro.vetmed.ufl.edu / Alt_med / Library / Research / research.html
http: / / neuro.vetmed.ufl.edu / Alt_med / Library / Research / Spice_sri.html
http: / / or.essortment.com / whatisturmeric_rxnm.htm
http: / / stuartxchange.com / OtherHerbals.html
http: / / www.allnaturalherbs.com / alpha-phypoic.htm
http: / / www.ann.com.au / herbs / Monographs / curcuma.htm
http: / / www.ars-grin.gov / duke / dictionary / tico / c.html
http: / / www.ars-grin.gov / duke / syllabus / module11.htm
http: / / www.ayurveda.com / materiamedica / Curcuma%20longa-Haridra-Turmeric2.htm
http: / / www.ayurveda.com / materiamedica / Curcuma%20longa-Haridra-Turmeric.htm
http: / / www.ayurvedahc.com / research.htm
http: / / www.borneofocus.com / vaic / R&D / article41.htm
http: / / www.botanical.com / botanical / mgmh / t / turmer30.html
http: / / www.botanichealth.com /
http: / / www.care2.com / channels / solutions / pets / 104
http: / / www.chakratunedbowls.com
http: / / www.dbbm.fiocruz.br / www-mem / 965 / 4040his.html
http: / / www.findarticles.com / cf_0 / g2603 / 0007 / 2603000715 / print.jhtml
http: / / www.geocities.com / nutriflip / Naturopathy / Turmeric.html
http: / / www.gnc.com / wellness / natpharm / Herb / Turmeric.htm
http: / / www.herb.com / materia.htm
http: / / www.herbmed.org / herbs / curcuma.htm
http: / / www.herbsecret.co.uk / pages / product.php3?idt=54&idw=2
http: / / www.herbsecret.co.uk / pages / product.php3?idt=56&idw=2
http: / / www.herbtrade.com / t-z.htm
http: / / www.herbweb.com / herbage / A161.htm
http: / / www.holisticonline.com / Herbal-Med / _Herbs / h27.htm
http: / / www.hookele.com / canoeplants / olena.html
http: / / www.ho-tinursery.com / hawaiian.html#Curcuma longa
http: / / www.humorscope.com / herbs / turmeric.html
http: / / www.ibiblio.org / herbmed / eclectic / felter / curcuma-long.html
http: / / www.ibiblio.org / herbmed / eclectic / kings / curcuma.html
http: / / www.indianherbs.com / cucum_95.htm
http: / / www.intelihealth.com / IH / ihtIH / WSIHW000 / 8513 / 29277.html#Overview
http: / / www.internethealthlibrary.com / Therapies / Ayurvedic-Medicine-Research.htm
http: / / www.joglosemar.co.id / jamu.html
http: / / www.k12.hi.us / ~kapunaha / olena.htm
http: / / www.kobakoba.co.uk / curcuma%20longa.htm
http: / / www.kohala.net / kaimalino / KMWC-4.html#anchor471944
http: / / www.komvet.at / english / issue0199 / xfiles0199.htm
http: / / www.laurasleanbeef.com /
http: / / www.liberherbarum.com / Pn0615.HTM
http: / / www.mahidol.ac.th / abstracts / annual2000 / 0306.htm
http: / / www.med.nagoya-u.ac.jp / Environderm / edj / vol3 / 34-357.htm
http: / / www.medicalmeals.com / zingiberaceaeC.htm
http: / / www.mercksource.com / pp / us / cns / cns_news_article.

jspzQzidzEz260879
http: / / www.mssrf.org / Fris9809 / fris1103.html
http: / / www.natmedpro.com / nmp / Refs-Peptulce.htm
http: / / www.naturalhealthnotebook.com / Herbs / Latin_Herbs / Genus-C / Curcuma_longa.htm
http: / / www.ncbi.nlm.nih.gov:80 / entrez / query. fcgi?CMD=Text&DB=PubMed
http: / / www.niam.com / corp-web / mediplnt.htm
http: / / www.nursing.uiowa.edu / sites / PedsPain / Nonpharm / Herbaltt.htm
http: / / www.nutrisana.com / html / Monograph-Curcuma.html
http: / / www.pacificholistics.com / in-ex.html
http: / / www.positivehealth.com / permit / Articles / Arthritis / kimbr52.htm
http: / / www.rain-tree.com / tumeric.htm
http: / / www.slowfood.com / Slowfood_UpLoad / Riviste / SLOW / EN / 21 / en_curcuma.html
http: / / www.swsbm.com / Constituents / Curcuma_longa.txt
http: / / www.turmeric.8m.com / about.html
http: / / www.umd.umich.edu / cgi-bin / herb /
http: / / www.vediccancer.com / herbal%20medicine24.htm
http: / / www.vshiva.net / biodiversity / pirate.htm
http: / / www.webhealthcentre.com / altmed / ayurveda / disease. asp
http: / / www.wholisticanimal.com / Herbs.html
http: / / www.wonderfulbuys.com /

Cymbopogon refractus References

Bista 1997(a); Carbajal 1989; Carlini 1986; De Lucca 1992; Govere 2000; Kishore 1993; Li 1976; Newman; Pattnaik 1995(a); Pattnaik 1995(b); Pattnaik 1999; Pukui 1986; Sarbhoy 1978; Seaforth 1985; Whistler 1992(b); Whistler 1992(c); Whistler 1996.

http: / / 202.139.254.149 / herbs / lemongrass.htm
http: / / 208.5.178.253 / products / lmngrass_content.htm
http: / / home.istar.ca / ~ddobie / jamie / right17.htm
http: / / medicinegarden.com / Library / herbssafety1.html
http: / / members.ozemail.com.au / ~frgntgar / cafe / thicook.html
http: / / members.tripod.com / ~mhassel / recepies / index.htm
http: / / thriveonline.oxygen.com / medical / library / herbs / ame0353.html
http: / / total.dufte.de / aromatherapie / Beschreibungen / aethoel / oele / Lemongras.htm&prev= / search%3Fq%3DCymbopogon%26 num%3D50%26hl%3Den%26safe%3Doff
http: / / www.abbeyessentials.co.uk / lemongrass.htm
http: / / www.amrita.net / aromatherapyinfo / lemongrass.html
http: / / www.ars-grin.gov / cgi-bin / duke / ethnobot.pl
http: / / www.ars-grin.gov / duke / dictionary / tico / c.html
http: / / www.botanical.com / botanical / mgmh / g / grasse34.html
http: / / www.botany.com / cymbopogon.html
http: / / www.dittmar.dusnet.de / english / suche-e. php?term=Cymbopogon
http: / / www.eclecticpaganshop.com / 52 / cat52.htm
http: / / www.essencefactory.com / oils / lemongrass.html
http: / / www.essenticsweb.com / References / Lemongrass%20 references.htm
http: / / www.fsmarketplace.co.uk / ubik.dll / store / sashascents / item / -aWQ9Njkmc2Vzc2lvbj0lMkQx-Ea
http: / / www.herbweb.com / herbage / A165.htm
http: / / www.i5ive.com / article.cfm / aromatherapy / 20929
http: / / www.ibiblio.org / herbmed / faqs / culi-2-19-lemong.html
http: / / www.medicine.cmu.ac.th / dept / biochem / ~rawiwan / CV.htm
http: / / www.msinp.com / herbs / lemongra.htm
http: / / www.myfavoriteherbs.net / Lemongrass.html
http: / / www.ncbi.nlm.nih.gov:80 / entrez / query. fcgi?CMD=Display&DB=PubMed
http: / / www.pennysfromheavensoaps.com / lemongrass.htm
http: / / www.roebourne.wa.edu.au / culture / bush.htm
http: / / www.tropilab.com / lemon-gras.html
http: / / www.uni-saarland.de / ~su13mwfs / med / i-medcym. html&prev= / search%3Fq%3DCymbopogon%26num%3D50%26 hl%3Den%26safe%3Doff

Cyperus rotundus References

Bensky 1986; Bensky 1993; Chang 1987; Chen 2004; Duke 1985; Gupta 1980; Haselwood 1983; Hsu 1986; Seo 2001; Translation of a Barefoot Doctor's Manual 1977; Weenen 1990; Xue 1993.

http: / / hcgvn.vps.org / west_au / cyperotu.htm
http: / / herbwalk.com / remedy / herb_Xiang_Fu_225.html
http: / / www.ars-grin.gov / duke / dictionary / tico / c.html
http: / / www.ayuvet-usa.com / Html / Press_Articles.htm
http: / / www.colostate.edu / Depts / Entomology / courses / en570 / papers_2000 / krompegel.html
http: / / www.cpreec.org / edu / medi-pln.htm
http: / / www.healthlibrary.com / reading / mother / chap5.htm
http: / / www.holisticonline.com / Herbal-Med / _Herbs / h171.htm
http: / / www.ibiblio.org / pfaf / cgi-bin / arr_ html?Cyperus+rotundus
http: / / www.immunesupport.com / library / showarticle. cfm?ID=2848
http: / / www.naturalhealthnotebook.com / Herbs / Latin_Herbs / Genus-C / Cyperus_rotundus.htm
http: / / www.ncbi.nlm.nih.gov:80 / entrez / query. fcgi?CMDΔsearch&DBΔPubMed
http: / / www.pjbs.org / ansinet / ojbs / journal / 2001 / toc1(1).htm
http: / / www.rain-tree.com / ethnic.htm
http: / / www.rain-tree.com / tiririca.htm
http: / / www.tropilab.com / nutgrass.html
http: / / www.umd.umich.edu / cgi-bin / herb /
http: / / www.users.globalnet.co.uk / ~ehpa / core8A.htm
http: / / www.vedahealth.com / abdomen_middle.html

Desmodium spp. References

Addy 1984; Addy 1986; Addy 1988; Addy 1990; Addy 1992; Bajracharya 1979; Barreto 2002; Bista 1997(a); Botta 2003; Chen 2004; De Lucca 1992; Duke; Foster 2000; Hirayama 1993; Hsu 1986; Jimenez 1979; Kirkbride; Li 1976; McManus 1993; Moerman 1986; Neal 1965; N'gouemo1996; Raj 1975; Sivarajan 1994; Taylor 1998; Translation of A Barefoot Doctor's Manual 1977; Tsanuo 2003; Wagner 1999.

http: / / hepatitis-c.de / useful.htm
http: / / seed.agron.ntu.edu.tw / ENG / ethno / ethnobot1e.htm
http: / / www.ambergriscaye.com / pages / medicine5.html
http: / / www.ars-grin.gov / duke / dictionary / tico / d.html
http: / / www.earthsbounty.com / products / bladderex / Bladderex_herbfunction.htm
http: / / www.ethnobotany.com / seeds / Seed_a-e.html
http: / / www.geocities.com / HotSprings / 5670 / tcmherb.html
http: / / www.gnosticgarden.com / seeds2.htm
http: / / www.herbalhealer.com / formulaone.html
http: / / www.herbsecret.co.uk / pages / product. php3?idt=15&idw=2
http: / / www.hort.purdue.edu / newcrop / proceedings1999 / v4-196.html
http: / / www.indena.it / fito / fito-598.htm
http: / / www.itmonline.org / arts / bidens.htm
http: / / www.itmonline.org / arts / legumes.htm
http: / / www.naturalhealthconsult.com / Monographs / desmodium.html

http: / / www.nutraceutic.com / Products / AmazonHerbs / WholeWorldBotanicals / desmodium.htm
http: / / www.objectivemedicine.com / liverherbs.htm
http: / / www.rain-tree.com / amorseco.htm
http: / / www.spearsmacleod.com / links / m / mastitis /
http: / / www.tropilab.com / desmodium-ad.html
http: / / www.weight-care.com / herb_manayupa.htm

Dodonaea viscosa References

Brooker 1987; Browner 1985; Cribb 1986; De Lucca 1992; Degener 1945; Duke; Getie 2003; Lamb 1981; Rojas 1992; Rojas 2003; Stone 1994; Wagner 1999; Whistler 1992(b).

http: / / www.darebin.vic.gov.au / Aboriginal / Early%20Spring.doc
http: / / farrer.riv.csu.edu.au / ASGAP / APOL27 / sep02-1.html
http: / / fig.cox.miami.edu / ~scofield / sofl_plants / med_dodo
http: / / forests.org / archive / samerica / medtrees.htm
http: / / gamma.mhpcc.edu / ulupalakua / auwahi / aalii / aalii.ht
http: / / herb.umd.umich.edu / herb / search.pl
http: / / hml.org / WWW / garden.html
http: / / itserver.footscray.vic.edu.au / ARCgrasslands / natural%20medicine.htm
http: / / kalama.doe.hawaii.edu / hern95 / pt009 / Ann / mcc_nativeplants.html
http: / / kms.kapalama.ksbe.edu / students / 2007 / 070469 / pl
http: / / www.accufind.com / bin / Redir=keywords=waltheria+indica=redir=http: / / www.kmxq.com / hrbmoore / Abstracts / Hyptis-AB.txt
http: / / www.ars-grin.gov / duke / dictionary / tico / d.html
http: / / www.botany.hawaii.edu / faculty / carr / natives.htm
http: / / www.bri.net.au / medicine.html
http: / / www.hawcc.hawaii.edu / hawcc / eday / garden.html
http: / / www.ibiblio.org / pfaf / cgi-bin / arr_html?Dodonaea+viscosa&CAN=LATIND
http: / / www.ncbi.nlm.nih.gov:80 / entrez / query.fcgi?CMD=Display&DB=PubMed
http: / / www.telmedpak.com / agricultures.asp=a=medplan
http: / / www.tlahui.com / libros / fitxo.htm
http: / / www.traffic.org / ecuadorworkshop /

Eclipta prostrata References

Bensky 1986; Bensky 1993; Cao 2000; Chen 2004; Chevallier 1996; Han 1998; Haselwood 1983; Lapulapu; Li 1976; Martz 1992; Melo 1994; Mors 1989; Mors 1991; Sawant 2004; Saxena 1993; Singh 2001; Sivarajan 1994; Translation of A Barefoot Doctor's Manual 1977; Wagner 1986; Wiart 2004; Zhang 2001.

http: / / attunement.com / ayur2.htm
http: / / cpreec.org / edu / medi-pln.htm
http: / / explorer.msn.com / intl.asp.
http: / / members.aol.com / _ht_a / godshaer / herbal-def.htm
http: / / secure-shopping-cart.com / niam / cart / cart58.html
http: / / webpages.charter.net / czar207196 / plants.htm
http: / / www.aetna.com / agb / documents / health-clinic.pdf.
http: / / www.ayurveda-herbs.com / 12.htm
http: / / www.biomedcentral.com / 1472-6882 / 1 / 10 / abstract
http: / / www.chakrapaniayurveda.com / news / march1.html
http: / / www.discoverayurveda.com / beauty / beautyninetips.html
http: / / www.discoverayurveda.com / massage / ayurvedicmassage.html
http: / / www.elixirfarm.com / chiherb2.htm
http: / / www.healthandage.com / html / res / com / ConsConditions / HepatitisViralcc.html
http: / / www.healthhelper.com / complementary / book_botanical / research.htm
http: / / www.healthy.net / library / journals / naturopathic / vol1no1 / cirrhosis.htm
http: / / www.healthy.net / library / journals / naturopathic / vol1no1 / news / liver.htm
http: / / www.herbmed.org / Herbs / Herb153.htm
http: / / www.holistic-online.com / Herbal-Med / _Herbs / h130.htm
http: / / www.ibiblio.org / pfaf / cgi-bin / arr_html?Eclipta+prostrata
http: / / www.itmonline.org / arts / itp.htm
http: / / www.lef.org / magazine / mag99 / oct99_report2a.html
http: / / www.ncbi.nlm.nih.gov:80 / entrez / query.fcgi?CMD=Text&DB=PubMed
http: / / www.niam.com / corp-web / eclipta.htm
http: / / www.niam.com / corp-web / TradUses.html#eclp
http: / / www.shamanictonics.com / tonics / antioxin.html#12.0
http: / / www.tropilab.com / eclipta.html

Emilia spp. References

Gao 1993; Li 1976; Muko 2000; Shylesh 2000.

http: / / www.ars-grin.gov / duke / dictionary / tico / e.html
http: / / www.ars-grin.gov / duke / syllabus / module9.htm
http: / / www.ibiblio.org / herbmed / PAs / PAs-plants.html
http: / / www.ibiblio.org / pfaf / cgi-bin / arr_html?Emilia+sonchifolia
http: / / www.mssrf.org / Fris9809 / Fris1135.html
http: / / www.ncbi.nlm.nih.gov:80 / entrez / query.fcgi?CMD=Display&DB=PubMed
http: / / www.plantatlas.usf.edu / main.asp?plantID=1801

Foeniculum vulgare References

Abdul-Ghani 1988; Albert-Puleo 1980; Bensky 1986; Bista 1997 (a); El Bardai 2001; Frawley 1988; Hoffman 1988; Holmes 1989; Hsu 1986; Hutchens 1983; Kowalchik 1987; Mabey 1988; Malini 1985; Medicinal Plants; Mindell 1992, 2000; Moerman 1986; Moore 1993; Muller-Limmroth 1980; Nielsen 1971; Ozbek 2003; Readers Digest Editors 1986; Reiter 1985; Ruberto 2000; Shah 1991; Tierra 1987.

http: / / BoDD.cf.ac.uk / BotDermFolder / BotDermU / UMBE.html
http: / / hcvn.com / health&healingz / K_Fennel /
http: / / www.bibliomania.com / 2 / 1 / 66 / 113 / frameset.html
http: / / www.botanical.com / botanical / mgmh / f / fennel01.html
http: / / www.dalkeyhomepage.ie / herb.html
http: / / www.dijon.inra.fr / malherbo / hyppa / hyppa-a / foevu_ah.htm
http: / / www.gnc.com / wellness / natpharm / Herb / Fennel.htm
http: / / www.healthy.net / asp / templates / article.asp?id=1583
http: / / www.healthy.net / asp / templates / Article.asp?PageType=Article&Id=1883
http: / / www.herbal-advisor.com / herbs / fennel.htm
http: / / www.herbmed.org / herbs / Foeniculum.htm
http: / / www.herbsociety.org / fennel.htm
http: / / www.herbweb.com / herbage / A213.htm
http: / / www.holisticonline.com / Herbal-Med / _Herbs / h55.htm
http: / / www.hort.purdue.edu / newcrop / med-aro / factsheets / FENNEL.html
http: / / www.ibiblio.org / herbmed / eclectic / kings / foeniculum.html
http: / / www.ibiblio.org / pfaf / cgi-bin / arr_html?Foeniculum+vulgare
http: / / www.joglosemar.co.id / jamu.html
http: / / www.naturalhealthnotebook.com / Herbs / Latin_Herbs / Genus-F / Foeniculum_vulgare.htm

http: / / www.ncbi.nlm.nih.gov:80 / entrez / query. fcgi?CMD=Display&DB=PubMed
http: / / www.nutritionfocus.com / nutrition_supplementation / herbs / Fennel.html
http: / / www.purplesage.org.uk / profiles / fennel.htm
http: / / www.swsbm.com / Constituents / Foeniculum_vulgare.txt
http: / / www.thehimalayadrugco.com / h-foeniculum.htm
http: / / www.tlahui.com / medic / medic7 / hinojo.htm

Hibiscus rosa-sinensis References

Bajracharya 1979; Bista 1997(a); Brinker 2001; Kawai'ae 1980; Kholkute 1977; Lapulapu; Nath 1992; Pakrashi 1986; Pal 1985; Prakash 1979; Sachdewa 2001; Sivarajan 1994; Telefo 1998; Whistler 1996; World Health Organization 1998; Zheng 1989.

http: / / b-and-t-world-seeds.com / Family.htm
http: / / bodd.cf.ac.uk / BotDermFolder / BotDermM / MALV.html
http: / / www.ars-grin.gov / cgi-bin / duke / ethnobot.pl
http: / / www.ars-grin.gov / duke /
http: / / www.ars-grin.gov / duke / dictionary / tico / h.html
http: / / www.ars-grin.gov / duke / ethnobot.html
http: / / www.ars-grin.gov / duke / plants.html
http: / / www.b-and-t-world-seeds.com / info.htm
http: / / www.botany.hawaii.edu / faculty / carr / images / hib_bra. jpg
http: / / www.findarticles.com / g2603 / 0004 / 2603000422 / p1 / article.jhtml
http: / / www.geobop.com / Symbols / plants / flowers / hibiscus /
http: / / www.healthcalls.net / flow2.html
http: / / www.healthy.net / asp / templates / article.asp?id=1207
http: / / www.herbmed.org / Herbs / Herb43.htm
http: / / www.hibiscus.org / toeat.php
http: / / www.hinduonnet.com / thehindu / mag / 2002 / 07 / 07 / stories / 2002070700210700.htm
http: / / www.ibiblio.org / pfaf / cgi-bin / arr_ html?Hibiscus+rosa%2dsinensis
http: / / www.ibiblio.org / pfaf / cgi-bin / arr_html?Hibiscus+rosa-sinensis&CAN=LATIND
http: / / www.lokvani.com / lokvani / article.php?article_id=980
http: / / www.magiclaser.com / html / herbalmedicine.htm
http: / / www.nutritionfocus.com / nutrition_supplementation / herbs / Hibiscus.html
http: / / www.phytomania.com / 2hibiscus.htm
http: / / www.samoalive.com / Ancient%20Samoan%20Herbal%20 Medicine.htm

Mimosa pudica References

Amalraj 2002; Duke; Joyamma 1990; Li 1976(a); Mahanta 2001; Ngo Bum 2004; Prasad 1975; Salgado 2004; Tiwari 1982; World Health Organization 1998;

http: / / BoDD.cf.ac.uk / BotDermFolder / BotDermL / LEGU.html
http: / / perso.infonie.fr / a.bohbot.infoni / english / LJ / ayurveda. htm
http: / / www.bio.miami.edu / Mimosa / Mimosa.html
http: / / www.borneofocus.com / vaic / R&D / article42.htm
http: / / www.corecom.net / ~gardener / NewsLetter / June01 / June01.html
http: / / www.drdeorio.com / ayruvedic.html
http: / / www.goinggreen.net / alternative / azherbs.htm
http: / / www.healingtherapies.info / ayurveda.htm
http: / / www.herbalmedicinebag.com / Salvia-Divinorum.htm
http: / / www.herb-man.com / catalog / hmongmedicine.html
http: / / www.mamiwata.com / hoodoo.html
http: / / www.mssrf.org / fris9809 / fris1151.html
http: / / www.ncbi.nlm.nih.gov:80 / entrez / query. fcgi?CMDΔDisplay&DBΔPubMed
http: / / www.niam.com / corp-web / mediplnt.htm
http: / / www.parentspitara.com / health / alternate / 4.htm
http: / / www.rain-tree.com / mimosa.htm
http: / / www.sertek.com.tw / temp / bmtcg / english / knowlodge / production.htm
http: / / www.tscwa.org / Elephants.html
http: / / www.users.globalnet.co.uk / ~ehpa / core8A.htm
http: / / www.vedamsbooks.com / no12297.htm
http: / / www.winternet.com / ~chuckg / dictionary / dictionary.159.html
http: / / www3.sk.sympatico.ca / becqr / 14.htm

Morinda citrifolia References

Abbott 1992; Fiurusawa 2002; Gutmanis 1987; Hirazumi 1999; Johnson 2002; Ka'alakea; Krauss; Li 2003; Maui Community College database McBride 1975; McClatchey 2002; Mueller 2000; Nelson 2002; Raj 1975; Ross; Saludes 2002; Sang 2001; Wang 2001; Whistler 1996; World Health Organization 1998; Xie; Xu 1993; Younos 1990; Zhong 1993.

http: / / marshall.csu.edu.au / html / plants / medicine.html
http: / / www.4-u-veges.com / noni_use.html
http: / / www.bamp.org.bb / getarticle.cfm?ID=33
http: / / www.healthwell.com / healthnotes / Herb / Noni.cfm
http: / / www.herbmed.org / Herbs / Herb107. htm#Category5Herb107
http: / / www.puresourcenoni.com / scientific.html#chem

Musa spp. References

Arvigo 2001; Best 1984; Bista 1997(b); Bliss 1973; Carper 1988; Chevallier 1996; Dunne 1983; Garcia-Moreno 1980; Goel 1986; Helander 1992; Kaaiakamanu 1922; Kawai'ae 1980; Krauss 2001; Krauss; Kuchel 1985; Lu 1994; Neal 1965; Pari 1999; Pari 2000; Prasad 1993; Richards; Translation of A Barefoot Doctor's Manual 1977; Wagner 2004; Whistler 1992(b); Whistler 1996; World Health Organization 1998; Xu 1993.

http: / / library.kcc.hawaii.edu / ~soma / krauss / maia.html
http: / / research.bmn.com / medline / search / record?uid=MDLN.20284076
http: / / weaving.about.com / hobbies / weaving / library / dyeplants / blmusa.htm?terms=musa
http: / / www.ars-grin.gov / cgi-bin / duke / ethnobot.pl
http: / / www.ars-grin.gov / duke / dictionary / tico / m.html
http: / / www.botanical.com / botanical / mgmh / p / plafru51.html
http: / / www.dittmar.dusnet.de / english / suche-e.php?term=musa
http: / / www.herbmed.org / herbs / Musa_Banana.htm
http: / / www.herbmed.org / herbs / Musa_Banana.htm#folk
http: / / www.ibiblio.org / pfaf / cgi-bin / arr_html?Musa+basjoo
http: / / www.medscape.com / server-java / MedLineApp? / member-search / getdoc.cgi?ord=30&searchid=3&have_local_holdings_file=0&local_journals_only=0
http: / / www.medscape.com / server-java / MedLineApp? / member-search / getdoc.cgi?ord=5&searchid=3&have_local_holdings_file=0&local_journals_only=0
http: / / www.mssrf.org / Fris9809 / fris1162.html
http: / / www.umd.umich.edu / cgi-bin / herb /

Opuntia spp. References

Ahmad 1996; Arvigo 2001; Bista 1997(a); Budinsky 2001; Butera 2002; Bwititi 2000; Bwititi 2001; Cardenas 1998; Chevallier 1996; Cunningham 1985; Dok-Go 2003; El Kossori 1998; Fernandez 1992; Fernandez 1994; Frati-Munari 1988; Frati-Munari 1989(a); Frati-Munari 1989(b); Frati-Munari 1989(c); Frati-Munari 1990; Frati-Munari 1992; Galati 2001; Galati 2002(a); Galati 2002(b);

Galati 2003; Han 2001; Haselwood 1983; Higgs 1993; Hoffman 1988; Hsu 1986; Huang 1993; Krochmal 1984; Lee 2002; Li 1976(a); Loro 1999; Meckes-Lozoya 1989; Moore 1989; Moore 1993; Moore Materia Medica; Palumbo 2003; Park 1998; Park 2001(a); Park 2001(b); Peterson 1999; Tesoriere 2004; Veronin 2000; Wagner 1999; Wiese 2004; Wolfram 2002; Wolfram 2003; Xie 1996; Zhong 1993.

http: / / chili.rt66.com / hrbmoore / AJP / AJP_1898_No_3.pdf
http: / / desertusa.com / magoct97 / oct_pear.html
http: / / hometown.aol.com / vanishwood / guild / brew1.htm
http: / / hv.greenspun.com / bboard / q-and-a-fetch-msg.tcl?msg_id=003mdv
http: / / tchester.org / fb / plants / na_uses.html
http: / / www.aaas.org / international / africa / moz / bandeira.html
http: / / www.al-fin.com / healthfitness.htm
http: / / www.arizonacactus.com / medicine.htm
http: / / www.ars-grin.gov / duke / dictionary / tico / o.html
http: / / www.herbalremedies.com / pricpearop.html
http: / / www.herbamed.co.il / prost1.html
http: / / www.herbvideos.com / global.P.htm#Prickly%20Pear
http: / / www.herbvideos.com / survivetips.htm
http: / / www.herbweb.com / herbage / A341.htm
http: / / www.ibiblio.org / herbmed / eclectic / kings / cereus.html
http: / / www.ibiblio.org / pfaf / cgi-bin / find_lat?LAT=opuntia&COM=&FAM=
http: / / www.mhhe.com / biosci / pae / botany / botany_map / articles / article_23.html
http: / / www.mssrf.org / Fris9809 / Fris1249.html
http: / / www.nybg.org / events / armdang.html
http: / / www.plantasmedicinales.org / abstract / feb2002 / Opuntia%20ficus-indica.htm
http: / / www.plantgenome.uga.edu / project-cactus.htm
http: / / www.rivenrock.com / rivenrocklinks.html
http: / / www.tamuk.edu / webuser / cactus / cac_med.html
http: / / www.tcisearch.com / articles.htm?storyid=18
http: / / www.umd.umich.edu / cgi-bin / herb /

Oxalis spp. References

Andoh 1986; Bista 1997; Darwin 1996; Foster 2000; Gruenwald; Joerg; ed 1998; Honychurch 1986; Krochmal 1984; Lewis 1977; Li Ninghan 1976; Mabey 1988; Miller 1988; Moerman 1986; Sivarajan1994; Whistler 1992(b); Whistler 1992(c).

http: / / botanical.com / botanical / mgmh / s / sorwoo68.html
http: / / kids.osd.wednet.edu / Marshall / homepage / temptrees.html
http: / / members.aol.com / FiberNews / janis.html
http: / / starbulletin.com / 2001 / 02 / 16 / features / garden.html
http: / / www.angelfire.com / journal / cathbodua / Herbal / HerbalS.html
http: / / www.ars-grin.gov / cgi-bin / npgs / html / taxon.pl?401793
http: / / www.ars-grin.gov / duke / .. / cgi-bin / duke / ethnobot.pl
http: / / www.ars-grin.gov / var / apache / cgi-bin / npgs / html / taxon.pl?401793 (01
http: / / www.dentalcomfortzone.com / archive / HerbalMedicine2.html
http: / / www.holistic-online.com / Herbal-Med / _Herbs / h138.htm
http: / / www.ibiblio.org / herbmed / eclectic / cook / OXALIS_ACETOSELLA.htm
http: / / www.ibiblio.org / herbmed / eclectic / kings / oxalis.html
http: / / www.ibiblio.org / pfaf / cgi-bin / arr_html?Oxalis+acetosella
http: / / www.ibiblio.org / pfaf / cgi-bin / arr_html?Oxalis+corniculata
http: / / www.magialuna.net / o.html
http: / / www.utopiasprings.com / agtibet.htm
http: / / www.utopiasprings.com / agtibet.htm
http: / / www.vetwork.org.uk / pune20.htm
http: / / www.webhealth.co.uk / Complementary_Health / Complementary_Therapies / Complementary_Therapy_Overview / Complementary_Therapy_Overview / complementary_therapy_overview.html

Pandanus tectorius References

Barrau 1958; Barrau 1962; Ching 2001; Englberger 2003; Hunt 2000; Hunt 2004; Krauss; Li 1976(a); Maui Community College database; Ooi 2004; Peungvicha 1996; Topics 2003; Whistler 1992(c); Xie 1996; Xu 1993; Zhong 1993.

http: / / cocos.arecaceae.com / 1958.html
http: / / cocos.arecaceae.com / 1962.html
http: / / marshall.csu.edu.au / html / plants / medicine.html
http: / / www.ars-grin.gov / duke / dictionary / tico / p.html
http: / / www.botany.hawaii.edu / faculty / carr / images / pan_tec_hab.jpg
http: / / www.deoxy.org / trypfaq.htm
http: / / www.ncbi.nlm.nih.gov / entrez / query.fcgi?CMD=Display&DB=pubmed http: / / www.winrock.org / FORESTRY / FACTPUB / AIS_web / AIS11.html
http: / / www-ang.kfunigraz.ac.at / ~katzer / engl / generic_frame.html?Pand_ama.html

Piper methysticum References

Backhauß 1992; Boonen 1998(a); Boonen 1998(b); Brooker 1987; Chevallier 1996; Dam-Bakker 1958; Davies 1992; Dragull 2003; Duffield 1989; Duffield 1991; Gleitz 1996; Gleitz 1997; Gruenwald 1988; Herberg 1993; Holm 1991; Hope 1993; Jamieson 1989; Jamieson 1990(a); Jamieson 1990(b); Jussofie 1994; Kaaiakamanu 1922; Ka'alakea; Kinzler 1991; Krauss; Leonard; Lewis 1977; Locher 1995; Mathews 1988; McKenna 2002; Mindell 1992, 2000; Munte 1993; Nerurkar 2004; Pittler 2000; Schelosky 1995; Schirmacher 1999; Schmitz1995; Singh 1983; Steiner 2000; Uebelhack 1998; Volz 1997; Walden 1997; Warnecke 1991; Whistler 1992(b).

http: / / alaike.lcc.hawaii.edu / millen / bot130 / learning_objectives / lo03 / list / awa.html
http: / / BoDD.cf.ac.uk / BotDermFolder / BotDermP / PIPE.html
http: / / chili.rt66.com / hrbmoore / Abstracts / Piper%20methysticum-AB.txt
http: / / hawaiianherbalteas.com / awa.html
http: / / hoolokahi.vizip.com / laau.html
http: / / library.kcc.hawaii.edu / ~soma / krauss / awa.html
http: / / members.aol.com / _ht_a / godshaer / herbal-opq.htm
http: / / nepenthes.lycaeum.org / Drugs / Misc / Kava.html
http: / / ohioline.osu.edu / hyg-fact / 5000 / 5406.html
http: / / staff-www.uni-marburg.de / ~akhaeber / H._Haberlein / Fields_of_intrestHanns / Natural_Subs._effecting_the_CN / Kava / body_kava.html
http: / / www.4-u-veges.com / kava_recipe.html
http: / / www.ann.com.au / herbs / Monographs / piper.htm
http: / / www.ayurveda.com / materiamedica / Piper%20methysticum--Kava%20Kava.htm
http: / / www.biopsychiatry.com / kava /
http: / / www.botanical.com / temp / mgmh-no-products / k / kavaka02.html
http: / / www.checkspace.com / ?RB=-ka14496.
http: / / www.christopherhobbs.com
http: / / www.coconutinfo.com
http: / / www.comfsm.fm / ~dleeling / botany / 1998 / vhp / sakau.

html
http: / / www.hawaii-nation.org / canoe / awa.html
http: / / www.healthy.net / asp / templates / article.
asp?PageType=Article&ID=305
http: / / www.healthy.net / hwlibrarynewsletters / update / kava.htm
http: / / www.herb.com / materia.htm
http: / / www.herbmed.org / herbs / piper.htm
http: / / www.herbweb.com / herbage / 8-P.htm
http: / / www.herbweb.com / herbage / A365.htm
http: / / www.holisticonline.com / Herbal-Med / _Herbs / h24.htm
http: / / www.hort.purdue.edu / newcrop / proceedings1999 / v4-442.html
http: / / www.ibiblio.org / herbmed / eclectic / kings / piper-meth.
html
http: / / www.immunesolutions.net / suggested_reading_resources / ingredient / Kava12_97ND.pdf.
http: / / www.itmonline.org / arts / kava.htm
http: / / www.k12.hi.us / ~kapunaha / awa.htm
http: / / www.k12.hi.us / ~kapunaha / TOJr.files / LiveLifeLiveLong / medicine%20files / hawaiian / hawaiian%20.htm
http: / / www.kavakauai.com / kava_info.html
http: / / www.kavakure.com / aboutKava.htm
http: / / www.motherearthherbs.com / tincture.html
http: / / www.naturalhealthnotebook.com / Herbs / Latin_Herbs / Genus-P / Piper_methysticum.htm
http: / / www.ncbi.nlm.nih.gov:80 / entrez / query.
fcgi?CMD=Text&DB=PubMed
http: / / www.phytotherapies.org / monograph_detail.cfm?id=168
http: / / www.pioneerherbs.com / piper_methysticum.htm
http: / / www.sbherbals.com / 1198HotM.html
http: / / www.stevenfoster.com / education / monograph / kava.html
http: / / www.supplementalmed.com / html / kava.htm
http: / / www.thorne.com / altmedrev / fulltext / kava2-5.html
http: / / www.tribalsite.com / nuka / kava.htm
http: / / www.umd.umich.edu / cgi-bin / herb /
http: / / www.vitacost.com / science / MedStudies / Kava.html

Pipturus spp. References

Abbott 1992; Ahuna 1978; Auwae; Gutmanis 1987; Kaaiakamanu 1922; Leonard 1992-2005; Leonard; Locher 1995; Maui Community College database; Whistler 1992(b).

http: / / hawaiianherbalteas.com / mamaki.html
http: / / hml.org / WWW / garden.html
http: / / www.airtahitimagazine.com / us_version / mag_32 / plants.
htm
http: / / www.ars-grin.gov / duke / syllabus / module14.htm
http: / / www.botany.hawaii.edu / gradstud / saxon / foo.htm
http: / / www.geocities.com / gdekinder / algemeen / betekenis_n_z.
htm
http: / / www.herbmed.org / Herbs / Herb36.htm
http: / / www.ho-tinursery.com / hawaiian.html
http: / / www.ncbi.nlm.nih.gov / entrez / query.fcgi?cmd=Retrieve&db=PubMed&list_uids=8786654&dopt=Abstract
http: / / www.spc.int / coastfish / News / WIF / WIF11 / WIF11-4.
pdf.

Plantago spp. References

Bensky 1986; Bernays 2000; Biere 2004; Chevallier 1996; Chiang 2003(a); Chiang 2003(b); Chiang 2003(c); Darwin 1996; Gomez-Flores 2000; Hetland 2000; Jenkins 2002; Karpilovskaia 1989; Lithander 1992; Murai 1995; Tamura 2002; Translation of A Barefoot Doctor's Manual 1977.

http: / / altnature.com / gallery / Plantain.htm
http: / / BoDD.cf.ac.uk / BotDermFolder / BotDermP / PLAN.html
http: / / home.t-online.de / home / 520097278994-0001 / yuthog / plants / 1.html
http: / / members.tripod.com / susana_x / plaintain-2.htm
http: / / www.ann.com.au / herbs / Monographs / plantago.htm
http: / / www.ann.com.au / herbs / Monographs / plantmaj.htm
http: / / www.bibliomania.com / 2 / 1 / 66 / 113 / frameset.html
http: / / www.botanical.com / botanical / mgmh / p / plarib48.html
http: / / www.findarticles.com / cf_0 / g2603 / 0005 / 2603000594 / print.jhtml
http: / / www.healthy.net / asp / templates / article.
asp?PageType=article&ID=1434
http: / / www.herbmed.org / herbs / Plantago_major.htm
http: / / www.herbweb.com / herbage / A368.htm
http: / / www.hsibaltimore.com / ea2004 / ea_040218.shtml
http: / / www.ibiblio.org / herbmed / eclectic / kings / plantago.
html
http: / / www.ibiblio.org / pfaf / cgi-bin / arr_
html?Plantago+asiatica
http: / / www.ibiblio.org / pfaf / cgi-bin / arr_
html?Plantago+lanceolata
http: / / www.ibiblio.org / pfaf / cgi-bin / arr_html?Plantago+major
http: / / www.magdalin.com / herbal /
http: / / www.ncbi.nlm.nih.gov:80 / entrez / query.
fcgi?CMD=Display&DB=PubMed

Sida rhombifolia References

Islam 2003; Li 1976; Rao 1997; Venkatesh 1999.

http / / www.ijp-online.com / archi
http: / / ultralingua.net / results.html?lookup_action=en%7Cenglish %7Cenglish&lookup_letters=hemp
http: / / www.ann.com.au / herbs / Monographs / sida.htm
http: / / www.arbec.com.my / pdf / art1janmar03.pdf.
http: / / www.ars-grin.gov / cgi-bin / duke / ethnobot.pl
http: / / www.ars-grin.gov / duke / dictionary / tico / s.html
http: / / www.ars-grin.gov / duke / syllabus / module8.htm
http: / / www.elsevier.com / cdweb / journals / 03788741 / viewer.
htt?viewtype=keywords&rangeselected=194
http: / / www.ethnictourism.com / ayurveda / trea_sashtika.asp
http: / / www.fs.fed.us / global / iitf / pdf / Sida%20rhombifolia.
pdf.
http: / / www.holistic-online.com / Herbal-Med / _Herbs / h_sida-rhombifolia.htm
http: / / www.holisticonline.com / Herbal-Med / _Herbs / h_sida-rhombifolia.htm
http: / / www.hyperdictionary.com / dictionary / Sida+rhombifolia
http: / / www.ibiblio.org / herbmed / eclectic / kings / althaea.html
http: / / www.ijp-online.com / archives / 1997 / 029 / 02 / r0110-0116ra.pdf
http: / / www.indiangyan.com / books / ayurvedabooks / ayurvedic_cures / diseases_urinary_reproductive_system.shtml
http: / / www.indmedplants-kr.org / Sida_acuta.htm
http: / / www.infinityfoundation.com / mandala / t_es / Himalayan_Materia_Medica_Table.pdf.
http: / / www.kamleshayurveda.com / top / k_k_yoga.htm
http: / / www.mothernature.com / Library / bookshelf / Books / 41 / 50.cfm
http: / / www.nadanherbcomp.com.au / herb-s.html
http: / / www.ncbi.nlm.nih.gov:80 / entrez / query.
fcgi?CMD=Display&DB=PubMed
http: / / www.nt.gov.au / dpif / pubcat / agnotes / 542.htm. 4 p.
http: / / www.pulsemans.com / proving1b.htm
http: / / www.samoalive.com / Ancient%20Samoan%20Herbal%20 Medicine.htm
http: / / www.swsbm.com / Constituents / Sida_rhombifolia.txt
http: / / www.teriin.org / biodiv / medicine.htm

http: / / www.thenaturalheritage.com / htmljune / articles6.htm
http: / / www.t-mag.com / articles / 206alt.html
http: / / www.tscwa.org / wildlife / elephant_remedies_full.html
http: / / www.wrc.net / phyto / Bala.html

Siegesbeckia orientalis References

Dong 1989; Hwang 2001; Kang 1997; Kim 2001; Li 1976; Translation of A Barefoot Doctor's Manual 1977; Whistler 1992(c);

http: / / natureproducts.net / Ecology / Biodiversity%20Products / biodiversity_products.html
http: / / www.angelfire.com / biz3 / nutramedic / magnolia.html
http: / / www.ars-grin.gov / duke / dictionary / tico / s.html
http: / / www.botanical.com / botanical / mgmh / s / sieges48.html
http: / / www.health-and-medical.com
http: / / www.holographichealth.com / listings / 14.html
http: / / int.clarins.com / main.cfm?PlanteID=293&lettre=S
http: / / www.itmonline.org / arts / millettia.htm
http: / / www.krouma.com / herbs.asp?id=280
http: / / www.nadanherbcomp.com.au / herb-s.html
http: / / www.scienceoflife.com / MedicalDiagnosis.asp
http: / / www.swsbm.com / AJP / AJP_1888_No_7.pdf.
http: / / www.tcmbasics.com / materiamedica / herba_siegesbeckiae.htm
http: / / www.ucmp.berkeley.edu / history / linnaeus.html
http: / / www.ummah.net.pk / dajjal / blood1.html

Solanum americanum References

Ahuna 1978; Akhtar 1989; Chestnut 1974; de Melo 1978; Hu 1999; Krauss 2001; Locher 1005; Perez 1998; Plants in Hawaiian Culture by Krauss; Sammon 1992; Sultana 1995; Vogel 1970.

http: / / 2bnthewild.com / phvsixn.htm
http: / / botany.about.com / library / weekly / aa041699c.htm
http: / / cal.nbc.upenn.edu / poison / Brett / AgBook / pg140161.htm
http: / / gateway.library.uiuc.edu / vex / toxic / nightsha / nightsh0.htm
http: / / home4.swipnet.se / ~w-47128 / Nights_ab.html
http: / / hoolokahi.vizip.com / laau.html
http: / / www.angelfire.com / journal2 / flowers / pcd24.html
http: / / www.ann.com.au / herbs / Monographs / solanum.htm
http: / / www.ayurvedahc.com / research.htm
http: / / www.botanical.com / botanical / mgmh / n / nighbl04.html
http: / / cal.nbc.upenn.edu / poison / Brett / AgBook / pg140161.htm http: / / www.elsevier.nl / inca / publications / store / 5 / 0 / 6 / 0 / 3 / 5 / ?menu=cont&label=Table
http: / / www.holisticonline.com / Herbal-Med / _Herbs / h155.htm
http: / / www.ibiblio.org / herbmed /
http: / / www.ibiblio.org / pfaf / cgi-bin / arr_html?Solanum+americanum
http: / / www.ibiblio.org / pfaf / cgi-bin / arr_html?Solanum+nigrum
http: / / www.inchem.org / documents / pims / plant / solanum.htm
http: / / www.koausa.org / SamsarChandKoul / flowers.html
http: / / www.kohala.net / kaimalino / KMWC-4.html#anchor473905
http: / / www.mssrf.org / Fris9809 / Fris1335.html
http: / / www.ncbi.nlm.nih.gov:80 / entrez / query.fcgi?CMDΔDisplay&DBΔPubMed
http: / / www.nhm.ac.uk / hosted_sites / schisto / prcschisto / abst / abst24.html
http: / / www.oneworld.org / ileia / newsletters / 11-3 / 11-3-6.htm
http: / / www.umd.umich.edu / cgi-bin / herb /
http: / / www.viable-herbal.com / herbdesc4 / 1woodyni.htm

Sonchus oleraceus References

Brooker 1987; El 2004; Haselwood 1983; Kaaiakamanu 1922; Kim 1996; Moerman 1986; Qu 1996;
Thomson 2002.

http: / / www.ars-grin.gov / duke / dictionary / tico / s.html
http: / / www.bibliomania.com / 2 / 1 / 66 / 113 / frameset.html
http: / / www.botanical.com / botanical / mgmh / s / sowthi71.html
http: / / www.csdl.tamu.edu / FLORA / cgi / ruled_html_query?colldir=kartesz%2Fmgdata&collname=bonap98&query=Sonchus
http: / / www.ibiblio.org / pfaf / cgi-bin / arr_html?Sonchus+arvensis
http: / / www.ibiblio.org / pfaf / cgi-bin / arr_html?Sonchus+oleraceus
http: / / www.magdalin.com / herbal /
http: / / www.mssrf.org / fris9809 / kadar-details.html
http: / / www.oardc.ohio-state.edu / scripts / weed.dll / getone.1050.htm#toxicity
http: / / www.sonic.net / melissk / plantp-t.html#s
http: / / www.wssa.net / subpages / weed / weedstoday / WT23.htm

Syzygium jambos References

Bajracharya 1979; Bista 1997(b); Djipa 2000; Honychurch 1986; Sivarajan 1994; Xie 1996; Zhong 1993.

http: / / health.yahoo.com / health / Alternative_Medicine / Herbal_Remedies_Tree / Herbal_Remedies / jambolan /
http: / / photos.msn.com / support / worldwide.aspx
http: / / www.ahdintl.com / specialtyreview2002.htm
http: / / www.ars-grin.gov / duke / dictionary / tico / e.html
http: / / www.crownhealthcareproducts.com / medhleen.html
http: / / www.diabetes-herbs.com / herbs1.html
http: / / www.godshaer.co.uk / monk.htm
http: / / www.haryana-online.com / Flora / jamun.htm
http: / / www.hear.org / pier / sycum.htm
http: / / www.herbmed.org / Herbs / Herb70.htm
http: / / www.hort.purdue.edu / newcrop / morton / jambolan.html
http: / / www.ibiblio.org / herbmed / eclectic / ellingwood / syzygium.html
http: / / www.journaloflongevity.com / JOLWeb / Archives / 80 / bloodsugar2.html
http: / / www.ncbi.nlm.nih.gov / entrez / query.fcgi?CMD=Text&DB=PubMed
http: / / www.space-age.com / herbs / home.html
http: / / www.thioxazobiotechlab.com / pharma.html
http: / / www.tibet-travel.com / e-Medicine-Renchen-Mangior.htm
http: / / www.tropilab.com / syzygium-jamun.html

Syzygium malaccense References

Abbott 1992; Brooker 1987; Gutmanis1987; Kaaiakamanu1922; Locher 1995; Mitchell 1992; Neal 1965; Wagner 1999; Whistler 1992(b); Whistler 1992(c); Whistler 1996; Xie 1996.

http: / / apdl.kcc.hawaii.edu / ~ahupuaa / botany / medicinal / ohiaai.htm
http: / / cpcp.ensearch.org / cpcp / smkdl / groupe / team5 / our%20science%20project%204.htm
http: / / hoolokahi.vizip.com / laau.html
http: / / www.ahdintl.com / specialtyreview2002.htm
http: / / www.hawaii-nation.org / canoe / ohia.html
http: / / www.hookele.com / canoeplants / ohia.html
http: / / www.ncbi.nlm.nih.gov / entrez / query.fcgi?cmd=Retrieve&db=PubMed&list_uids=8786654&dopt=Abstract
http: / / www.samoalive.com / Ancient%20Samoan%20Herbal%20Medicine.htm
http: / / www.soton.ac.uk / ~icuc / adbib / ad-u-m2.htm

http: / / www.tradewindsfruit.com / malay_apple.htm
http: / / www.tropilab.com / syzygium-malaccense.html
http: / / www.umd.umich.edu / cgi-bin / herb /

Taraxacum spp. References

Bensky 1986; Chakurski 1981; Cheong 1998; Chevallier 1996; Chivato 1996; Choi 2002; Darwin 1996; Holmes 1989; Hu 2003; Hussain 2004; Jeong 1991; Kim 2000; Koo 2004; Luo 1993; Takasaki 1999(b); Takasaki 1999(a); Translation of A Barefoot Doctor's Manual 1977; Williams 1996; Yun 2002; Zheng 1990; Zhu 1999.

http: / / www.ann.com.au / herbs / Monographs / taraxacu.htm http: / / altnature.com / gallery / Dandelion.htm
http: / / www.ayurveda.com
http: / / www.bibliomania.com / 2 / 1 / 66 / 113 / frameset.html
http: / / www.botanical.com / temp / mgmh-no-products / d / dandel08.html
http: / / www.herbweb.com / herbage / A478.htm
http: / / www.holisticonline.com / Herbal-Med / _Herbs / h48.htm
http: / / www.ibiblio.org / herbmed / eclectic / kings / taraxacum. html
http: / / www.ibiblio.org / pfaf / cgi-bin / arr_ html?Taraxacum+officinale www.pfaf.org
http: / / www.magdalin.com / herbal /
http: / / www.ncbi.nlm.nih.gov:80 / entrez / query. fcgi?CMD=Display&DB=PubMed
http: / / www.odont.aau.dk / LibHerb2 / Pn0108.HTM
http: / / www.umd.umich.edu / cgi-bin / herb /
http: / / www.ars-grin.gov / duke / syllabus / module12.htm
http: / / www3.allherb.com / consumer / default.asp?j=dandelion

Trametes versicolor References

Collins 1997; Ebina 1987; Ebina 1989; Farghali 1998; Habelhah 1998(a); Habelhah 1998(b); Hobbs; Hsieh 2001; Iino 1995; Kidd 2000; Kobayashi 1993; Kobayashi 1994; Li 1990; Matsunaga 1986; Mitomi 1992; Nagao 1981; Nakazato 1994; Ng 1997; Oguchi 1986; Ohmura 2003; Sakamaki 1992; Taniguchi 1984; Torisu 1990; Tsuru 1984(a); Tsuru 1984(b).

http: / / 216.239.51.100 / search?q=cache:LOnfE6tCzoAC:www.devonian.ualberta.ca / uamh / ar00ff2.PDF+Trametes+medicine&hl=en&start=44&ie=UTF-8&e=42
http: / / botit.botany.wisc.edu / toms_fungi / polypore.html
http: / / health.pon.net / nmh.html
http: / / psp.bc.ca / Cancer-and-ulcers / trametes.htm
http: / / www.bastyr.edu / academic / botmed / coriolus_versicolor. asp?reform=pf&
http: / / www.blueboyherbs.com / herbs_eclectic.htm
http: / / www.cancer.org / eprise / main / docroot / ETO / content / ETO_5_3X_Coriolous_Versicolor?sitearea=ETO
http: / / www.dracoherbs.com / Exfax%209906%20final%20 new%20addr.PDF
http: / / www.geocities.com / VoyagerServiceSoftware / artemiev / mushroom / Trametes_versicolor.htm
http: / / www.haworthpressinc.com / store / Toc / J044v06n04_ TOC.pdf
http: / / www.healthy.net / asp / templates / article. asp?PageType=Article&ID=865
http: / / www.hort.purdue.edu / newcrop / duke_energy / Aleurites_moluccana.html
http: / / www.jhsnp.com / store / about_coriolus.html
http: / / www.munchkinsoftware.com / mycology / 2000_abstracts. html
http: / / www.mushroomcompany.com / books / hobbs.html
http: / / www.mushroomscience.com / msstore / about_mushrooms. htm
http: / / www.nammex.com / MushroomArticles / healthBenefit-Mushrooms.html
http: / / www.naturelink.net / hair.htm
http: / / www.ncbi.nlm.nih.gov:80 / entrez / query. fcgi?CMD=Text&DB=PubMed
http: / / www.new-chapter.com / medicinal_mushrooms.html
http: / / www.newhope.com / nfm-online / nfm_backs / Jan_99 / mushrooms.cfm
http: / / www.nutraceutic.com / Products / NativeAmericanHerbals / eternalprotection.htm
http: / / www.orst.edu / dept / botany / mycology / bot461 / class / lecture11.html
http: / / www.prohealthsolutions.com / RM-10.html
http: / / www.purehealthsystems.com / coriolus_versicolor.html
http: / / www.springboard4health.com / notebook / health_agaricus_1.html
http: / / www.zeri.org / news / 1999 / march / mar_muli.htm

Tropaeolum majus References

Chevallier 1996; De Lucca 1992; de Medeiros 2000; Gruenwald 1998; Hoffman 1988; Johns 1982; Kowalchik 1987; Mabey 1988; McIntyre 1996; Montagna; Pintao 1995; Poblete 1992; Thomson 1983.

http: / / health.yahoo.com / health / Alternative_Medicine / Herbal_Remedies_Tree / Herbal_Remedies / nasturtium /
http: / / www.angelfire.com / journal2 / flowers / n.html
http: / / www.ann.com.au / herbs / Monographs / tropaeol.htm
http: / / www.healthy.net / asp / templates / article. asp?pageType=article&Id=1590
http: / / www.i5ive.com / article.cfm / herbal_lore / 44947
http: / / www2.cba.unige.it / 01polm / polm07.htm

Usnea spp. References

Aalto-Korte 2005; Bezivin 2004; Bian 2002; Campanella 2002; Carreras 2002; Caviglia 2001; Cocchietto 2002; Dobrescu 1993; Durazo 2004; Figueira 2002; Fournet 1997; Francolini 2004; Garcia 1999; Ghione 1988; Goncalo 1987; Han 2004; Ingolfsdottir 2002; Lauterwein 1995; Mitchell 1965; Odabasoglu 2004; Okuyama 1995; Periera 1994; Poblet 1997; Pramyothin 2004; Proksa 1999; Rancan 2002; Ribeiro-Costa 2004; Rossbach 1999; Rowe 1989; Scirpa 1999; Takani 2002; Vijayakumar 2000; Vijayan 2004; Wu 1995; Yamamoto 1995.

http: / / altnature.com / gallery / usnea.htm
http: / / bodd.cf.ac.uk /
http: / / webmd.lycos.com / content / article / 3187.13312
http: / / www.healthwell.com / hnbreakthroughs / aug98 / usnealomatium.cfm
http: / / www.lichen.com / people.html
http: / / www.mothernature.com / ency / Herb / Usnea.asp
http: / / www.umd.umich.edu / cgi-bin / herb /
http: / / www.wisetouch.com / usnea.html

Vitex rotundifolia References

Alam 2002; Bensky 1986; Brooker 1987; De Lucca 1992; Fahs 2003; Hossain 2001; Hsu 1986; Huang 1993; Ikawati 2001; Kawazoe 2001; Ko 2000; Ko 2001; Ko 2002; Li 1976; Merlin 1999; Okuyama 1998; Shin 2000; Wagner 1999; Watanabe 1995; Whistler 1992(a); Whistler 1992(b); Whistler 1992(c); You 1998.

http: / / bodd.cf.ac.uk / BotDermFolder / BotDermV / VERB.html
http: / / bpi.da.gov.ph / websitemedicinal / all / l / lagunding-dagat. htm
http: / / chinhnghia.org / tailieu / duocthao.htm
http: / / herb.umd.umich.edu / herb / search.pl

http: / / mobot.mobot.org / cgi-bin / search_pick
http: / / www.ars-grin.gov / cgi-bin / duke / ethnobot.pl
http: / / www.asaphair.com / pages / products.html
http: / / www.botony.hawaii.edu / faculty / carr / images / vit_rot.jpg vit_rot_hab.jpg
http: / / www.happyherbalist.com / aphordiacs_herbs.htm
http: / / www.hawaii.edu / scb / scinativ_mycor.html
http: / / www.healthy.net / asp / templates / article.asp?PageType=article&ID=1583
http: / / www.herb.com / materia.htm
http: / / www.holisticonline.com / Herbal-Med / _Herbs / h211.htm
http: / / www.islandvisions.com / biology / hawaiian.html
http: / / www.ncbi.nlm.nih.gov:80 / entrez / query.fcgi?CMD=Display&DB=PubMed
http: / / www.tcmbasics.com / materiamedica / fructus_viticis.htm
http: / / www.winternet.com / ~chuckg / dictionary / dictionary.173.html
http: / / www.yohea.com / plants.shtml

Waltheria indica References

Haselwood 1983; Honychurch 1986; Kaaiakamanu 1922; Maui Community College database; McBride 1975; Miyashiro 1994; Pukui 1986.

http: / / www.bvet.admin.ch / info-service / e / publikationen / magazin / 2003 / 45_28_31.pdf.
http: / / www.kohala.net / kaimalino / KMWC-2.html
http: / / www.ars-grin.gov / duke / dictionary / tico / w.html
http: / / www.ncbi.nlm.nih.gov:80 / entrez / query.fcgi?CMD=Display&DB=PubMed
http: / / www.tropilab.com / sleepy-waltheria.html
http: / / www.umd.umich.edu / cgi-bin / herb /

Youngia japonica References

Li Ninghan 1976; Whistler 1995; Yang 1995.

http: / / www.ibiblio.org / pfaf / cgi-bin / arr_html?Youngia+japonica
http: / / www.ibiblio.org / pfaf / cgi-bin / find_lat?LAT=Youngia&COM=&FAM=
http: / / www.levity.com / alchemy / afrm0050.html
http: / / www.plantatlas.usf.edu / main.asp?plantID=235

Zingiber officinale References

Altman 2001; al-Yahya 1989; Bensky 1986; Bensky 1993; Bista 1997(a); Bliss 1973; Bode 2001; Bordia 1997; Brinker 2001; Carper 1988; Carper 1994; Castleman 1991; Chevallier 1996; Choi 2000; Denyer 1994; Fischer-Rasmussen 1991; Flynn 1986; Foster 1997; Frawley 1988; Fuhrman 2000; Futrell 1993; Gonlachanvit 2003; Gruenwald 1998; Guh 1995; Hashimoto 2002; Heck 2000; Herb Research Publications 1995; Hobbs 1998; Honychurch 1986; Hsu 1986; Hutchens 1983; Jagetia 2003; Janssen 1996; Kamtchouing 2002; Katiyar 1996; Keating 2002; Keys 1976; Kiuchi 1992; Kobayashi 1988; Koo 2001; Kowalchik1987; Krueth 2004; Lee 1998; Lewis 1977; Lien 2003; Liu 2002; Liu 2003; Lu 1994; Lu 2003; Mahady 2003; Martins 2001; Mascolo 1989; McIntyre 1996; Meyer 1995; Mindell 2000; Moriarty 2003; Mowrey 1986; Murakami 2002; Murakami 2003; Murakami 2004; Nagasawa 2002; Niebyl 992; Ody 1993; Patro 2002; Pongrojpaw 2003; Qian 1992; Qureshi 1989; Sanderson 2002; Schmid 1994; Shen 2003; Sohni 1996; Srivastava 1984; Srivastava 1986; Stewart 1991; Suekawa 1986; Surh 1998; Surh 1999; Surh 2002; Thomson2002; Tjendraputra 2001; Translation of A Barefoot Doctor's Manual 1977; Vimala 1999; Weidner 2001; Whistler 1991(b); Wu 1990; Wu 1998; Yamahara 1985; Yamahara 1988; Yamahara 1992; Yoshikawa 1994.

http: / / cpreec.org / edu / medi-pln.htm
http: / / de.essortment.com / gingerzingiber_rmgc.htm
http: / / health.yahoo.com / health / Alternative_Medicine / Herbal_Remedies_Tree / Herbal_Remedies / Ginger_Root /
http: / / medicinegarden.com / Library / herbsginger1.html
http: / / vitalvillage.net / nmc / nmc-pages / ginger.htm
http: / / www.acaom.edu /
http: / / www.aromaassociates.com /
http: / / www.bayho.com / MM011.ASP?pageno=258
http: / / www.botgard.ucla.edu / html / botanytextbooks / economicbotany / Zingiber /
http: / / www.calloftheraven.com /
http: / / www.childrenshospital.org / holistic /)
http: / / www.eclecticphysician.com / herbs / ginger.shtml
http: / / www.erowid.org / herbs / ginger / ginger.shtml
http: / / www.esys.org / seekrank / sekrnk11.html
http: / / www.farmradio.org / english / 53-5script.html
http: / / www.friedli.com / herbs / ginger.html
http: / / www.gnc.com / wellness / natpharm / Herb / Ginger.htm
http: / / www.goldentemple.com / Clients / KIIT / GT / Ingredients.nsf / Ingredients / *OG+Ginger+Root+(Zingiber+officinale)?OpenDocument
http: / / www.greenntrade.com / rbfe.htm
http: / / www.healthyelements.com / ca / encyclo / Herb / Ginger.html
http: / / www.herbalinsights.com / article1003.html
http: / / www.herbmed.org / herbs / zingiber.htm
http: / / www.herbphoto.com / education / monograph / ginger.html
http: / / www.herbsandcandles.com / herbs / thaiherbs / ginger.htm
http: / / www.holisticonline.com / Herbal-Med / _Herbs / h61.htm
http: / / www.ibiblio.org / herbmed / eclectic / felter / zingiber.html
http: / / www.indianherbs.com / z_offi20.htm
http: / / www.indmedplants-kr.org / ZINGIBER_OFFICINALE.HTM
http: / / www.intelihealth.com / IH / ihtIH / WSIHW000 / 8513 / 28300.html
http: / / www.internethealthlibrary.com / Plant-Remedies / Ginger.htm
http: / / www.liberherbarum.com / Pn0610.HTM
http: / / www.mcp.edu / herbal / default.htm
http: / / www.mcp.edu / herbal / ginger / ginger.cis.pdf
http: / / www.mcp.edu / herbal / herbal / ginger / ginger.pdf
http: / / www.motherearthherbs.com / tincture.html
http: / / www.mothernature.com / library / books / natmed / ginger.asp
http: / / www.naturesgift.com /
http: / / www.pccnaturalmarkets.com / health / Herb / Ginger.htm
http: / / www.positivehealth.com / permit / Articles / Regular / butlin60.htm
http: / / www.puritan.com / healthnotes / Herb / Ginger.htm
http: / / www.purplesage.org.uk / profiles / ginger.htm
http: / / www.rootgrafix.com / herbalnexus / h_ginger.htm
http: / / www.sciencedaily.com / releases / 2003 / 10 / 031029064357.htm
http: / / www.thedacare.org / healthinfo / Herb / Ginger.htm
http: / / www.vedahealth.com / abdomen_middle.html
https: / / www.joinonespirit.com /

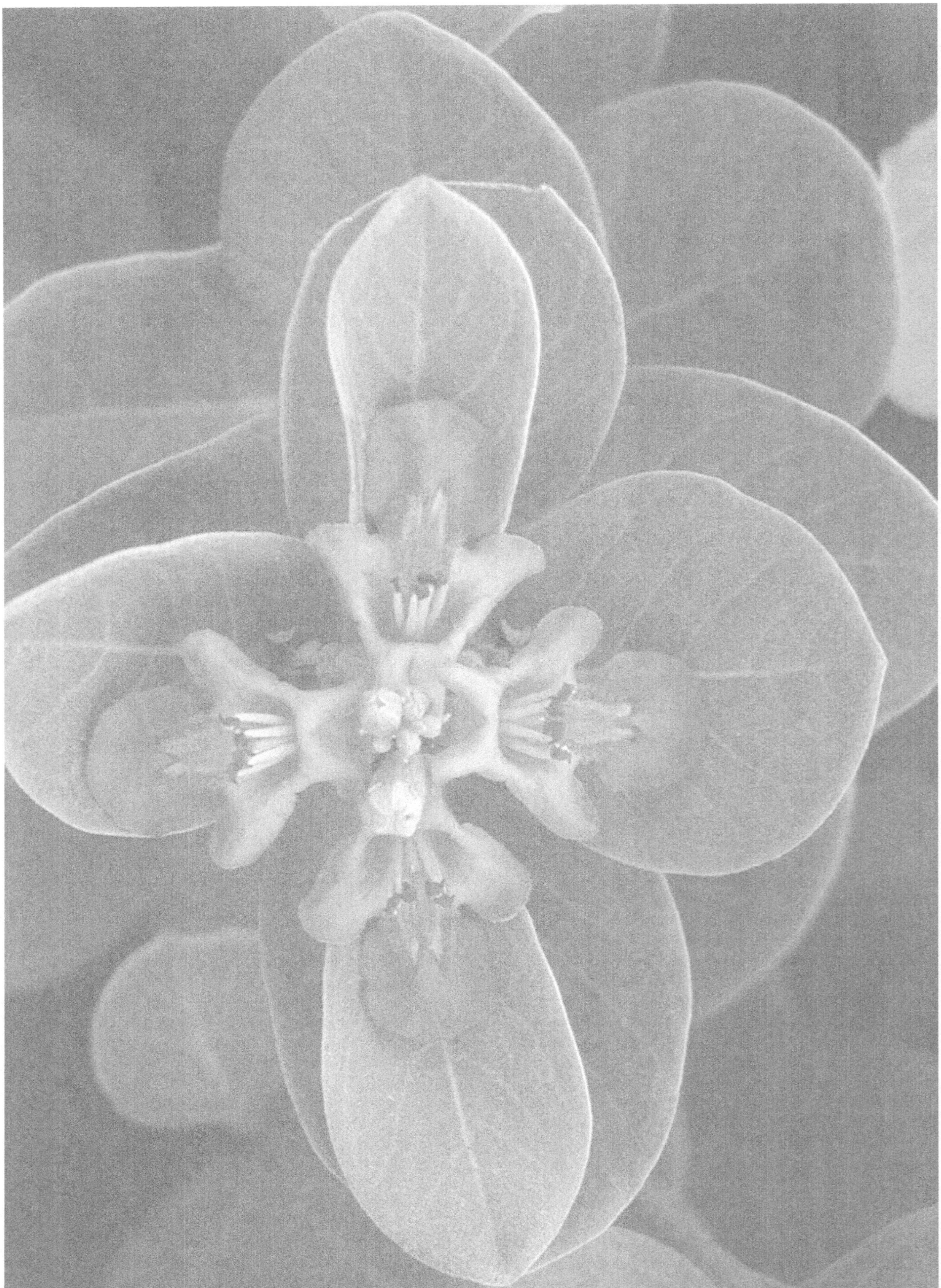

BIBLIOGRAPHY BY AUTHOR

Aalto-Korte K, Lauerma A, Alanko K. 2005. Occupational allergic contact dermatitis from lichens in present-day Finland. *Contact Dermatitis.* Jan;52(1):36-8.

Abbott, Isabel Aiona.1992. *La'au Hawai'i. Traditional Hawaiian Uses of Plants.* Honolulu: Bishop Museum Press

Abdul-Ghani AS, Amin R. 1988. The vascular action of aqueous extracts of *Foeniculum vulgare* leaves. *J Ethnopharmacol* Dec;24(2-3):213-218

Addy ME, et al. 1984. Effects of the extracts of *Desmodium adscendens* on anaphylaxis. *J Ethnopharmacol.* Aug;11(3):283-92.

Addy ME, et al. 1986. Dose-response effects of *Desmodium adscendens* aqueous extract on histamine response, content and anaphylactic reactions in the guinea pig. *J Ethnopharmacol.* Oct;18(1):13-20.

Addy ME, et al. 1988. Effect of *Desmodium adscendens* fractions on antigen- and arachidonic acid-induced contractions of guinea pig airways. *Can J Physiol Pharmacol.* Jun;66(6):820-5.

Addy ME, et al. 1990. Effect of *Desmodium adscendens* fraction 3 on contractions of respiratory smooth muscle. *J Ethnopharmacol.* Jul;29(3):325-35.

Addy ME. 1992. Some secondary plant metabolites in *Desmodium adscendens* and their effects on arachidonic acid metabolism. *Prostaglandins Leukot Essent Fatty Acids.* Sep;47(1):85-91.

Agarwal KC, Russo FX, Parks RE Jr. 1982. Inhibition of human and rat platelet aggregation by extracts of Mo-er (*Auricularia auricula*). *Thromb Haemost.* Oct 29;48(2):162-5.

Aggarwal BB, Kumar A, Bharti AC. 2003. Anticancer potential of curcumin: preclinical and clinical studies. *Anticancer Res.* Jan-Feb;23(1A):363-98.

Agrawal RC, Sarode AV, et al. 1985 Chilli extract treatment and induction of eye lesions in hamsters. *Toxicol Lett.* Oct;28(1):1-7.

Agrawal RC, Wiessler M, Hecker E, Bhide SV. 1986. Tumour-promoting effect of chilli extract in BALB / c mice. *Int J Cancer.* Nov 15;38(5):689-9

Ahmad A, Davies J, et al. 1996. Antiviral properties of extract of *Opuntia streptacantha. Antiviral Res.* May;30(2-3):75-85.

Ahuna, Moses H. 1978. Notes from an herb walk on Kauai.

Akagi A, Sano N, et al. 1998 Non-carcinogenicity of capsaicinoids in B6C3F1 mice. *Food Chem Toxicol.* Dec;36(12):1065-71.

Akhtar MS, Munir M. 1989. Evaluation of the gastric antiulcerogenic effects of *Solanum nigrum, Brassica oleracea,* and *Ocimum basilicum* in rats. *J Ethnopharmacol* Nov;27(1-2):163-176

Alam G, Wahyuono S, et al. 2002 Tracheospasmolytic activity of viteosin-A and vitexicarpin isolated from vitex trifolia. *Planta Med.* Nov;68(11):1047-9.

Albert-Puleo M. 1980. Fennel and anise as estrogenic agents. *J Ethnopharmacol* Dec;2(4):337-344

Altman RD, Marcussen KC. Effects of a ginger extract on knee pain in patients with osteoarthritis. *Arthritis Rheum.* 2001 Nov;44(11):2531-8.

Amalraj T, Ignacimuthu S. 2002. Hyperglycemic effect of leaves of *Mimosa pudica* Linn. *Fitoterapia.* Jul;73(4):351-2.

al-Yahya MA, Rafatullah S, et al. 1989. Gastroprotective activity of ginger *Zingiber officinale* rosc., in albino rats. *Am J Chin Med.*;17(1-2):51-6.

Ambegaokar SS, Wu L, Alamshahi K, Lau J, Jazayeri L, Chan S, Khanna P, Hsieh E, Timiras PS. 2003. Curcumin inhibits dose-dependently and time-dependently neuroglial cell proliferation and growth. *Neuro Endocrinol Lett.* Dec;24(6):469-73.

Andoh, Anthony K. 1986. The Science and Romance of Selected Herbs Used in Medicine and Religious Ceremony. San Francisco: North Scale Institute

Antony S, et al. 1999. Immunomodulatory activity of curcumin. *Immunol Invest* Sep-Dec;28(5-6):291-303

Arpaia MR, Ferrone R, et al. 1990. Effects of *Centella asiatica* extract on mucopolysaccharide metabolism in subjects with varicose veins. *Int J Clin Pharmacol Res* 10:4 229-33

Arvigo, Rosita and Nadine Epstein. 2001. *Rainforest Home Remedies: The Maya Way To Heal Your Body and Replenish Your Soul.* San Francisco: Harper.

Auntie Marie Place

Auwae. Conversations with students of Papa Henry Auwae.

Babineau TJ, Hackford A, et al. 1994. A phase II multicenter, double-blind, randomized, placebo-controlled study of three dosages of an immunomodulator (PGG-glucan) in high-risk surgical patients. *Arch Surg.* Nov;129(11):1204-10.

Babu TD, Kuttan G, Padikkala J. 1995. Cytotoxic and anti-tumour properties of certain taxa of Umbelliferae with special reference to *Centella asiatica* (L.) Urban. *J Ethnopharmacol.* Aug 11;48(1):53-7.

Backhauß C, Krieglstein J. 1992. Extract of kava (*Piper methysticum*) and its methysticin constituents protect brain tissue against ischemic damage in rodents. *Eur J Pharmacol* May 14;215(2-3):265-9

Bajracharya, M. B. 1979. *Ayurvedic Medicinal Plants and General Treatment.* Kathmandu: Jore Ganesh Press.

Baldwin, Roger E. 1979. *Hawai'i's Poisonous Plants.* Hilo, HI: Petroglyph Press.

Barrau, Jacques. 1958. *Subsistence agriculture in Melanesia.* B.P. Bishop Museum Bulletin No. 219. Honolulu.

Barrau, Jacques. 1962. Plant exploration and introduction in the improvement of the coconut palm. *Ind. Coconut.* J. 15, 91-93.

Barreto GS. 2002. Effect of butanolic fraction of *Desmodium adscendens* on the anococcygeus of the rat. *Braz J Biol.* May;62(2):223-30.

Barthelemy S, Vergnes L, et al. 1998. Curcumin and curcumin derivatives inhibit Tat-mediated transactivation of type 1 human immunodeficiency virus long terminal repeat. *Res Virol.* Jan-Feb;149(1):43-52.

Belcaro GV, Rulo A, Grimaldi R. 1990. Capillary filtration and ankle edema in patients with venous hypertension treated with TTFCA. *Angiology.* Jan;41(1):12-8.

Bensky, Dan, & Andrew Gamble. 1986. *Chinese Herbal Medicine: Materia Medica.* Seattle: Eastland Press.

Bensky, Dan, & Andrew Gamble. 1993. *Chinese Herbal Medicine: Materia Medica,* revised edition. Seattle: Eastland Press.

Beppu H, Koike T, et al. 2003. Radical-scavenging effects of *Aloe arborescens* Miller on prevention of pancreatic islet B-cell destruction in rats. *J Ethnopharmacol.* Nov;89(1):37-45.

Berger A, Gremaud G, et al. 2003. Cholesterol-lowering properties of amaranth grain and oil in hamsters. *Int J Vitam Nutr Res.* Feb;73(1):39-47.

Bernays EA, Chapman RF, Singer MS. 2000. Sensitivity to chemically diverse phagostimulants in a single gustatory neuron of a polyphagous caterpillar. *J Comp Physiol* [A]. Jan;186(1):13-9.

Bernstein, J.E., Parish, L.C., Rapaport, M., Rosenbaum, M.M. and Roenigk, H.H., Jr. 1986. Effects of topically applied capsaicin on moderate and severe psoriasis vulgaris. *Journal of the American Academy of Dermatology* 15: 504-507.

Best R, Lewis DA, Nasser N. 1984. The anti-ulcerogenic activity of the unripe plantain banana (*Musa* species). *Br J Pharmacol.* May;82(1):107-16.

Bezivin C, Tomasi S, Rouaud I, Delcros JG, Boustie J. 2004. Cytotoxic activity of compounds from the lichen: *Cladonia convoluta. Planta Med.* Sep;70(9):874-7.

Bian X, Jin J, et al. 2002. Study on the scavenging action of polysaccharide of *Usnea longissima* to oxygen radical and its anti-lipi peroxidation effects. (Article in Chinese) Zhong Yao Cai. Mar;25(3):188-9.

Biere A, Marak HB, Van Damme JM. 2004. Plant chemical defense against herbivores and pathogens: generalized defense or trade-offs? *Oecologia.* Aug;140(3):430-41. Epub 2004 May 14.

Biggs, D.F. and Ladenius, R.C. (1990). Capsaicin selectively reduced airway responses to histamine, substance P, and vagal stimulation. *European Journal of Pharmacology* 175: 29-33.

Bista, M. S., director. 1997(a). *Medicinal Plants of Nepal.* 5th ed. Kathmandu: His Majesty's Government, Ministry of Forests and Soil Conservation, Department of Natural Resources.

Bista, M. S., director. 1997(b). *Medicinal Plants of Nepal.* (Supplement Volume). 2nd ed. Kathmandu: His Majesty's Government, Ministry of Forests and Soil Conservation, Department of Natural Resources.

Blanco C, Ortega N, Castillo R, Alvarez M, Dumpierrez AG, Carrillo T. 1998. *Carica papaya* pollen allergy. *Ann Allergy Asthma Immunol.* Aug;81(2):171-5.

Bliss, Beatrice. 1973. *Chinese Medicinal Herbs* (Li Zi-Shen's Ben Cao). San Francisco: Georgetown Press.

Bode AM, Ma WY, et al. 2001. Inhibition of epidermal growth factor-induced cell transformation and activator protein 1 activation by [6]-gingerol. *Cancer Res.* Feb 1;61(3):850-3.

Bonte F, Dumas M, et al. 1994. Influence of asiatic acid, madecassic acid, and asiaticoside on human collagen I synthesis. *Planta Med.* Apr;60(2):133-5.

Bonte F, Dumas M, et al. 1995. Comparative activity of asiaticoside and madecassoside on type I and III collagen synthesis by cultured human fibroblasts. (Article in French) *Ann Pharm Fr.*;53(1):38-42.

Boonen G, Ferger B, Kuschinsky K, Haberlein H. 1998(b). In vivo effects of the kavapyrones (+)-dihydromethysticin and (+ / -)-kavain on dopamine, 3,4-dihydroxyphenylacetic acid, serotonin and 5-hydroxyindoleacetic acid levels in striatal and cortical brain regions. *Planta Med.* Aug;64(6):507-10.

Boonen G, Haberlein H. 1998(a). Influence of genuine kavapyrone enantiomers on the GABA-A binding site. *Planta Med.* Aug;64(6):504-6.

Bordia A, Verma SK, etc. 1997. Effect of ginger (*Zingiber officinale* Rosc.) and fenugreek (Trigonella foenumgraecum L.) on blood lipids, blood sugar and platelet aggregation in patients with coronary artery disease. *Prostaglandins Leukot Essent Fatty Acids.* May;56(5):379-84

Bosse JP, Papillon J, et al. 1979. Clinical study of a new antikeloid agent. *Ann Plast Surg.* Jul;3(1):13-21.

Botta B, et al. 2003. Three isoflavanones with cannabinoid-like moieties from *Desmodium canum. Phytochemistry.* Sep;64(2):599-602.

Bouraoui A, Toumi A, Ben Mustapha H, Brazier JL. 1988. Effects of capsicum fruit on theophylline absorption and bioavailability in rabbits. *Drug Nutr Interact*;5(4):345-50.

Brandao MG, et al. 1997. Antimalarial activity of extracts and fractions from *Bidens pilosa* and other *Bidens* species (Asteraceae) correlated with the presence of acetylene and flavonoid compounds. *J Ethnopharmacol* Jul; 57(2):131-8

Bresciani LF, Priebe JP, et al. 2003 Pharmacological and phytochemical evaluation of *Adiantum ceneatum* growing in Brazil. *Z Naturforsch* [C]. Mar-Apr;58(3-4):191-4.

Brinker, Francis. 2001. *Herb Contraindications and Drug Interactions.* Sandy, OR: Eclectic Medical Publications.

Brinkhaus B, Lindner M, Schuppan D, et al. 2000. Chemical, pharmacological and clinical profile of the East Asian medicial plant *Centella asiatica. Phytomedicine* 7(5): 427-448.

Brooker, S. G., et al. 1987. *New Zealand Medicinal Plants.* Rev. ed. Aukland: Reed Books.

Brown, Tom, Jr., 1989. Tom Brown's Field Guide to Wilderness Survival. Berkley Pub Group.

Browner CH. 1985. Plants used for reproductive health in Oaxaca, Mexico. *Econ Bot.* Oct-Dec;39(4):482-504.

Budinsky A, Wolfram R, et al. 2001. Regular ingestion of *Opuntia* robusta lowers oxidation injury. *Prostaglandins Leukot Essent Fatty Acids.* Jul;65(1):45-50.

Butera D, Tesoriere L, et al. 2002. Antioxidant activities of sicilian prickly pear (*Opuntia ficus indica*) fruit extracts and reducing properties of its betalains: betanin and indicaxanthin. *J Agric Food Chem.* Nov 6;50(23):6895-901.

Bwititi P, Musabayane CT, Nhachi CF. 2000. Effects of *Opuntia megacantha* on blood glucose and kidney function in streptozotocin diabetic rats. *J Ethnopharmacol.* Mar;69(3):247-52.

Bwititi PT, Machakaire T, et al. 2001. Effects of *Opuntia megacantha* leaves extract on renal electrolyte and fluid handling in streptozotocin (STZ)-diabetic rats. *Ren Fail.* Mar;23(2):149-58.

Calabrese V, Butterfield DA, Stella AM. 2003. Nutritional antioxidants and the heme oxygenase pathway of stress tolerance: novel targets for neuroprotection in Alzheimer's disease. *Ital J Biochem.* Dec;52(4):177-81.

Cambie RC, Ferguson LR. 2003. Potential functional foods in the traditional Maori diet. *Mutat Res.* Feb-Mar;523-524:109-17.

Campanella L, Delfini M, Ercole P, Iacoangeli A, Risuleo G. 2002. Molecular characterization and action of usnic acid: a drug that inhibits proliferation of mouse polyomavirus in vitro and whose main target is RNA transcription. *Biochimie.* Apr;84(4):329-34.

Cao H, et al. 2000. Study on erzhi pill effects on neuro-endocrinologic-immuno network of animal of deficiency of yin. (article in Chinese) *Zhong Yao Cai.* Mar;23(3):164-6.

Carbajal D, et al. 1989. Pharmacological study of *Cymbopogon citratus* leaves. *J Ethnopharmacol* Feb;25(1):103-7.

Cardenas Medellin ML, Serna Saldivar SO, Velazco de la Garza J. 1998. Effect of raw and cooked nopal (*Opuntia ficus indica*) ingestion on growth and profile of total cholesterol, lipoproteins, and blood glucose in rats. (Article in Spanish) *Arch Latinoam Nutr.* Dec;48(4):316-23.

Carlini EA, et al. 1986. Pharmacology of lemongrass (*Cymbopogon citratus* Stapf). I. Effects of teas prepared from the leaves on laboratory animals. *J Ethnopharmacol* Jul;17(1):37-64

Carlquist, Sherwin. 1980. *Hawai'i a Natural History.* Lawai, HI: Pacific Tropical Botanical Garden.

Carper, Jean. 1988. *The Food Pharmacy.* New York: Bantam Books.

Carper, Jean. 1994. *Food Your Miracle Medicine.* Perennial.

Carreras HA, Pignata ML. 2002. Biomonitoring of heavy metals and air quality in Cordoba City, Argentina, using transplanted lichens. *Environ Pollut.*;117(1):77-87.

Castleman, Michael & Sheldon Saul Hendler. 1991. *The Healing Herbs: The Ultimate Guide to the Curative Power of Nature's Medicines.* Emmaus, Pennsylvania: Rodale Press

Caviglia AM, Nicora P, Giordani P, Brunialti G, Modenesi P. 2001. Oxidative stress and usnic acid content in *Parmelia caperata* and *Parmelia soredians* (Lichenes). *Farmaco.* May-Jul;56(5-7):379-82.

Cesarone MR, Belcaro G, Rulo A, et al 2001(a). Microcirculatory effects of total triterpenic fraction of *Centella asiatica* in chronic venous hypertension: measurement by laser Doppler, TcPO2-CO2, and leg volumetry. *Angiology.* Oct;52 Suppl 2:S45-8.

Cesarone MR, Incandela L, De Sanctis MT, Bavera P, et al. 2001(b). Evaluation of treatment of diabetic microangiopathy with total triterpenic fraction of *Centella asiatica*: a clinical prospective randomized trial with a microcirculatory model. *Angiology.* Oct;52 Suppl 2:S49-54.

Cesarone MR, Incandela L, De Sanctis MT, Belcaro G, et al. 2001(c). Flight microangiopathy in medium- to long-distance flights: prevention of edema and microcirculation alterations with total triterpenic fraction of *Centella asiatica. Angiology.* Oct;52 Suppl 2:S33-7.

Chainani-Wu N. 2003. Safety and anti-inflammatory activity of curcumin: a component of tumeric (*Curcuma longa*). *J Altern Complement Med.* Feb;9(1):161-8.

Chakurski I, Matev M, et al. 1981. Treatment of chronic colitis with an herbal combination of *Taraxacum officinale, Hipericum perforatum, Melissa officinaliss, Calendula officinalis* and *Foeniculum vulgare.* Vutr Boles.;20(6):51-4.

Chandan BK, Sharma AK, Anand KK. 1991. *Boerhaavia diffusa*: a study of its hepatoprotective activity. *J Ethnopharmacol.* Mar;31(3):299-307.

Chang H.C., et al. 2003. Antiproliferative and chemopreventive effects of adlay seed on lung cancer in vitro and in vivo. *J Agric Food Chem.* Jun 4;51(12):3656-60.

Chang, But. 1987. *Pharmacology and application of Chinese materia medica.*

Chang, Yishiang. 1996. Notes from herb walks with Yishiang Chang,

Charles V, Charles SX. 1992. The use and efficacy of *Azadirachta indica* ADR ('Neem') and *Curcuma longa* ('Turmeric') in scabies. A pilot study. *Trop Geogr Med* Jan;44(1-2):178-81

Chatterjee TK, Chakraborty A, et al. 1992. Effects of plant extract *Centella asiatica* (Linn.) on cold restraint stress ulcer in rats. *Indian J Exp Biol.* Oct;30(10):889-91.

Chaturvedi A, Sarojini G, Devi NL. 1993. Hypocholesterolemic effect of amaranth seeds (*Amaranthus esculantus*). *Plant Foods Hum Nutr.* Jul;44(1):63-70.

Chen CF, et al. 1981. Protective effects of *Carica papaya* Linn on the exogenous gastric ulcer in rats. *American Journal of Chinese Medicine* 9(3):205-12

Chen H, Zhang ZS, Zhang YL, Zhou DY. 1999. Curcumin inhibits cell proliferation by interfering with the cell cycle and inducing apoptosis in colon carcinoma cells. *Anticancer Res.* Sep-Oct;19(5A):3675-80.

Chen, John K., and Tina T. Chen. 2004. *Chinese Medical Herbology and Pharmacology.* City of Industry CA: Art of Medicine Press, Inc.

Cheng AL, Hsu CH, Lin JK, Hsu MM, Ho YF, Shen TS, Ko JY, Lin JT, Lin BR, Ming-Shiang W, Yu HS, Jee SH, Chen GS, Chen TM, Chen CA, Lai MK, Pu YS, Pan MH, Wang YJ, Tsai CC, Hsieh CY. 2001. Phase I clinical trial of curcumin, a chemopreventive agent, in patients with high-risk or pre-malignant lesions. *Anticancer Res.* Jul-Aug;21(4B):2895-900.

Cheng CL, Guo JS, et al. 2004. The healing effects of *Centella* extract and asiaticoside on acetic acid induced gastric ulcers in rats. *Life Sci.* Mar 19;74(18):2237-49.

Cheng CL, Koo MW. 2000. Effects of *Centella asiatica* on ethanol induced gastric mucosal lesions in rats. *Life Sci.* Oct 13;67(21):2647-53.

Cheng Z, et al. 2001. Broussochalcone A, a potent antioxidant and effective suppressor of inducible nitric oxide synthase in lipopolysaccharide-activated macrophages. *Biochem Pharmacol* 61(8):939-46

Cheong H, Choi EJ, et al. 1998. Desacetylmatricarin, an anti-allergic component from *Taraxacum platycarpum. Planta Med.* Aug;64(6):577-8.

Chestnut, V. K. 1974. *Plants Used by the Indians of Mendicino County, California.* Fort Bragg, CA: Mendicino County Historical Society.

Chevallier, Andrew. 1996. *The Encyclopedia of Medicinal Plants.* New York: DK Publishing Inc.

Chiang LC, Chiang W, et al. 2003(b) In vitro cytotoxic, antiviral and immunomodulatory effects of *Plantago major* and *Plantago asiatica. Am J Chin Med.*;31(2):225-34.

Chiang LC, Chiang W, et al. 2003(c). Antileukemic activity of selected natural products in Taiwan. *Am J Chin Med.*;31(1):37-46.

Chiang LC, Ng LT, et al. 2003(a). Immunomodulatory activities of flavonoids, monoterpenoids, triterpenoids, iridoid glycosides and phenolic compounds of Plantago species. *Planta Med.* Jul;69(7):600-4.

Chin HW, et.al., 1995. Anti-inflammatory activity of Taiwan folk medicine "ham-hong-chho" in rats. *Am J Chin Med* 23(3-4), 273-278

Chin HW, et.al., 1996. The hepatoprotective effects of Taiwan folk medicine ham-hong-chho in rats. *Am J Chin Med* 24(3-4), 231-240

Ching LS, Mohamed S. 2001. Alpha-tocopherol content in 62 edible tropical plants. *J Agric Food Chem.* Jun;49(6):3101-5.

Chithra P, Sajithlal GB, et al 1998. Influence of *Aloe vera* on collagen turnover in healing of dermal wounds in rats. *Indian J Exp Biol.* Sep;36(9):896-901.

Chivato T, Juan F, et al. 1996. Anaphylaxis induced by ingestion of a pollen compound. *J Investig Allergol Clin Immunol.* May-Jun;6(3):208-9.

Choi JH, Shin KM, et al. 2002. Taraxinic acid, a hydrolysate of sesquiterpene lactone glycoside from the *Taraxacum coreanum* NAKAI, induces the differentiation of human acute promyelocytic leukemia HL-60 cells. Biol Pharm Bull. Nov;25(11):1446-50.

Choi KH, Laursen RA. 2000. Amino-acid sequence and glycan structures of cysteine proteases with proline specificity from ginger rhizome *Zingiber officinale*. Eur J Biochem. Mar;267(5):1516-26.

Choi SW, Son BW, et al. 2001. The wound-healing effect of a glycoprotein fraction isolated from *Aloe vera*. *Br J Dermatol.* Oct;145(4):535-45.

Ciolino HP, Daschner PJ, et al. 1998. Effect of curcumin on the aryl hydrocarbon receptor and cytochrome P450 1A1 in MCF-7 human breast carcinoma cells. *Biochem Pharmacol.* Jul 15;56(2):197-206.

Cleghorn F, Battoo K, Diaz C, Balbosa S, Jack N, Blattner W, and Bartholomew C. *Update on the epidemiology of AIDS in Trinidad.* International Conference on AIDS, San Francisco, June 20-23, 1990

Cocchietto M, Skert N, Nimis PL, Sava G. 2002. A review on usnic acid, an interesting natural compound. *Naturwissenschaften.* Apr;89(4):137-46.

Collins RA, Ng TB. 1997 Polysaccharopeptide from *Coriolus versicolor* has potential for use against human immunodeficiency virus type 1 infection. *Life Sci*; 60(25):PL383-7

Commonwealth. *Medicinal Plants of Trinidad & Tobago.*

Corsi MM, Bertelli AA, et al. 1998. The therapeutic potential of *Aloe vera* in tumor-bearing rats. *Int J Tissue React.*;20(4):115-8.

Cribb, Alan Bridson, and Joan Winifred Cribb. 1986. *Wild Medicine in Australia.* Sydney, Australia: Fontana Books.

Cruz, G. L. *Dicionario Das Plantas Uteis Do Brasil.* 4th ed. Rio de Janiero: Bertrand Brasil.

Cunningham, Scott. 1985. *Cunningham's Encyclopedia of Magical Herbs.* 2nd ed. Llewellyn Publications.

Dam-Bakker AW, van de Groot AP Luyken R. 1958. Influence of wati (*Piper methysticum*) on the fertility of male rats. *Tropical and Geographical Medicine* 10: 68-70.

Darwin, Tess. 1996. *The Scots Herbal.* The Plant Lore of Scotland. Edinburgh: Mercat Press.

Davies LP, Drew CA, et al. 1992. Kava pyrones and resin: studies on GABAA, GABAB and benzodiazepine binding sites in rodent brain. *Pharmacol Toxicol.* Aug;71(2):120-6.

Davis RH, Leitner MG, et al. 1989(a). Anti-inflammatory activity of *Aloe vera* against a spectrum of irritants. *J Am Podiatr Med Assoc.* Jun;79(6):263-76.

Davis RH, Leitner MG, Russo JM, et al. 1989(c). Wound healing. Oral and topical activity of *Aloe vera. J Am Podiatr Med Assoc.* Nov;79(11):559-62.

Davis RH, Rosenthal KY, et al. 1989(b). Processed *Aloe vera* administered topically inhibits inflammation. *J Am Podiatr Med Assoc.* Aug;79(8):395-7.

De Lucca, Manuel, Jaime Zalles. 1992. *Flora Medicinal Boliviana: Diccionario Enciclopedico.* La Paz, Bolivia: Editorial Los Amigos Del Libro.

de Medeiros JM, Macedo M, Contancia JP, Nguyen C, Cunningham G, Miles DH. 2000. Antithrombin activity of medicinal plants of the Azores. *J Ethnopharmacol.* Sep;72(1-2):157-65.

de Melo AC, et al. 1978. Acetylcholine-like activity in the fruit of the black nightshade (Solanaceae). *Acta Physiol Lat Am*;28(4-5):19-26

Degener, Otto. 1945. *Plants of Hawaii National Park Illustrative of Plants and Customs of the South Seas.* Pub by Otto Degener.

Denyer CV, Jackson P, et al. 1994. Isolation of antirhinoviral sesquiterpenes from ginger (*Zingiber officinale*). *J Nat Prod.* May;57(5):658-62.

Dikshit M, Rastogi L, et al. 1995. Prevention of ischaemia-induced biochemical changes by curcumin & quinidine in the cat heart. *Indian J Med Res.* Jan;101:31-5.

Dimo T, et al., 1999. Hypotensive effects of a methalol extract of *Bidens pilosa* on hypertensive rats, *CR Academy of Sciences III*; 322(4): 323-329.

Djipa CD, et al. 2000. Antimicrobial activity of bark extracts of *Syzygium jambos* (L.) alston (Myrtaceae). *J Ethnopharmacol* Jul;71(1-2):307-13.

Dobrescu D, Tanasescu M, Mezdrea A, Ivan C, Ordosch E, Neagoe F, Rizeanu A, Trifu L, Enescu V. 1993. Contributions to the complex study of some lichens-*Usnea* genus. Pharmacological studies on *Usnea barbata* and *Usnea hirta* species. *Rom J Physiol.* Jan-Jun;30(1-2):101-7.

Dok-Go H, Lee KH, et al. 2003. Neuroprotective effects of antioxidative flavonoids, quercetin, (+)-dihydroquercetin and quercetin 3-methyl ether, isolated from *Opuntia ficus-indica var. saboten.* Brain Res. Mar 7;965(1-2):130-6.

Dong XY, Chen M, Jin W, Huang DX, Shen SM, Li HT. 1989. Studies on antifertility constituents of *Siegesbeckia glabrescens* Mak (Article in Chinese)Yao Xue Xue Bao.;24(11):833-6.

Dragull K, Yoshida WY, Tang CS. 2003. Piperidine alkaloids from *Piper methysticum. Phytochemistry.* May;63(2):193-8.

Duansak D, Somboonwong J, Patumraj S. 2003. Effects of *Aloe vera* on leukocyte adhesion and TNF-alpha and IL-6 levels in burn wounded rats. *Clin Hemorheol Microcirc.*;29(3-4):239-46.

Duffield PH, et al. 1991. Development of tolerance to kava in mice. *Clin Exp Pharmacol Physiol* Aug;18(8):571-8

Duffield PH, Jamieson DD, Duffield AM. 1989. Effect of aqueous and lipid-soluble extracts of kava on the conditioned avoidance response in rats. *Arch Int Pharmacodyn* Ther. Sep-Oct;301:81-90.

Duke, J.A. 1984. *Borderline herbs.* CRC Press. Boca Raton, FL.

Duke, James. The author's correspondence with James Duke.

Duke. J. A. and Ayensu. E. S., 1985. *Medicinal Plants of China.* Reference Publications, Inc.

Dunne JW, Davidson L, Vandongen R, Beilin LJ, Rogers P. 1983. The effect of ascorbic acid on plasma sulfate conjugated catecholamines after eating bananas. *Life Sci.* Oct 10;33(15):1511-7.

Durazo FA, Lassman C, Han SH, Saab S, Lee NP, Kawano M, Saggi B, Gordon S, Farmer DG, Yersiz H, Goldstein RL, Ghobrial M, Busuttil RW. 2004. Fulminant liver failure due to usnic acid for weight loss. *Am J Gastroenterol.* May;99(5):950-2.

Ebina T, Kohya H, Ishikawa K. 1989. Antitumor effect of PSK: role of regional lymph nodes and enhancement of concomitant and sinecomitant immunity in the mouse. Jpn J *Cancer Res.* Feb;80(2):158-66.

Ebina T, Kohya H. 1987. Antitumor effect of PSK (2): effector mechanism of the antimetastatic effect in the "double grafted tumor system. (Article in Japanese) *Gan To Kagaku Ryoho*. Jun;14(6 Pt 1):1847-53.

Egan M.E., et al. 2004. Curcumin, a major constituent of turmeric, corrects cystic fibrosis defects. *Science*. Apr 23;304(5670):600-2.

El Bardai S, Lyoussi B, et al. 2001 Pharmacological evidence of hypotensive activity of *Marrubium vulgare* and *Foeniculum vulgare* in spontaneously hypertensive rat. *Clin Exp Hypertens* May;23(4):329-343

El Kossori et al. 1998. Composition of pulp, skin and seeds of prickly pears fruit (*Opuntia ficus indica* sp.). *Plant Foods Hum Nutr*;52(3):263-70

El SN, Karakaya S. 2004. Radical scavenging and iron-chelating activities of some greens used as traditional dishes in Mediterranean diet. *Int J Food Sci Nutr*. Feb;55(1):67-74.

El-Abyad MS, et al. 1990. Preliminary screening of some Egyptian weeds for antimicrobial activity. *Microbios* 62(250):47-57

Elattar TM, Virji AS. 2000. The inhibitory effect of curcumin, genistein, quercetin and cisplatin on the growth of oral cancer cells in vitro. *Anticancer Res*. May-Jun;20(3A):1733-8.

Elpel, Thomas J. 2000. *Botany in a Day*. 4th ed. Pony, MT.: HOPS Press.

Emergency Food Plants and Poisonous Plants of the Islands of the Pacific. 1943. Washington: United States Government Printing Office

Emeruwa AC. 1982. Antibacterial substance from *Carica papaya* fruit extract. *Journal of Natural Products* 45(2):123-7

Englberger L, Fitzgerald MH, Marks GC. 2003. Pacific pandanus fruit: an ethnographic approach to understanding an overlooked source of provitamin A carotenoids. *Asia Pac J Clin Nutr*.;12(1):38-44.

Eno, A.E. et al. 2000. Blood pressure depression by the fruit juice of *Carica papaya* (L.) in renal and DOCA-induced hypertension in the rat. *Phytother Res* Jun;14(4):235-9

Fahs, Barbara. 2003. Notes from Hi'iaka's Healing Herb Garden.

Farghali H, Masek K. 1998 Immunopharmacologic agents in the amelioration of hepatic injuries. *Int J Immunopharmacol* Apr-May;20(4-5):125-39

Farnsworth NR, Bingel AS, et al. 1975. Potential value of plants as sources of new antifertility agents I. *J Pharm Sci*. Apr;64(4):535-98.

Fernandez ML, Lin EC, et al. 1992. Prickly pear (*Opuntia* sp.) pectin reverses low density lipoprotein receptor suppression induced by a hypercholesterolemic diet in guinea pigs. *J Nutr*. Dec;122(12):2330-40.

Fernandez ML, Lin EC, et al. 1994. Prickly pear (*Opuntia* sp.) pectin alters hepatic cholesterol metabolism without affecting cholesterol absorption in guinea pigs fed a hypercholesterolemic diet. *J Nutr*. Jun;124(6):817-24.

Ferreira LA, Henriques OB, et al. 1992. Antivenom and biological effects of ar-turmerone isolated from *Curcuma longa* (Zingiberaceae). *Toxicon* 1992 Oct;30(10):1211-8. Erratum in: *Toxicon* Dec;30(12):1637

Figueira R, Pacheco AM, Sousa AJ, Catarino F. 2002. Development and calibration of epiphytic lichens as saltfall biomonitors--dry-deposition modelling. *Environ Pollut*.;120(1):69-78.

Fischer-Rasmussen W, Kjaer SK, Dahl C, Asping U. 1991. Ginger treatment of hyperemesis gravidarum. *Eur J Obstet Gynecol Reprod Biol*; 38:19-24.

Furusawa, Eiichi. *Anti-cancer Activity of Noni Fruit Juice Against Tumors in Mice*. Proceedings of the 2002 Hawai'i Noni Conference. Scot C. Nelson, ed. University of Hawai'i at Manoa. 2002.

Flynn D, Rafferty M, Boctor A. 1986. Inhibition of human neutrophil 5-liopxygenase activity by gingerdione, shogaol, capsaicin and related pungent compounds. *Prostaglandins Leukot Med*; 24:195-8.

Foster, Steven, and James A. Duke. 2000. *A Field Guide to Medicinal Plants and Herbs of Eastern and Central North America*. 2nd ed. New York: Houghton Mifflin Company

Foster, Steven, and Yue Chongxi. 1997. *Herbal Emissaries*. Rochester, VT: Healing Arts Press.

Fournet A, Ferreira ME, Rojas de Arias A, Torres de Ortiz S, Inchausti A, Yaluff G, Quilhot W, Fernandez E, Hidalgo ME. 1997. Activity of compounds isolated from Chilean lichens against experimental cutaneous leishmaniasis. *Comp Biochem Physiol C Pharmacol Toxicol Endocrinol*. Jan;116(1):51-4.

Francolini I, Norris P, Piozzi A, Donelli G, Stoodley P. 2004. Usnic acid, a natural antimicrobial agent able to inhibit bacterial biofilm formation on polymer surfaces. *Antimicrob Agents Chemother*. Nov;48(11):4360-5.

Frati-Munari AC, Altamirano-Bustamante E, et al. 1989(a). Hypoglycemic action of *Opuntia streptacantha* Lemaire: study using raw extracts [Article in Spanish]. *Arch Invest Med* (Mex). Oct-Dec;20(4):321-5.

Frati-Munari AC, Del Valle-Martinez LM, et al. 1989(c). Hypoglycemic action of different doses of nopal (*Opuntia streptacantha* Lemaire) in patients with type II diabetes mellitus [Article in Spanish] *Arch Invest Med* (Mex). Apr-Jun;20(2):197-201.

Frati-Munari AC, Gordillo BE, et al. 1988. Hypoglycemic effect of *Opuntia streptacantha* Lemaire in NIDDM. *Diabetes Care*. Jan;11(1):63-6.

Frati-Munari AC, Licona-Quesada R, et al. 1990. Activity of *Opuntia streptacantha* in healthy individuals with induced hyperglycemia [Article in Spanish] *Arch Invest Med* (Mex). Apr-Jun;21(2):99-102.

Frati-Munari AC, Rios Gil U, et al. 1989(b). Duration of the hypoglycemic action of *Opuntia streptacantha* Lem [Article in Spanish]. *Arch Invest Med* (Mex). Oct-Dec;20(4):297-300.

Frati-Munari AC, Vera Lastra O, Ariza Andraca CR. 1992. Evaluation of nopal capsules in diabetes mellitus. (Article in Spanish) *Gac Med Mex*. Jul-Aug;128(4):431-6.

Frautschy SA, Hu W, Kim P, Miller SA, Chu T, Harris-White ME, Cole GM. 2001. Phenolic anti-inflammatory antioxidant reversal of Abeta-induced cognitive deficits and neuropathology. *Neurobiol Aging*. Nov-Dec;22(6):993-1005.

Frawley, David, and Vasant Lad. 1988. *The Yoga of Herbs*. 2nd ed. Santa Fe: Lotus Press.

Fuhrman B, Rosenblat M, et al. 2000. Ginger extract consumption reduces plasma cholesterol, inhibits LDL oxidation and attenuates development of atherosclerosis in atherosclerotic, apolipoprotein E-deficient mice. *J Nutr*. May;130(5):1124-31.

Fujisawa S, Atsumi T, Ishihara M, Kadoma Y. 2004. Cytotoxicity, ROS-generation activity and radical-scavenging activity of curcumin and related compounds. *Anticancer Res*. Mar-Apr;24(2B):563-9.

Furukawa F, Nishikawa A, et al. 2002. Chemopreventive effects of *Aloe arborescens* on N-nitrosobis(2-oxopropyl)amine-induced pancreatic carcinogenesis in hamsters. *Cancer Lett*. Apr 25;178(2):117-22.

Futrell JM, Rietschel RL. 1993. Spice allergy evaluated by results of patch tests. *Cutis.* Nov;52(5):288-90.

Galati EM, Mondello MR, et al. 2003. Chemical characterization and biological effects of Sicilian *Opuntia ficus indica* (L.) mill. Fruit juice: antioxidant and antiulcerogenic activity. *J Agric Food Chem.* Aug 13;51(17):4903-8.

Galati EM, Monforte MT, et al. 2001. Antiulcer activity of *Opuntia ficus indica* (L.) Mill. (Cactaceae): ultrastructural study. *J Ethnopharmacol.* Jun;76(1):1-9.

Galati EM, Pergolizzi S, et al. 2002(b). Study on the increment of the production of gastric mucus in rats treated with *Opuntia ficus indica* (L.) Mill. cladodes. *J Ethnopharmacol.* Dec;83(3):229-33.

Galati EM, Tripodo MM, et al. 2002(a). Biological effect of *Opuntia ficus indica* (L.) Mill. (Cactaceae) waste matter. Note I: diuretic activity. *J Ethnopharmacol.* Jan;79(1):17-21.

Gao JJ, et al. 1993. Chemical constituents of *Emilia sonchifolia* L. DC *Zhongguo Zhong Yao Za Zhi* Feb;18(2):102-103.

Garcia Rowe J, Garcia Gimenez MD, Saenz Rodriguez MT. 1999. Some lichen products have antimicrobial activity. *Z Naturforsch* [C]. Jul-Aug;54(7-8):605-9.

Garcia-Moreno C, Nogales-Alarcon A, Gomez-cerro A, Marine-Font A. 1980 Spectrofluorometric determination and thin layer chromatographic identification of serotonin in foods. *J Assoc Off Anal Chem.* Jan;63(1):19-21.

Geissberger P, et al., 1991. Constituents of *Bidens pilosa* L.: do the components found so far explain the use of this plant in traditional medicine? *Acta Trop* 48(4):251-61

Getie M, et al. 2003 Evaluation of the anti-microbial and anti-inflammatory activities of the medicinal plants *Dodonaea viscosa, Rumex nervosus* and *Rumex abyssinicus. Fitoterapia.* Feb;74(1-2):139-43.

Ghannam N, Kingston M, et al. 1986. The antidiabetic activity of aloes: preliminary clinical and experimental observations. *Horm Res.*;24(4):288-94.

Ghione M, Parrello D, Grasso L. 1988. Usnic acid revisited, its activity on oral flora. *Chemioterapia.* Oct;7(5):302-5.

Gibbons, Euell. 2000. *Euell Gibbons' Beach Combers Handbook.* David McKay Co.

Giordani R., et al. 1996. Fungicidal activity of latex sap from *Carica papaya* and antifungal effect of D(+)-glucosamine on *Candida albicans* growth. Mycoses 39(3-4):103-10

Gleitz J, Beile A, et al. 1997. Antithrombotic action of the kava pyrone (+)-kavain prepared from *Piper methysticum* on human platelets. *Planta Med.* Feb;63(1):27-30.

Gleitz J, Tosch C, et al. 1996. The protective action of tetrodotoxin and (+ / -)-kavain on anaerobic glycolysis, ATP content and intracellular Na+ and Ca2+ of anoxic brain vesicles. *Neuropharmacology*;35(12):1743-52.

Goel RK, Gupta S, Shankar R, Sanyal AK. 1986. Anti-ulcerogenic effect of banana powder (*Musa sapientum var. paradisiaca*) and its effect on mucosal resistance. *J Ethnopharmacol.* Oct;18(1):33-44.

Gomez-Flores R, Calderon CL, Scheibel LW, Tamez-Guerra P, Rodriguez-Padilla C, Tamez-Guerra R, Weber RJ. 2000. Immunoenhancing properties of *Plantago major* leaf extract. *Phytother Res* Dec;14(8):617-622

Gomita Y, et al. 1981. Behavioral and EEG effects of coixol (6-methoxybenzoxazolone), one of the components in *Coix Lachryma-Jobi* L. var. ma-yuen Stapf (article in Japanese) Nippon Yakurigaku Zasshi. Mar;77(3):245-59

Goncalo S. 1987. Contact sensitivity to lichens and compositae in Frullania dermatitis. *Contact Dermatitis.* Feb;16(2):84-6.

Gonlachanvit S, Chen YH, et al. 2003. Ginger reduces hyperglycemia-evoked gastric dysrhythmias in healthy humans: possible role of endogenous prostaglandins. *J Pharmacol Exp Ther.* Dec;307(3):1098-103.

Govere J, et al. 2000. Local plants as repellents against *Anopheles arabiensis*, in Mpumalanga Province, South Africa. *Cent Afr J Med* Aug;46(8):213-6

Grieve, M. 1971. *A Modern Herbal. Volumes 1 & 2.* New York: Dover Publications Inc.

Gross, Ann. *La'au Lapa'au: An Introductory Guide to Hawaiian Medicinal Plants.* Revised Ed.

Gruenwald, Joerg, ed. 1998. *PDR for Herbal Medicines.* Montvale, NJ: Medical Economics Company, Inc.

Guh JH, Ko FN, et al. 1995. Antiplatelet effect of gingerol isolated from *Zingiber officinale. J Pharm Pharmacol.* Apr;47(4):329-32.

Gupta YK, Veerendra Kumar MH, Srivastava AK. 2003. Effect of *Centella asiatica* on pentylenetetrazole-induced kindling, cognition and oxidative stress in rats. *Pharmacol Biochem Behav.* Feb;74(3):579-85.

Gupta, MB et al. 1980. Anti-inflammatory and anti-pyretic activities of B-sitosterol. *Planta Medica.* 39, 157-163,

Gutmanis, Jane. 1987. *Kahuna La'au Lapa'au.* 4th ed. Honolulu: Island Heritage.

Habelhah H, Okada F, et al. 1998(b). Polysaccharide K induces Mn superoxide dismutase (Mn-SOD) in tumor tissues and inhibits malignant progression of QR-32 tumor cells: possible roles of interferon alpha, tumor necrosis factor alpha and transforming growth factor beta in Mn-SOD induction by polysaccharide K. *Cancer Immunol Immunother.* Aug;46(6):338-44.

Habelhah H. 1998(a) Induction of manganese superoxide dismutase by an immunopotentiator as a mechanism of inhibiting of malignant progression of murine tumor cells. (Article in Japanese) *Hokkaido Igaku Zasshi.* Sep;73(5):519-29.

Han D, Matsumaru K, Rettori D, Kaplowitz N. 2004. Usnic acid-induced necrosis of cultured mouse hepatocytes: inhibition of mitochondrial function and oxidative stress. *Biochem Pharmacol.* Feb 1;67(3):439-51.

Han et al. 2001. Monoamine oxidase B inhibitors from the fruits of *Opuntia ficus-indica var. saboten. Arch Pharm Res* Feb;24(1):51-4

Han SS, Keum YS, Seo HJ, Chun KS, Lee SS, Surh YJ. 2001. Capsaicin suppresses phorbol ester-induced activation of NF-kappaB / Rel and AP-1 transcription factors in mouse epidermis. *Cancer Lett.* Mar 26;164(2):119-26

Han Y, et al. 1998. Preliminary studies on chemical constituents and pharmacological action of *Eclipta prostrata* L. (article in Chinese) *Zhongguo Zhong Yao Za Zhi.* Nov;23(11):680-2, 703.

Handy, E. S. C., Mary Kawena Pukui and Katherine Livermore. 1934. *Outline of Hawaiiian Physical Therapeutics.* Bernice P. Bishop Museum Bulletin 126. Honolulu: Bernice P. Bishop Museum

Hargreaves, Dorothy, and Bob Hargreaves. 1964. *Tropical Trees of Hawai'i.* Lāhainā HI: Ross Hargreaves

Haselwood, E.L. and G. G. Motter, eds. 1983. *Handbook of Hawaiian Weeds.* 2nd ed. Honolulu: University of Hawai'i Press.

Hashimoto K, Satoh K, et al. 2002. Component of *Zingiber officinale* that improves the enhancement of small intestinal transport. *Planta Med.* Oct;68(10):936-9.

Heck AM, DeWitt BA, Lukes AL. 2000. Potential interactions between alternative therapies and warfarin. *Am J Health Syst Pharm.* Jul 1;57(13):1221-7; quiz 1228-30.

Heinerman, John. 1996. *Heinerman's Encyclopedia of Healing Herbs & Spices.* Paramus, NJ: Prentice Hall.

Helander A, Wikstrom T, Lowenmo C, Jacobsson G, Beck O. 1992. Urinary excretion of 5-hydroxyindole-3-acetic acid and 5-hydroxytryptophol after oral loading with serotonin. *Life Sci.*;50(17):1207-13.

Henderson, D.E., Slickman, A.M. and Henderson, S.K. 1999. Quantitative HPLC determination of the antioxidant activity of capsaicin on the formation of lipid hydroperoxides of linoleic acid: a comparative study against BHT and melatonin. *Journal of Agricultural and Food Chemistry* 47: 2563-2570.

Herb Research Publications. 1995. *Naturopathic Handbook of Herbal Formulas.* 4th ed. Ayer, MA: Herb Research Publications, Inc.

Herberg KW. 1993. Effect of Kava-Special Extract WS 1490 combined with ethyl alcohol on safety-relevant performance parameters. (Article in German) *Blutalkohol*;30:96-105.

Hetland G, Samuelsen AB, et al. 2000. Protective effect of *Plantago major* L. Pectin polysaccharide against systemic *Streptococcus pneumoniae* infection in mice. *Scand J Immunol* Oct;52(4):348-355

Hewitt H, et al. 2000. Topical use of papaya in chronic skin ulcer therapy in Jamaica. *West Indian Med J.* 49(1):32-3.

Higgs, Leslie. 1993. *Bush Medicine in the Bahamas.* Nassau, Bahamas: Leslie Higgs

Hirayama H, et al. 1993. Effect of *Desmodium styracifolium*-triterpenoid on calcium oxalate renal stones. *Br J Urol.* Feb;71(2):143-7.

Hirazumi A, Furusawa E. 1999. An immunomodulatory polysaccharide-rich substance from the fruit juice of *Morinda citrifolia* (noni) with antitumour activity. *Phytother Res.* Aug;13(5):380-7.

Hiruma-Lima CA, Gracioso JS, et al. 2000. The juice of fresh leaves of *Boerhaavia diffusa* L. (Nyctaginaceae) markedly reduces pain in mice. *J Ethnopharmacol.* Jul;71(1-2):267-74.

Hobbs, Christopher, 1995. *Medicinal Mushrooms.* An Exploration of Tradition, Healing, and Culture. Summertown, TN: Botanica Press

Hobbs, Christopher. 1998. *Herbal Remedies for Dummies.* Foster City, CA: IDG Books Worldwide, Inc.

Hobbs, Christopher. Author's correspondence with Christopher Hobbs.

Hoffman, David. 1988. *The Holistic Herbal.* 2nd ed. Longmead, Shaftesbury, Dorset: Element Books Ltd.

Holm E, Staedt U, et al. 1991. The action profile of D,L-kavain. Cerebral sites and sleep-wakefulness-rhythm in animals (Article in German) *Arzneimittelforschung.* Jul;41(7):673-83.

Holmes, Peter. 1989. *The Energetics of Western Herbs.* Volumes I & II. Boulder, CO: Artemis Press Inc.

Holmes, Peter. 1996. *Jade Remedies: A Chinese Herbal Reference for the West.* Vol. 1. Boulder, CO: Snow Lotus Press.

Holzer P, Pabst MA, Lippe IT. 1989. Intragastric capsaicin protects against aspirin-induced lesion formation and bleeding in the rat gastric mucosa. *Gastroenterology.* Jun;96(6):1425-33.

Honychurch, Penelope N. 1986. *Caribbean Wild Plants & their Uses.* London: Macmillan Education Limited.

Hope BE, Massey DG, Fournier-Massey G. 1993. Hawaiian materia medica for asthma. *Hawaii Med J.* Jun;52(6):160-6.

Hossain MM, Paul N, et al. 2001 Antibacterial activity of *Vitex trifolia. Fitoterapia.* Aug;72(6):695-7.

Hsieh TC, Wu JM. 2001. Cell growth and gene modulatory activities of Yunzhi (Windsor Wunxi) from mushroom *Trametes versicolor* in androgen-dependent and androgen-insensitive human prostate cancer cells. *Int J Oncol.* Jan;18(1):81-8.

Hsu Hong-Yen et al. 1986. *Oriental Materia Medica A Concise Guide.* Long Beach, CA: Oriental Healing Arts Institute

Hu C, Kitts DD. 2003. Antioxidant, prooxidant, and cytotoxic activities of solvent-fractionated dandelion (*Taraxacum officinale*) flower extracts in vitro. *J Agric Food Chem.* Jan 1;51(1):301-10.

Hu K, Kobayashi H, et al. 1999. Antineoplastic agents. III: Steroidal glycosides from *Solanum nigrum. Planta Med* Feb;65(1):35-38.

Huang, Bing Shan. 1993. *Thousand Formulas and Thousand Herbs of Traditional Chinese Medicine. Volume One: Materia Medica.* Harbin, People's Republic of China: Heilongjiang Education Press.

Hudson, J.B., et al. 1986. Investigation of the antiviral actions of the photoactive compound phenylheptatriyne. *Photochem Photobio* 43(1):27-33

Hung, W.C., et al. 2003. Methanolic extract of adlay seed suppresses COX-2 expression of human lung cancer cells via inhibition of gene transcription. *J Agric Food Chem.* Dec 3;51(25):7333-7

Hunt GR, Gray RD. 2004. Direct observations of pandanus-tool manufacture and use by a New Caledonian crow *Corvus moneduloides. Anim Cogn.* Apr;7(2):114-20. Epub 2003 Nov 28.

Hunt GR. 2000. Human-like, population-level specialization in the manufacture of pandanus tools by New Caledonian crows *Corvus moneduloides. Proc R Soc Lond B Biol Sci.* Feb 22;267(1441):403-13.

Hussain MS, Chandrasekhara N. 1992. Effect on curcumin on cholesterol gall-stone induction in mice. *Indian J Med Res.* Oct;96:288-91.

Hussain MS, Chandrasekhara N. 1994. Biliary proteins from hepatic bile of rats fed curcumin or capsaicin inhibit cholesterol crystal nucleation in supersaturated model bile. *Indian J Biochem Biophys.* Oct;31(5):407-12.

Hussain Z, Waheed A, et al. 2004. The effect of medicinal plants of Islamabad and Murree region of Pakistan on insulin secretion from INS-1 cells. *Phytother Res.* Jan;18(1):73-7.

Hutchens, Alma R. 1983. *Indian Herbology of North America.* 9th ed. Windsor, Ontario, Canada: Merco.

Huxley. A. 1992. The New RHS Dictionary of Gardening. MacMillan Press

Hwang WJ, Park EJ, Jang CH, Han SW, Oh GJ, Kim NS, Kim HM. 2001. Inhibitory effect of immunoglobulin E production by jin-deuk-chal (*Siegesbeckia orientalis*). *Immunopharmacol Immunotoxicol.* Nov;23(4):555-63.

Iino Y, Yokoe T, Maemura M, Horiguchi J, Takei H, Ohwada S, Morishita Y. 1995. Immunochemotherapies versus chemotherapy as adjuvant treatment after curative resection of operable breast cancer. *Anticancer Res.* Nov-Dec;15(6B):2907-11.

Ikawati Z, Wahyuono S, et al. 2001 Screening of several Indonesian medicinal plants for their inhibitory effect on histamine release from RBL-2H3 cells. *J Ethnopharmacol.* May;75(2-3):249-56.

Ikezaki S, Nishikawa A, Furukawa F, Kudo K, Nakamura H, Tamura K, Mori H. 2001. Chemopreventive effects of curcumin on glandular stomach carcinogenesis induced by N-methyl-N'-nitro-N-nitrosoguanidine and sodium chloride in rats. *Anticancer Res.* Sep-Oct;21(5):3407-11.

Incandela L, Belcaro G, De Sanctis MT, et al. 2001(a). Total triterpenic fraction of *Centella asiatica* in the treatment of venous hypertension: a clinical, prospective, randomized trial using a combined microcirculatory model. *Angiology.* Oct;52 Suppl 2:S61-7.

Incandela L, Belcaro G, Nicolaides AN et al. 2001(b). Modification of the echogenicity of femoral plaques after treatment with total triterpenic fraction of *Centella asiatica*: a prospective, randomized, placebo-controlled trial. *Angiology.* Oct;52 Suppl 2:S69-73.

Incandela L, Cesarone MR, et al. 2001(c). Total triterpenic fraction of *Centella asiatica* in chronic venous insufficiency and in high-perfusion microangiopathy. *Angiology.* Oct;52 Suppl 2:S9-13.

Ingolfsdottir K. 2002. Usnic acid. *Phytochemistry.* Dec;61(7):729-36.

Islam ME, Haque ME, Mosaddik MA. 2003. Cytotoxicity and antibacterial activity of *Sida rhombifolia* (Malvaceae) grown in Bangladesh. *Phytother Res.* Sep;17(8):973-5.

Jāger AK, et al., 1996. Screening of Zulu medicinal plants for prostaglandin-synthesis inhibitors. *J Ethnopharmacol* 52(2):95-100

Jagetia GC, Baliga MS, et al. 2003. Influence of ginger rhizome (*Zingiber officinale* Rosc) on survival, glutathione and lipid peroxidation in mice after whole-body exposure to gamma radiation. *Radiat Res.* Nov;160(5):584-92.

Jamieson DD, Duffield PH, et al. 1989. Comparison of the central nervous system activity of the aqueous and lipid extract of kava (*Piper methysticum*). *Arch Int Pharmacodyn* Ther. Sep-Oct;301:66-80.

Jamieson DD, Duffield PH. 1990(a). The antinocioceptive actions of kava components in mice. *Clin Exp Pharmacol Physiol*;17:495-507.

Jamieson DD, Duffield PH. 1990(b). Positive interaction of ethanol and kava resin in mice. *Clin Exp Pharmacol Physiol*;17:509-514.

Jang JJ, Cho KJ, Lee YS, Bae JH. 1991. Different modifying responses of capsaicin in a wide-spectrum initiation model of F344 rat. *J Korean Med Sci.* Mar;6(1):31-6.

Janssen PL, Meyboom S, et al. 1996. Consumption of ginger (*Zingiber officinale* Roscoe) does not affect ex vivo platelet thromboxane production in humans. *Eur J Clin Nutr.* Nov; 50(11):772-4.

Jenkins DJ, Kendall CW, et al. 2002. Soluble fiber intake at a dose approved by the US Food and Drug Administration for a claim of health benefits: serum lipid risk factors for cardiovascular disease assessed in a randomized controlled crossover trial. *Am J Clin Nutr.* May;75(5):834-9.

Jeong JY, Chung YB, et al. 1991. Studies on immunopotentiating activities of antitumor polysaccharide from aerial parts of *Taraxacum platycarpum. Arch Pharm Res.* Mar;14(1):68-72.

Jimenez Misas CA, et al. 1979. Biological evaluation of Cuban plants (Article in Spanish). *Rev Cubana Med Trop.* Jan-Apr; 31(1):5-12.

Johns T, Kitts WD, Newsome F, Towers GH. 1982. Anti-reproductive and other medicinal effects of *Tropaeolum tuberosum. J Ethnopharmacol.* Mar;5(2):149-61.

Johnson, A., S. T. Hemscheidt, et al. 2002. *Cytotoxicity of Water and Ethanol Extracts of Morinda citrifolia (L.) Against Normal Epithelial and Breast Cancer Cell Lines.* Proceedings of the 2002 Hawai'i Noni Conference. Scot C. Nelson, ed. University of Hawai'i at Manoa.

Johnson, P.B., et al. 1999. *Euphorbia hirta* leaf extracts increase urine output and electrolytes in rats. *J Ethnopharmacol* Apr;65(1):63-9

Johnston, Hannah Will. 1997. *Mo'omomi, West Moloka'i: A Coastal Treasure.* Honolulu: University of Hawai'i Sea Grant College Program, Extension Service.

Jones NL, Shabib S, Sherman PM. 1997 Capsaicin as an inhibitor of the growth of the gastric pathogen *Helicobacter pylori. FEMS Microbiol Lett.* Jan 15;146(2):223-7

Jordon, Peter and Steven Wheeler. 2003. *The Practical Mushroom Encyclopedia: Identifying, picking and cooking with mushrooms.* London. Arness Publishing Limited.

Joyamma V, et al. 1990. Biochemical mechanisms and effects of *Mimosa pudica* (Linn) on experimental urolithiasis in rats. *Indian J Exp Biol* Mar 28:3 237-40

Jussofie A, Schmiz A, Hiemke C. 1994. Kavapyrone enriched extract from *Piper methysticum* as modulator of the GABA binding site in different regions of rat brain. *Psychopharmacology* (Berl). Dec;116(4):469-74.

Kaaiakamanu, D. M. 1922. *Hawaiian Herbs of Medicinal Value.* (Trans. by Akaiko Akana) Rutland, VT: Charles E. Tuttle Company

Ka'alakea. Conversations with Kupuna Hulu Kawika Ka'alakea

Kamtchouing P, et al. 2002. Evaluation of androgenic activity of *Zingiber officinale* and *Pentadiplandra brazzeana* in male rats. *Asian J Androl.* Dec;4(4):299-301.

Kandarkar SV, et al. 1998. Subchronic oral hepatotoxicity of turmeric in mice - - histopathological and ultrastructural studies. *Indian J Exp Biol.* Jul;36(7):675-9.

Kaneakua, Kaipo. Conversations with Kaipo Kaneakua.

Kang BK, Lee EH, Kim HM. 1997. Inhibitory effects of Korean folk medicine 'Hi-Chum' on histamine release from mast cells in vivo and in vitro. *J Ethnopharmacol.* Jul;57(2):73-9.

Kang JY, Teng CH, et al. 1995. Effect of capsaicin and chilli on ethanol induced gastric mucosal injury in the rat. *Gut.* May;36(5):664-9.

Karpilovskaia ED, Gorban' GP, et al. 1989. Inhibiting effect of the polyphenolic complex from *Plantago major* (plantastine) on the carcinogenic effect of endogenously synthesized nitrosodimethylamine. (Article in Russian) *Farmakol Toksikol.* Jul-Aug;52(4):64-7.

Katiyar SK. Agarwal R. Mukhtar H. 1996. Inhibition of tumor promotion in SENCAR mouse skin by ethanol extract of *Zingiber officinale* rhizome. *Cancer Research.* Mar 56(5):1023-30,.

Kato S, et al. 2003. Expression of vanilloid receptors in rat gastric epithelial cells: role in cellular protection. *Biochem Pharmacol.* 66(6):1115-21.

Kawada T, Sakabe S, Watanabe T, Yamamoto M, Iwai K. 1988. Some pungent principles of spices cause the adrenal medulla to secrete catecholamine in anesthetized rats. *Proc Soc Exp Biol Med.* Jun;188(2):229-33.

Kawada, T., Hagihara, K.I. and Iwai, K. 1986. Effects of capsaicin on lipid metabolism in rats fed a high fat diet. *Journal of Nutrition* 116: 1272-1278.

Kawai'ae, Keiki K. C. 1980. Hawaiian Pathological Terms. Author's collection.

Kawamori T, Lubet R, et al. 1999. Chemopreventive effect of curcumin, a naturally occurring anti-inflammatory agent, during the promotion / progression stages of colon cancer. *Cancer Res* Feb 1;59(3):597-601

Kawazoe K, Yutani A, et al. 2001 Phenylnaphthalene compounds from the subterranean part of *Vitex rotundifolia* and their antibacterial activity against methicillin-resistant Staphylococcus aureus. *J Nat Prod.* May;64(5):588-91.

Keating A, Chez RA. 2002. Ginger syrup as an antiemetic in early pregnancy. *Altern Ther Health Med.* Sep-Oct;8(5):89-91.

Kepler, Angela Kay. 1990. *Trees of Hawai'i.* Hononlulu: University of Hawai'i Press.

Kermanshai R, McCarry BE, Rosenfeld J, Summers PS, Weretilnyk EA, Sorger GJ. 2001. Benzyl isothiocyanate is the chief or sole anthelmintic in papaya seed extracts. *Phytochemistry.* Jun;57(3):427-35.

Keys, John D., 1976. *Chinese Herbs. Their Botany, Chemistry, and Pharmacodynamics.* Rutland, VT.: Charles E. Tuttle Company, Inc.

Kholkute SD, et al. 1977. Studies on the antifertility potentiality of *Hibiscus rosa sinensis.* Parts of medicinal value; selection of species and seasonal variations. *Planta Med.* Feb;31(1):35-9.

Kidd PM. 2000. The use of mushroom glucans and proteoglycans in cancer treatment. *Altern Med Rev.* Feb;5(1):4-27.

Kim CS, Kawada T, Kim BS, Han IS, Choe SY, Kurata T, Yu R. 2003. Capsaicin exhibits anti-inflammatory property by inhibiting IkB-a degradation in LPS-stimulated peritoneal macrophages. *Cell Signal.* Mar;15(3):299-306.

Kim CS, Park WH, Park JY, Kang JH, Kim MO, Kawada T, Yoo H, Han IS, Yu R. 2004. Capsaicin, a spicy component of hot pepper, induces apoptosis by activation of the peroxisome proliferator-activated receptor gamma in HT-29 human colon cancer cells. *J Med Food.* Fall;7(3):267-73.

Kim HM, Lee JH, Won JH, Park EJ, Chae HJ, Kim HR, Kim CH, Baek SH. 2001. Inhibitory effect on immunoglobulin E production in vivo and in vitro by *Siegesbeckia glabrescens. Phytother Res.* Nov;15(7):572-6.

Kim HM, Shin HY, et al. 2000. *Taraxacum officinale* inhibits tumor necrosis factor-alpha production from rat astrocytes. *Immunopharmacol Immunotoxicol.* Aug;22(3):519-30.

Kim JP, Park JG, Lee MD, Han MD, Park ST, Lee BH, Jung SE. 1985. Co-carcinogenic effects of several Korean foods on gastric cancer induced by N-methyl-N'-nitro-N-nitrosoguanidine in rats. *Jpn J Surg.* Nov;15(6):427-37.

Kim KM, Kawada T, Ishihara K, Inoue K, Fushiki T. 1997. Increase in swimming endurance capacity of mice by capsaicin-induced adrenal catecholamine secretion. *Biosci Biotechnol Biochem.* Oct;61(10):1718-23.

Kim KM, Kawada T, Ishihara K, Inoue K, Fushiki T. 1998. Swimming capacity of mice is increased by oral administration of a nonpungent capsaicin analog, stearoyl vanillylamide. *J Nutr.* Nov;128(11):1978-83.

Kim SC, Crawford DJ, Francisco-Ortega J, Santos-Guerra A. 1996. A common origin for woody *Sonchus* and five related genera in the Macaronesian islands: molecular evidence for extensive radiation. *Proc Natl Acad Sci* U S A. Jul 23;93(15):7743-8.

Kinzler E, Kromer J, Lehmann. 1991. Effect of a special kava extract in patients with anxiety-, tension-, and excitation states of non-psychotic genesis. Double blind study with placebos over 4 weeks. (Article in German) *Arzneimittelforschung*; 41:584-588.

Kirkbride, Joseph H. The author's correspondence with Joseph H. Kirkbride, Jr.

Kishore N, et al. 1993. Fungitoxicity of essential oils against dermatophytes. *Mycoses.* May-Jun;36(5-6):211-5.

Kiuchi F et al, 1992. Inhibition of prostaglandin and leukotriene biosynthesis by gingerols and diarylheptanoids, *Chem Pharm Bull* (Tokyo);40(2):387-91

Klimczak I, Malecka M, et al. 2002. Antioxidant activity of ethanolic extracts of amaranth seeds. *Nahrung.* Jun;46(3):184-6.

Ko WG, Kang TH, et al. 2000 Polymethoxyflavonoids from *Vitex rotundifolia* inhibit proliferation by inducing apoptosis in human myeloid leukemia cells. *Food Chem Toxicol.* Oct;38(10):861-5.

Ko WG, Kang TH, et al. 2001 Rotundifuran, a labdane type diterpene from *Vitex rotundifolia*, induces apoptosis in human myeloid leukaemia cells. *Phytother Res.* Sep;15(6):535-7.

Ko WG, Kang TH, et al. 2002 Effects of luteolin on the inhibition of proliferation and induction of apoptosis in human myeloid leukaemia cells. *Phytother Res.* May;16(3):295-8.

Kobayashi H, et al. 1993 PSK as a chemopreventive agent. *Cancer Epidemiol Biomarkers Prev* May-Jun;2(3):271-6

Kobayashi M, Ishida Y, Shoji N, Ohizumi Y. 1988. Cardiotonic action of [8]-gingerol, an activator of the Ca++-pumping adenosine triphosphatase of sarcoplasmic reticulum, in guinea pig atrial muscle. *J Pharmacol Exp Ther.* Aug;246(2):667-73.

Kobayashi Y, Kariya K, et al. 1994. Oxidative stress relief for cancer-bearing hosts by the protein-bound polysaccharide of *Coriolus versicolor* QUEL with SOD mimicking activity. *Cancer Biother.* Spring;9(1):55-62.

Kogure K, et al. 2002. Mechanism of potent antiperoxidative effect of capsaicin. *Biochim Biophys Acta.* 1573(1):84-92.

Koo HN, Hong SH, et al. 2004. *Taraxacum officinale* induces cytotoxicity through TNF-alpha and IL-1alpha secretion in Hep G2 cells. *Life Sci.* Jan 16;74(9):1149-57.

Koo KL, Ammit AJ, et al. Gingerols and related analogues inhibit arachidonic acid-induced human platelet serotonin release and aggregation. *Thromb Res.* 2001 Sep 1;103(5):387-97.

Koshihara Y, Fujimoto Y, Inoue H. 1988. A new 5-lipoxygenase selective inhibitor derived from *Artocarpus communis* strongly inhibits arachidonic acid-induced ear edema. *Biochem Pharmacol.* Jun 1; 37(11): 2161-5.

Kowalchik, Claire & William H. Hylton, ed. 1987. *Rodale's Illustrated Encyclopedia of Herbs.* Emmaus, Pennsylvania: Rodale Press

Krauss, Beatrice H., 2001. *Plants in Hawaiian Medicine.* Honolulu: The Bess Press.

Krauss, Beatrice. Notes from Beatrice Krauss' Ethnobotany class at the University of Hawai'i. Author's collection.

Krauss, Beatrice. *Plants in Hawaiian Culture*

Krochmal, Arnold, and Connie Krochmal. 1984. *A Field Guide to Medicinal Plants.* New York: Times Books.

Krompegel, K., *Ethnobotany of Two Contrasting American Ecosystems: Amazonia and the Sonoran Desert.*

Krueth, P; Brosi, E; et al. 2004. Ginger-associated over-anticoagulation by phenprocoumon. *Annals of Pharmacotherapy* 38 (2): 257-260.

Kuchel O, Hausser C, Buu NT, Tenneson S. 1985. CSF sulfoconjugated catecholamines in man: their relationship with plasma catecholamines. *J Neural Transm.*;62(1-2):91-7.

Kuroda K, et al., 1976. Inhibitory effect of *Capsella bursa-pastoris* extract on growth of Ehrlich solid tumor in mice. *Cancer Res* Jun;36(6):1900-3

Kuroda K, et al.1975. Effect of *Capsella bursa-pastoris* on liver catalase activity in rats fed 3'-methyl-4-(dimethylamino) azobenzene. *Gann* 66(4):461-462

Kuttan R, Bhanumathy P, et al. 1985. Potential anticancer activity of turmeric (*Curcuma longa*). *Cancer Lett* Nov;29(2):197-202

Lamb, Samuel H. 1981. *Native Trees & Shrubs of the Hawaiian Islands.* Santa Fe: Sunstone Press

Lamoureaux, Charles H. 1976. *Trailside Plants of Hawai'i's National Parks.* Volcano HI: Hawai'i Natural History Association.

Lanhers, M.C., et al. 1990. Behavioral effects of *Euphorbia hirta* L.: sedative and anxiolytic properties. *Journal of Ethnopharmacology* May;29(2):189-98

Lanhers, M.C., et al. 1991. Analgesic, antipyretic and anti-inflammatory properties of *Euphorbia hirta. Planta Med* 1991 Jun;57(3):225-31

Lans C, Brown G. 1998. Ethnoveterinary medicines used for ruminants in Trinidad and Tobago. *Prev Vet Med* Jun 1;35(3):149-63

Lapulapu, Darrell and Barbara Ota. Student notes from the Traditional Chinese Medical College of Hawai'i - Darrell Lapulapu, L.Ac. and Barbara Ota, L.Ac.

Lapulapu, Darrell. The author's conversations with practitioner of traditional Chinese and Hawaiian medicine, Darrell Lapulapu.

Larsen T, Thilsted SH, et al. 2003. The leafy vegetable amaranth (*Amaranthus gangeticus*) is a potent inhibitor of calcium availability and retention in rice-based diets. Br *J Nutr.* Sep;90(3):521-7.

Lauterwein M, Oethinger M, Belsner K, Peters T, Marre R. 1995. In vitro activities of the lichen secondary metabolites vulpinic acid, (+)-usnic acid, and (-)-usnic acid against aerobic and anaerobic microorganisms. *Antimicrob Agents Chemother.* Nov;39(11):2541-3.

Lee CK, Han SS, et al. 1997. *Immunopharmacology.* Oct;37(2-3):153-62. Prevention of ultraviolet radiation-induced suppression of accessory cell function of Langerhans cells by *Aloe vera* gel components. *Immunopharmacology.* 1997 Oct;37(2-3):153-62.

Lee E, Surh Y. 1998. Induction of apoptosis in HL-60 cells by pungent vanilloids, 6-gingerol and 6-paradol. *Cancer Lett.* 1998 Dec 25;134(2):163-8.

Lee JC, Kim HR, et al. 2002. Antioxidant property of an ethanol extract of the stem of *Opuntia ficus-indica var. saboten. J Agric Food Chem.* Oct 23;50(22):6490-6.

Lee KH, Hong HS, et al. 2000(a). Induction of apoptosis in human leukaemic cell lines K562, HL60 and U937 by diethylhexylphthalate isolated from *Aloe vera* Linne. *J Pharm Pharmacol.* Aug;52(8):1037-41.

Lee KH, Kim JH, et al. 2000(b). Anti-leukaemic and anti-mutagenic effects of di(2-ethylhexyl)phthalate isolated from *Aloe vera* Linne. *J Pharm Pharmacol.* May;52(5):593-8.

Lee MK, Kim SR, et al. 2000(c). Asiatic acid derivatives protect cultured cortical neurons from glutamate-induced excitotoxicity. *Res Commun Mol Pathol Pharmacol.* Jul-Aug;108(1-2):75-86.

Lejeune MP, et al. 2003. Effect of capsaicin on substrate oxidation and weight maintenance after modest body-weight loss in human subjects. Br *J Nutr.*90(3):651-59.

Leonard, David Bruce. 2003. Author's conversations with cancer survivors.

Leonard, David Bruce. 1992-2005. Conversations with Na Kupuna, my teachers.

Leonard, David Bruce. Anecdotal clinical perceptions of the author.

Lewis, Walter Hepworth. 1977. *Medical Botany: Plants Affecting Man's Health.* New York: John Wily & Sons.

Li Ninghan, et al. 1976. *Chinese Medicinal Herbs of Hong Kong. Volumes 1-5.* Hong Kong: Hong Kong Commercial Press, Ltd. (Shang Wu Yin Shu Guan, Xiang Gang You Xian Gong Si)

Li Ninghan, et al. 1994. *Chinese Medicinal Herbs of Hong Kong. Volume 6.* Hong Kong: Hong Kong Commercial Press, Ltd. (Shang Wu Yin Shu Guan, Xiang Gang You Xian Gong Si)

Li Qingdong, 1989. Effects of *Bidens* species on experimental hyperlipemia and thrombosis. *Chinese Journal of Integrated Traditional and Western Medicine*; 9(1): 33.

Li RW, Myers SP, et al. 2003. A cross-cultural study: anti-inflammatory activity of Australian and Chinese plants. *J Ethnopharmacol.* Mar;85(1):25-32.

Li XY, Wang JF, et al. 1990 Immune enhancement of a polysaccharides peptides isolated from *Coriolus versicolor. Zhongguo Yao Li Xue Bao* Nov;11(6):542-5

Lien HC, Sun WM, et al. 2003. Effects of ginger on motion sickness and gastric slow-wave dysrhythmias induced by circular vection. *Am J Physiol Gastrointest Liver Physiol.* Mar;284(3):G481-9.

Life Extension Magazine December 2004 pp 36-42

Lim BO, Seong NS, et al. 2003. Efficacy of dietary *Aloe vera* supplementation on hepatic cholesterol and oxidative status in aged rats. *J Nutr* Sci Vitaminol (Tokyo). Aug;49(4):292-6.

Lim GP, Chu T, Yang F, Beech W, Frautschy SA, Cole GM. 2001. The curry spice curcumin reduces oxidative damage and amyloid pathology in an Alzheimer transgenic mouse. *J Neurosci.* Nov 1;21(21):8370-7.

Liontas A, Yeger H. 2004. Curcumin and resveratrol induce apoptosis and nuclear translocation and activation of p53 in human neuroblastoma. *Anticancer Res.* Mar-Apr;24(2B):987-98.

Lithander A. 1992. Intracellular fluid of waybread (*Plantago major*) as a prophylactic for mammary cancer in mice. *Tumour Biol.*;13(3):138-41.

Liu H, Zhu Y. 2002. Effect of alcohol extract of *Zingiber officinale* rosc on immunologic function of mice with tumor. (Article in Chinese) *Wei Sheng Yan Jiu.* Jun;31(3):208-9.

Liu N, Huo G, et al. 2003. Effect of *Zingiber officinale* Rosc on lipid peroxidation in hyperlipidemia rats. (Article in Chinese) *Wei Sheng Yan Jiu.* Jan;32(1):22-3.

Locher CP, Burch MT, Mower HF, Berestecky J, Davis H, Van Poel B, Lasure A, Vanden Berghe DA, Vlietinck AJ. 1995. Anti-microbial activity and anti-complement activity of extracts obtained from selected Hawaiian medicinal plants. *J Ethnopharmacol.* Nov 17;49(1):23-32.

Lohiya NK, et al. 1994. Antifertility effects of aqueous extract of *Carica papaya* seeds in male rats. *Planta Med* 60(5):400-4

Lohiya NK, et al. 1999. Reversible contraception with chloroform extract of *Carica papaya* Linn. seeds in male rabbits. *Reprod Toxicol* 13(1):59-66.

Lohiya NK, et al. 2000. Human sperm immobilization effect of *Carica papaya* seed extracts: an in vitro study. *Asian J Androl* 2(2):103-9

Lopez-Carrillo L, Hernandez Avila M, Dubrow R. 1994. Chili pepper consumption and gastric cancer in Mexico: a case-control study. *Am J Epidemiol.* Feb 1;139(3):263-71.

Loro JF, del Rio I, Perez-Santana L. 1999. Preliminary studies of analgesic and anti-inflammatory properties of *Opuntia* dillenii aqueous extract. *J Ethnopharmacol.* Nov 1;67(2):213-8.

Lu P, Lai BS, et al. 2003. Antioxidation activity and protective effection of ginger oil on DNA damage in vitro. (Article in Chinese) *Zhongguo Zhong Yao Za Zhi.* Sep;28(9):873-5.

Lu, Henry C. 1990. *Chinese Foods for Longevity.* New York: Sterling Publishing Company, Inc.

Lu, Henry C. 1994. *Chinese Natural Cures.* New York: Sterling Publishing Company, Inc.

Lundberg JM, Martling CR, Saria A, Folkers K, Rosell S. 1983(a). Cigarette smoke-induced airway oedema due to activation of capsaicin-sensitive vagal afferents and substance P release. *Neuroscience.* Dec;10(4):1361-8.

Luo ZH. 1993. The use of Chinese traditional medicines to improve impaired immune functions in scald mice. (Article in Chinese) *Zhonghua Zheng Xing Shao Shang Wai Ke Za Zhi.* Jan;9(1):56-8, 80.

Lust, John B. 2001. *The Herb Book.* Benedict Lust Publications Inc

Mabey, Richard. 1988. *The New Age Herbalist.* London: Gaia Books Ltd.

Macias CA, Kameneva MV, et al. 2004. Survival in a rat model of lethal hemorrhagic shock is prolonged following resuscitation with a small volume of a solution containing a drag-reducing polymer derived from *Aloe vera. Shock.* Aug;22(2):151-156.

Mahady GB, Pendland SL, Yun G, Lu ZZ. 2002. Turmeric (*Curcuma longa*) and curcumin inhibit the growth of Helicobacter pylori, a group 1 carcinogen. *Anticancer Res.* Nov-Dec;22(6C):4179-81.

Mahady GB, Pendland SL, Yun GS, Lu ZZ, Stoia A. 2003. Ginger (*Zingiber officinale* Roscoe) and the gingerols inhibit the growth of Cag A+ strains of Helicobacter pylori. *Anticancer Res.* Sep-Oct;23(5A):3699-702.

Mahanta M, et al. 2001 Neutralisation of lethality, myotoxicity and toxic enzymes of *Naja kaouthia* venom by *Mimosa pudica* root extracts. *J Ethnopharmacol* Apr;75(1):55-60

Malini T, Vanithakumari G, et al. 1985. Effect of *Foeniculum vulgare* Mill. seed extract on the genital organs of male and female rats. *Indian J Physiol Pharmacol* Jan;29(1):21-26

Malterud KE, Farbrot TL, et al. 1993. Antioxidant and radical scavenging effects of anthraquinones and anthrones. *Pharmacology.* Oct;47 Suppl 1:77-85.

Maquart FX, Bellon G, et al. 1990. Stimulation of collagen synthesis in fibroblast cultures by a triterpene extracted from *Centella asiatica. Connect Tissue Res.*;24(2):107-20.

Martins AP, Salgueiro L, et al. 2001. Essential oil composition and antimicrobial activity of three Zingiberaceae from S.Tome e Principe. *Planta Med.* Aug;67(6):580-4.

Martz W. 1992. Plants with a reputation against snakebite. *Toxicon.* Oct;30(10):1131-42.

Mascolo N, Jain R, et al. 1989. Ethnopharmacologic investigation of ginger (*Zingiber officinale*). *J Ethnopharmacol.* Nov;27(1-2):129-40.

Mathews JD, Riley MD, et al. 1988. Effects of the heavy usage of kava on physical health: summary of a pilot survey in an aboriginal community. *Med J Aust.* Jun 6;148(11):548-55.

Matsunaga H, Katano M, Yamamoto H, Fujito H, Mori M, Takata K. 1990. Cytotoxic activity of polyacetylene compounds in *Panax ginseng* C. A. Meyer. *Chem Pharm Bull* (Tokyo). Dec;38(12):3480-2.

Matsunaga K, Morita I, et al. 1986. Restoration of immunologic responsiveness by PSK in tumor-bearing animals. (Article in Japanese) *Gan To Kagaku Ryoho.* Dec;13(12):3468-75.

Matthews. V. 1994. *The New Plantsman. Volume 1,* 1994. Royal Horticultural Society

Maui Community College database

McBride, L. R. 1975. *Practical Folk Medicine of Hawai'i.* Petroglyph Press.

McClatchey, Will C. *Diversity of Growth Forms and Uses in the Morinda citrifolia L. Complex.* Proceedings of the 2002 Hawai'i Noni Conference. Scot C. Nelson, ed. University of Hawai'i at Manoa. 2002.

McIntyre, Ann. 1996. *Flower Power.* New York: Henry Holt and Company, Inc.

McKenna Dennis J., Kerry Hughes, Kenneth Jones (coauthors & editors) 2002. *Botanical Medicines: The Desk Reference for Major Herbal Supplements.* Haworth Herbal Press.

McManus OB, et al. 1993. An activator of calcium-dependent potassium channels isolated from a medicinal herb. *Biochemistry.* Jun 22;32(24):6128-33.

Meckes-Lozoya M, Ibanez-Camacho R. 1989. Hypoglucaemic activity of *Opuntia streptacantha* throughout its annual cycle. *Am J Chin Med.*;17(3-4):221-4.

Medda S, Das N, Mahato SB, et al. 1995. Glycoside-bearing liposomal delivery systems against macrophage-associated disorders involving *Mycobacterium leprae* and *Mycobacterium tuberculosis. Indian J Biochem Biophys.* Jun;32(3):147-51.

Medicinal Plants and Old Time Remedies of Bermuda

Mehrotra S, Mishra KP, et al. 2002. Immunomodulation by ethanolic extract of *Boerhaavia diffusa* roots. *Int Immunopharmacol.* Jun;2(7):987-96

Melo PA, et al. 1994. Inhibition of the myotoxic and hemorrhagic activities of crotalid venoms by *Eclipta prostrata* (Asteraceae) extracts and constituents. *Toxicon* May;32(5):595-603.

Merlin, Mark. 1999. *Hawaiian Coastal Plants. An Illustrated Field Guide.* 4th rev. ed. Honolulu: Pacific Guide Books.

Meyer K, Schwartz J, et al. 1995. *Zingiber officinale* (ginger) used to prevent 8-Mop associated nausea. *Dermatol Nurs.* Aug;7(4):242-4.

Miller MS, Brendel K, Burks TF, Sipes IG. 1983. Interaction of capsaicinoids with drug-metabolizing systems. Relationship to toxicity. *Biochem Pharmacol.* Feb 1;32(3):547-51.

Miller, Amy Bess. 1988. *Shaker Medicinal Herbs.* Pownal, VT.: Storey Books.

Mindell, Earl. 1992, 2000. *Earl Mindell's New Herb Bible.* Rev ed. New York: Fireside.

Miquel J, Bernd A, Sempere JM, Diaz-Alperi J, Ramirez A. 2002. The curcuma antioxidants: pharmacological effects and prospects for future clinical use. A review. *Arch Gerontol Geriatr.* Feb;34(1):37-46.

Mirvish SS, Rose EF, Sutherland DM. 1979. Studies on the esophagus. ii. enhancement of [3h]thymidine incorporation in rat esophagus by *Bidens pilosa* (a plant eaten in South Africa) and by Croton oil. *Cancer Lett* 6(3):159-165

Misaki A, Kakuta M, Sasaki T, Tanaka M, Miyaji H. 1981. Studies on interrelation of structure and antitumor effects of polysaccharides: antitumor action of periodate-modified, branched (1 goes to 3)-beta-D-glucan of *Auricularia auricula-judae,* and other polysaccharides containing (1 goes to 3)-glycosidic linkages. *Carbohydr Res.* May 18;92(1):115-29.

Mitchell JC. 1965. Allergy to lichens. Allergic contact dermatitis from usnic acid produced by lichenized fungi. *Arch Dermatol.* Aug;92(2):142-6.

Mitchell, Donald D. Kiolani. 1992. *Resource units in Hawaiian Culture.* Revised edition. Honolulu: Kamehameha Schools.

Mitomi T, Tsuchiya S, Iijima N, Aso K, Suzuki K, Nishiyama K, Amano T, Takahashi T, Murayama N, Oka H, et al. 1992. Randomized, controlled study on adjuvant immunochemotherapy with PSK in curatively resected colorectal cancer. The Cooperative Study Group of

Surgical Adjuvant Immunochemotherapy for Cancer of Colon and Rectum (Kanagawa). *Dis Colon Rectum.* Feb;35(2):123-30.
Miyashiro H, Lim JA, et al. 1994 Inhibitory effects of tropical plants on HIV-protease. *Int Conf AIDS* (Aug 7-12) 10(2):112
Modly CE, Das M, Don PS, Marcelo CL, Mukhtar H, Bickers DR. 1986. Capsaicin as an in vitro inhibitor of benzo(a)pyrene metabolism and its DNA binding in human and murine keratinocytes. Drug Metab Dispos. Jul-Aug;14(4):413-6.
Moerman, Daniel E. 1986. *Medicinal Plants of Native America.* Volumes 1 & 2. Ann Arbor, MI.: University of Michigan Museum of Anthropology.
Monsereenusorn Y, Cassidy SS, Coast JR. 1985 Sensitivity of pulmonary chemo reflexes and lung inflation reflexes to repetitive stimulation and to inhibition with lidocaine and morphine. *Naunyn Schmiedebergs Arch Pharmacol.* Nov;331(2-3):166-74
Monsereenusorn Y. 1983. Subchronic toxicity studies of capsaicin and capsicum in rats. *Res Commun Chem Pathol Pharmacol.* Jul;41(1):95-110.
Montagna, F. Joseph. *P. D. R. People's Desk Reference.* Volumes 1 & 2. Library of Congress #80-52954.
Moore, Michael. Plant tincture brochure.
Moore, Michael. 1989. *Medicinal Plants of the Desert and Canyon West.* Santa Fe: Museum of New Mexico Press.
Moore, Michael. 1993. *Medicinal Plants of the Pacific West.* Santa Fe: Red Crane Books.
Moore, Michael. Herbal Materia Medica
Moore, Michael. Herbal-Medical Contraindications.
Moriarty, Michael. 2003, 2004. Author's conversations with Michael Moriarty
Mors WB, et al. 1989. Neutralization of lethal and myotoxic activities of South American rattlesnake venom by extracts and constituents of the plant *Eclipta prostrata* (Asteraceae). *Toxicon.*;27(9):1003-9.
Mors WB. 1991. Plants against snake-bites. *Mem Inst Oswaldo Cruz.*;86 Suppl 2:193.
Mowrey, Daniel B. 1986. *The Scientific Validation of Herbal Medicine.* Daniel B. Mowrey.
Mueller BA, Scott MK, et al. 2000. Noni juice (*Morinda citrifolia*): hidden potential for hyperkalemia? *Am J Kidney Dis.* Feb;35(2):330-2.
Muko KN, et al. 2000. A preliminary study on the anti-inflammatory properties of *Emilia sonchifolia* leaf extracts. *Fitoterapia* Feb;71(1):65-68.
Muller-Limmroth W, Frohlich HH. 1980. Effect of various phytotherapeutic expectorants on mucociliary transport. (Article in German) *Fortschr Med.* Jan 24;98(3):95-101.
Munte TF, Heinze HJ, et al. 1993. Effects of oxazepam and an extract of kava roots (*Piper methysticum*) on event-related potentials in a word recognition task. *Neuropsychobiology*; 27:46-53.
Murai M, Tamayama Y, Nishibe S. 1995. Phenylethanoids in the herb of *Plantago lanceolata* and inhibitory effect on arachidonic acid-induced mouse ear edema. *Planta Med.* Oct;61(5):479-80.
Murakami A, Hayashi R, et al. 2003. Suppression of dextran sodium sulfate-induced colitis in mice by zerumbone, a subtropical ginger sesquiterpene, and nimesulide: separately and in combination. *Biochem Pharmacol.* Oct 1;66(7):1253-61.
Murakami A, Takahashi D, et al. 2002. Zerumbone, a Southeast Asian ginger sesquiterpene, markedly suppresses free radical generation, proinflammatory protein production, and cancer cell proliferation accompanied by apoptosis: the alpha,beta-unsaturated carbonyl group is a prerequisite. *Carcinogenesis.* May;23(5):795-802.
Murakami A, Tanaka T, et al. 2004. Zerumbone, a sesquiterpene in subtropical ginger, suppresses skin tumor initiation and promotion stages in ICR mice. *Int J Cancer.* Jul 1;110(4):481-90.
Nagao T, Komatsuda M, Yamauchi K, Nozaki H, Watanabe K, Arimori S. 1981. Chemoimmunotherapy with Krestin in acute leukemia. *Tokai J Exp Clin Med.* Apr;6(2):141-6.
Nagasawa H, et al. 2002. Effects of bitter melon (*Momordica charantia* l.) or ginger rhizome (*Zingiber offifinale* rosc) on spontaneous mammary tumorigenesis in SHN mice. *Am J Chin Med.*;30(2-3):195-205.
Nakazato H, Koike A, Saji S, Ogawa N, Sakamoto J. 1994. Efficacy of immunochemotherapy as adjuvant treatment after curative resection of gastric cancer. *Lancet.* May 7;343(8906):1122-6.
Naone, Lyons Kapi'ioho. Conversations with Lyons Kapi'ioho Naone.
Nath D, Sethi N, et al. 1992. Commonly used Indian abortifacient plants with special reference to their teratologic effects in rats. *J Ethnopharmacol.* Apr;36(2):147-54.
Neal, Marie C. 1965. *In Gardens of Hawai'i.* Honolulu: Bishop Museum Press.
Nelson, Scott C. *Noni Cultivation and Production in Hawai'i. Proceedings of the 2002 Hawai'i Noni Conference.* Scot C. Nelson, ed. University of Hawai'i at Manoa. 2002.
Nerurkar PV, Dragull K, Tang CS. 2004. In vitro toxicity of kava alkaloid, pipermethystine, in HepG2 cells compared to kavalactones. *Toxicol Sci.* May;79(1):106-11. Epub 2004 Jan 21.
Newman, Robert. Author's conversations and correspondence with Robert Newman.
Ng TB, Chan WY. 1997 Polysaccharopeptide from the mushroom *Coriolus versicolor* possesses analgesic activity but does not produce adverse effects on female reproductive or embryonic development in mice. *Gen Pharmacol* Aug;29(2):269-73
Ngo Bum E, Dawack DL, Schmutz M, Rakotonirina A, Rakotonirina SV, Portet C, Jeker A, Olpe HR, Herrling P. 2004. Anticonvulsant activity of *Mimosa pudica* decoction. *Fitoterapia* Jun;75(3-4):309-14.
N'gouemo P, et al. 1996. Effects of an ethanolic extract of *Desmodium adscendens* on central nervous system in rodents. *J Ethnopharmacol.* Jun;52(2):77-83.
Niebyl JR. 1992. Drug therapy during pregnancy. *Curr Opin Obstet Gynecol.* Feb;4(1):43-7.
Nielsen BE, Larsen PK, Lemmich J. 1971. Constituents of umbelliferous plants. XVII. Coumarins from Seseli gummiferum Pall. The structure of two new coumarins. *Acta Chem Scand.*;25(2):529-33.
Norikura T, Kennedy DO, et al. 2002. Protective effect of aloe extract against the cytotoxicity of 1,4-naphthoquinone in isolated rat hepatocytes involves modulations in cellular thiol levels. *Pharmacol Toxicol.* May;90(5):278-84.
Notani PN, Jayant K. 1987. Role of diet in upper aerodigestive tract cancers. *Nutr Cancer.*;10(1-2):103-13.
Odabasoglu F, Aslan A, Cakir A, Suleyman H, Karagoz Y, Halici M, Bayir Y. 2004. Comparison of antioxidant activity and phenolic content of three lichen species. *Phytother Res.* Nov;18(11):938-41.
Ody, Penelope. 1993. *The Complete Medicinal Herbal.* New York: Dorling Kinnersley, Inc.

Oguchi Y, Morita I, et al. 1986. Involution of the thymus in tumor-bearing mice and its restoration by PSK (2). (Article in Japanese) *Gan To Kagaku Ryoho.* Aug;13(8):2645-52.

Oh TW, et al. 2003. Capsaicin increases endurance capacity and spares tissue glycogen through lipolytic function in swimming rats. *J Nutr Sci Vitaminol* 49(2):107-11.

Ohmura Y, Matsunaga K, et al. 2003. Protective effects of a protein-bound polysaccharide, PSK, against *Candida albicans* infection in syngeneic tumor-bearing mice via Th1 cell functions. *Cancer Biother Radiopharm.* Oct;18(5):769-80.

Okuyama E, Fujimori S, et al. 1998. Pharmacologically active components of viticis fructus (*Vitex rotundifolia*). II. The components having analgesic effects. *Chem Pharm Bull* (Tokyo). Apr;46(4):655-62.

Okuyama E, Umeyama K, Yamazaki M, Kinoshita Y, Yamamoto Y. 1995. Usnic acid and diffractaic acid as analgesic and antipyretic components of *Usnea* diffracta. *Planta Med.* Apr;61(2):113-5.

Okyar A, et al. 2001. Effect of *Aloe vera* leaves on blood glucose level in type I and type II diabetic rat models. *Phytother Res.* 15(2): 157-61

Oladosu LA, Case AA. 1979. Large animal hepatotoxic and nephrotoxic plants. *Vet Hum Toxicol.* Oct;21(5):363-5.

Ono K, Hasegawa K, Naiki H, Yamada M. 2004(a). Anti-amyloidogenic activity of tannic acid and its activity to destabilize Alzheimer's beta-amyloid fibrils in vitro. *Biochim Biophys Acta.* Nov 5;1690(3):193-202.

Ono K, Hasegawa K, Naiki H, Yamada M. 2004(b). Curcumin has potent anti-amyloidogenic effects for Alzheimer's beta-amyloid fibrils in vitro. *J Neurosci Res.* Mar 15;75(6):742-50.

Ono K, Yoshiike Y, Takashima A, Hasegawa K, Naiki H, Yamada M. 2003. Potent anti-amyloidogenic and fibril-destabilizing effects of polyphenols in vitro: implications for the prevention and therapeutics of Alzheimer's disease. *J Neurochem.* Oct;87(1):172-81.

Ooi LS, Sun SS, Ooi VE. 2004. Purification and characterization of a new antiviral protein from the leaves of *Pandanus amaryllifolius* (Pandanaceae). *Int J Biochem Cell Biol.* Aug;36(8):1440-6.

Ooi SO, Sim KY, et al. 1993. Selective antiproliferative effects of thymidine. *Experientia.* Jul 5;49(6-7):576-81.

Osato JA et al. 1993. Antimicrobial and antioxidant activities of unripe papaya. *Life Sci*;53(17):1383-9.

Otsuka H, et al. 1988. Anti-inflammatory activity of benzoxazinoids from roots of *Coix lachryma-jobi var. ma-yuen. J Nat Prod.* Jan-Feb;51(1):74-9.

Ozbek H, Ugras S, et al. 2003. Hepatoprotective effect of *Foeniculum vulgare* essential oil. *Fitoterapia.* Apr;74(3):317-9.

Page Linda R. 1998. *How to Be Your Own Herbal Pharmacist.* 2nd ed. Healthy Healing Publications

Pakrashi A, et al. 1986. Flowers of Hibiscus rosa-sinensis, a potential source of contragestative agent. III: Interceptive effect of benzene extract in mouse. *Contraception.* Nov;34(5):523-36.

Pal AK, Bhattacharya K, et al. 1985. Flowers of Hibiscus rosa-sinensis, a potential source of contragestative agent: II. Possible mode of action with reference to anti-implantation effect of the benzene extract. *Contraception.* Nov;32(5):517-29.

Palmer, Daniel D. 2003. *Hawai'i's Ferns and Fern Allies.* Honolulu: University of Hawai'i Press.

Palumbo B, Efthimiou Y, et al. 2003. Prickly pear induces upregulation of liver LDL binding in familial heterozygous hypercholesterolemia. *Nucl Med Rev Cent East Eur.*;6(1):35-9.

Pari L, Maheswari JU. 1999. Hypoglycaemic effect of *Musa sapientum* L. in alloxan-induced diabetic rats. *J Ethnopharmacol.* Dec 15;68(1-3):321-5.

Pari L, Umamaheswari J. 2000. Antihyperglycaemic activity of *Musa sapientum* flowers: effect on lipid peroxidation in alloxan diabetic rats. *Phytother Res.* Mar;14(2):136-8.

Park EH, Chun MJ. 2001(a). Wound healing activity of *Opuntia ficus-indica. Fitoterapia.* Feb;72(2):165-7.

Park EH, Kahng JH, et al. 2001(b). An anti-inflammatory principle from cactus. *Fitoterapia.* Mar;72(3):288-90.

Park EH, Kahng JH, Paek EA. 1998. Studies on the pharmacological action of cactus: identification of its anti-inflammatory effect. *Arch Pharm Res.* Feb;21(1):30-4.

Park JY, Kawada T, et al. 2004. Capsaicin inhibits the production of tumor necrosis factor alpha by LPS-stimulated murine macrophages, RAW 264.7: a PPARgamma ligand-like action as a novel mechanism. *FEBS Lett.* Aug 13;572(1-3):266-70. Erratum in: FEBS Lett. 2004 Sep 24;575(1-3):141.

Park KK, Surh YJ. 1997. Effects of capsaicin on chemically-induced two-stage mouse skin carcinogenesis. *Cancer Lett.* Mar 19;114(1-2):183-4.

Park Y, et al. 1988. Effect of coix on plasma, liver, and fecal lipid components in the rat fed on lard- or soybean oil-cholesterol diet. *Biochem Med Metab Biol.* Feb;39(1):11-7

Patro BS, Rele S, et al. 2002. Protective activities of some phenolic 1,3-diketones against lipid peroxidation: possible involvement of the 1,3-diketone moiety. *Chembiochem.* Apr;3(4):364-70.

Pattnaik S, et al. 1995(a). Antibacterial activity of essential oils from *Cymbopogon*: inter- and intra-specific differences. *Microbios* 84(341):239-45.

Pattnaik S, et al. 1995(b). Effect of essential oils on the viability and morphology of Escherichia coli (SP-11). *Microbios* 84(340):195-9.

Pattnaik S, et al. 1999. Antifungal activity of essential oils from *Cymbopogon*: inter- and intraspecific differences. Cytobios 97(386):153-9.

Pecere T, Gazzola MV, et al. 2000. Aloe-emodin is a new type of anticancer agent with selective activity against neuroectodermal tumors. *Cancer Res.* Jun 1;60(11):2800-4.

Pendell, Deke. 1995. *Pharmako/Poeia: Plant Powers, Poisons, and Herbcraft.* San Francisco: Mercury House.

Pedrosa RC, Meyre-Silva C, et al. 2002. Hypolipidaemic activity of methanol extract of Aleurites moluccana. *Phytother Res.* Dec;16(8):765-8.

Pereira RL, et al. 1999. Immunosuppressive and anti-inflammatory effects of methanolic extract and the polyacetylene isolated from *Bidens pilosa* L. *Immunopharmacology* 1999 Jun; 43(1):31-7

Perez RM, Perez JA, Garcia LM, Sossa H. 1998. Neuropharmacological activity of *Solanum nigrum* fruit. *J Ethnopharmacol.* Aug;62(1):43-8.

Periera EC, Nascimento SC, et al. 1994. Analysis of *Usnea* fasciata crude extracts with antineoplastic activity. Tokai J Exp Clin Med. Sep;19(1-2):47-52.

Peterson, Lee Allen with Roger Tory Peterson. 1999. *A Field Guide to Edible Wild Plants: Eastern and central North America.* Houghton Mifflin Co.

Peungvicha P, Thirawarapan SS, Watanabe H. 1996. Hypoglycemic effect of water extract of the root of *Pandanus odorus* RIDL. *Biol Pharm Bull.* Mar;19(3):364-6.

Pintao AM, Pais MSS, Coley H, Kelland LR, Judson IR. 1995. In vitro and in vivo antitumor activity of benzyl isothiocyanate: a natural product from *Tropaeolum majus. Planta-Medica.* 61: 3, 233-236; 19 ref.

Pitchford, Paul. 1993. *Healing with Whole Foods.* Revised ed. Berkeley, CA: North Atlantic Books.

Pittler MH, Ernst E. 2000. Efficacy of kava extract for treating anxiety: systematic review and meta-analysis. *J Clin Psychopharmacol.* Feb;20(1):84-9.

Poblet A, Andrade S, et al. 1997. The use of epilithic Antarctic lichens (*Usnea aurantiacoatra* and *U. antartica*) to determine deposition patterns of heavy metals in the Shetland Islands, Antarctica. *Sci Total Environ.* Nov 27;207(2-3):187-94.

Poblete, Enrique Oblitas. 1992. *Plantas Medicinales de Bolivia (Farmacopea Callawaya).* 2nd ed. Cochabamba, Bolivia: Los Amigos Del Libro

Polasa K., et al. 1992. Effect of turmeric on urinary mutagens in smokers. *Mutagenesis*; Mar;7(2):107-9.

Pongrojpaw D, Chiamchanya C. 2003. The efficacy of ginger in prevention of post-operative nausea and vomiting after outpatient gynecological laparoscopy. *J Med Assoc Thai.* Mar;86(3):244-50.

Prakash AO. 1979. Glycogen contents in the rat uterus: response to Hibiscus rosa-sinensis Linn. extracts. *Experientia.* Aug 15;35(8):1122-3.

Pramyothin P, Janthasoot W, Pongnimitprasert N, Phrukudom S, Ruangrungsi N. 2004. Hepatotoxic effect of (+)usnic acid from *Usnea siamensis* Wainio in rats, isolated rat hepatocytes and isolated rat liver mitochondria. *J Ethnopharmacol.* Feb;90(2-3):381-7.

Prasad GC, Khanna RP, et al. 1975. Effect of Lajjawanti (*Mimosa pudica*) on Regeneration of Nerve. *Jur. Res. Ind. Med.*10: 4, pp.37-44.

Prasad KV, Bharathi K, Srinivasan KK. 1993. Evaluation of *Musa paradisiaca* Linn. cultivar--"Puttubale" stem juice for antilithiatic activity in albino rats. *Indian J Physiol Pharmacol.* Oct;37(4):337-41.

Proksa B, Proksova A. 1999. Preparation and antineoplastic activity of acylhydrazones of R- and S-usnic acid. (Article in Slovak) *Ceska Slov Farm.* Sep;48(5):233-6.

Pukui, Mary Kawena, and Samuel H. Elbert. 1986. *Hawaiian Dictionary.* Honolulu: University of Hawai'i Press.

Qian DS, Liu ZS. 1992. Pharmacologic studies of antimotion sickness actions of ginger. (Article in Chinese) *Zhongguo Zhong Xi Yi Jie He Za Zhi.* Feb;12(2):95-8, 70.

Qiu Z, Jones K, et al. 2000. Modified *Aloe barbadensis* polysaccharide with immunoregulatory activity. *Planta Med.* Mar;66(2):152-6.

Qu G, Li X, Liu J. 1996. Flavonol glycosides of *Sonchus arvensis* L. (Article in Chinese) *Zhongguo Zhong Yao Za Zhi.* May;21(5):292-4, 319.

Quinones D, Alonso S, Lopez R, Sanchez I, Rodriguez F, Fernandez L, Jerez J. 1999. Contact urticaria, rhinoconjunctivitis and bronchial asthma from occupational use of papain. (Article in Spanish) *Allergol Immunopathol* (Madr). Sep-Oct;27(5):273-5.

Qureshi S, Shah AH, Ageel AM. 1992. Toxicity studies on *Alpinia galanga* and *Curcuma longa. Planta Med* Apr;58(2):124-7

Qureshi S, Shah AH, et al. 1989. Studies on herbal aphrodisiacs used in Arab system of medicine. *Am J Chin Med.*;17(1-2):57-63.

Rabe T, et al. 1997. Antibacterial activity of South African plants used for medicinal purposes. *J Ethnopharmacol.* Mar; 56(1):81-7

Rafatullah S, Tariq M, et al. 1990. Evaluation of turmeric (*Curcuma longa*) for gastric and duodenal antiulcer activity in rats. *J Ethnopharmacol* Apr;29(1):25-34

Raj RK. 1975. Screening of indigenous plants for anthelmintic action against human *Ascaris lumbricoides*: Part--II. *Indian J Physiol Pharmacol.* Jan-Mar;19(1)

Rajakrishnan V, Viswanathan P, et al. 1999. Neuroprotective role of curcumin from curcuma longa on ethanol-induced brain damage. *Phytother Res* Nov;13(7):571-4

Ramakrishna Rao R, et al. 2003. In vitro influence of spices and spice-active principles on digestive enzymes of rat pancreas and small intestine. *Nahrung.* 47(6):408-12.

Ramirez-Tortosa MC, Mesa MD, et al. 1999. Oral administration of a turmeric extract inhibits LDL oxidation and has hypocholesterolemic effects in rabbits with experimental atherosclerosis. *Atherosclerosis* Dec;147(2):371-8

Rancan F, Rosan S, Boehm K, Fernandez E, Hidalgo ME, Quihot W, Rubio C, Boehm F, Piazena H, Oltmanns U. 2002. Protection against UVB irradiation by natural filters extracted from lichens. *J Photochem Photobiol B.* Nov;68(2-3):133-9

Rao KS, SH Mishra. 1997. Anti-inflammatory and Hepatoprotective Activities of *Sida rhombifolla* Linn. *Indian Journal of Pharmacology*; 29: 110-116

Rawat AK, Mehrotra S, et al. 1997. Hepatoprotective activity of *Boerhaavia diffusa* L. roots--a popular Indian ethnomedicine. *J Ethnopharmacol.* Mar;56(1):61-6.

Readers Digest Editors. 1986. *Magic and Medicine of Plants.* Publisher: Readers Digest

Reddy AC, Lokesh BR. 1994. Effect of dietary turmeric (*Curcuma longa*) on iron-induced lipid peroxidation in the rat liver. *Food Chem Toxicol* Mar;32(3):279-83

Reid, Daniel P. 1987. *Chinese Herbal Medicine.* Boston: Shambala Publications, Inc.

Reilly CA, Taylor JL, Lanza DL, Carr BA, Crouch DJ, Yost GS. 2003. Capsaicinoids cause inflammation and epithelial cell death through activation of vanilloid receptors. *Toxicol Sci.* May;73(1):170-81.

Reiter M, Brandt W. 1985. Relaxant effects on tracheal and ileal smooth muscles of the guinea pig. *Arzneimittelforschung.*;35(1A):408-14.

Ribeiro-Costa RM, Alves AJ, Santos NP, Nascimento SC, Goncalves EC, Silva NH, Honda NK, Santos-Magalhaes NS. 2004. In vitro and in vivo properties of usnic acid encapsulated into PLGA-microspheres. *J Microencapsul.* Jun;21(4):371-84.

Richards. Conversations with Uncle Butch Richards

Richeux F, Cascante M, Ennamany R, Saboureau D, Creppy EE. 1999. Cytotoxicity and genotoxicity of capsaicin in human neuroblastoma cells SHSY-5Y. *Arch Toxicol.* Sep;73(7):403-9.

Richeux F, Cascante M, Ennamany R, Sanchez D, Sanni A, Saboureau D, Creppy EE. 2000. Implications of oxidative stress and inflammatory process in the cytotoxicity of capsaicin in human endothelial cells: lack of DNA strand breakage. *Toxicology.* May 19;147(1):41-9.

Rojas A, et al. 1992 Smooth muscle relaxing compounds from *Dodonaea viscosa. J Ethnopharmacol.* Jan;35(3):275-83.

Rojas A, et al. 2003 Screening for antimicrobial activity of crude drug extracts and pure natural products from Mexican medicinal plants. *Fitoterapia.* Feb;74(1-2):139-43.

Roman R.R, et al. 1992. Hypoglycemic effect of plants used in Mexico as antidiabetics. *Arch Med Res.* Spring;23(1):59-64.

Rosa A, et al. 2002. Antioxidant activity of capsinoids. *J Agric Food Chem.* 50(25):7396-401.

Ross, Virginia M. Author's conversations with Virginia M. Ross

Rossbach M, Jayasekera R, et al. 1999. Large scale air monitoring: lichen vs. air particulate matter analysis. *Sci Total Environ.* Jul 15;232(1-2):59-66.

Rowe JG, Saenz MT, Garcia MD. 1989. Antibacterial activity of some lichens from southern Spain. (Article in French) *Ann Pharm Fr.*;47(2):89-94.

Ruberto G, Baratta MT, et al. 2000. Antioxidant and antimicrobial activity of *Foeniculum vulgare* and *Crithmum maritimum* essential oils. *Planta Med* Dec;66(8):687-693.

Saada HN, Ussama ZS, Mahdy AM. 2003. Effectiveness of *Aloe vera* on the antioxidant status of different tissues in irradiated rats. *Pharmazie.* Dec;58(12):929-31.

Sachdewa A, et al. 2001. Hypoglycemic effect of *Hibiscus rosa sinensis* L. leaf extract in glucose and streptozotocin induced hyperglycemic rats. *Indian J Exp Biol.* Mar;39(3):284-6.

Sairam K, Rao CV, Goel RK. 2001. Effect of *Centella asiatica* Linn on physical and chemical factors induced gastric ulceration and secretion in rats. *Indian J Exp Biol.* Feb;39(2):137-42.

Sakagami T, Satoh K, Ishihara M, Sakagami H, Takeda F, Kochi M, Takeda M. 2000. Effect of cobalt ion on radical intensity and cytotoxic activity of antioxidants. *Anticancer Res.* Sep-Oct;20(5A):3143-50.

Sakamaki S, Kohgo Y, et al. 1992. Effect of Krestin (PSK) on the induction of IL-2 activated killer cells. *Jpn J Clin Oncol.* Apr;22(2):79-83.

Salgado CG, da Silva JP, Diniz JA, da Silva MB, da Costa PF, Teixeira C, Salgado UI. 2004. Isolation of *Fonsecaea pedrosoi* from thorns of *Mimosa pudica*, a probable natural source of chromoblastomycosis. *Rev Inst Med Trop Sao Paulo.* Jan-Feb;46(1):33-6. Epub 2004 Mar 29.

Saludes JP, Garson MJ, et al. 2002. Antitubercular constituents from the hexane fraction of *Morinda citrifolia* Linn. (Rubiaceae). *Phytother Res.* Nov;16(7):683-5.

Sammon AM. 1992. A case-control study of diet and social factors in cancer of the esophagus in Transkei. *Cancer* Feb 15;69(4):860-865

Sanderson L, Bartlett A, Whitfield PJ. 2002. In vitro and in vivo studies on the bioactivity of a ginger (*Zingiber officinale*) extract towards adult schistosomes and their egg production. *J Helminthol.* Sep;76(3):241-7.

Sang S, Cheng X, et al. 2001. Flavonol glycosides and novel iridoid glycoside from the leaves of *Morinda citrifolia. J Agric Food Chem.* Sep;49(9):4478-81.

Sarbhoy AK, et al. 1978. Efficacy of some essential oils and their constituents on few ubiquitous molds. *Zentralbl Bakteriol Naturwiss.*133(7-8):723-5.

Savinelli, Alfred. 1997. *Plants of Power.* Taos NM.: Alfred Savinelli.

Sawant M, et al. 2004. Analgesic studies on total alkaloids and alcohol extracts of *Eclipta alba* (Linn.) Hassk. *Phytother Res.* Feb;18(2):111-3.

Saxena AK, et al. 1993. Hepatoprotective effects of *Eclipta alba* on subcellular levels in rats. *J Ethnopharmacol.* Dec;40(3):155-61.

Schamber GJ, Misek AR. 1985 Amaranthus retroflexus (redroot pigweed): inability to cause renal toxicosis in rabbits. Am J Vet Res. Jan;46(1):266-7

Schelosky, L., Raffauf, C., Jendroska, K., Poewe, W. 1995. Kava and dopamine antagonism. *Journal of Neurology, Neurosurgery and Psychiatry* 58: 639-640.

Schirrmacher K, Busselberg D, Langosch JM, Walden J, Winter U, Bingmann D. 1999. Effects of (+ / -)-kavain on voltage-activated inward currents of dorsal root ganglion cells from neonatal rats. *Eur Neuropsychopharmacol.* Jan;9(1-2):171-6.

Schmid R, Schick T, Steffen R, Tschopp A, Wilk T. 1994. Comparison of Seven Commonly Used Agents for Prophylaxis of Seasickness. *J Travel* Med; 1:203-206.

Schmitz D, Zhang CL, et al. 1995. Effects of methysticin on three different models of seizure like events studied in rat hippocampal and entorhinal cortex slices. *Naunyn Schmiedebergs Arch Pharmacol*;351:348-355.

Scirpa P, Scambia G, Masciullo V, Battaglia F, Foti E, Lopez R, Villa P, Malecore M, Mancuso S. 1999. A zinc sulfate and usnic acid preparation used as post-surgical adjuvant therapy in genital lesions by Human Papillomavirus. (Article in Italian) *Minerva Ginecol.* Jun;51(6):255-60.

Scott, Susan, and Craig Thomas. 2000. *Poisonous Plants of Paradise.* Honolulu: University of Hawai'i Press.

Seaforth, C. E., C. D. Adams, and Y. Sylvester. 1985. *A Guide to the Medicinal Plants of Trinidad and Tobago.* Rev. ed. Cariri.

Selvam R, Subramanian L, et al. 1995. The anti-oxidant activity of turmeric (*Curcuma longa*). *J Ethnopharmacol* Jul 7;47(2):59-67

Seo W.G., et al. 2000. Inhibitory effects of methanol extract of seeds of Job's Tears (*Coix lachryma-jobi* L. var. ma-yuen) on nitric oxide and superoxide production in RAW 264.7 macrophages. *Immunopharmacol Immunotoxicol.* Aug;22(3):545-54.

Seo WG, et al. 2001. Inhibitory effects of methanol extract of *Cyperus rotundus* rhizomes on nitric oxide and superoxide productions by murine macrophage cell line, RAW 264.7 cells. *J Ethnopharmacol.* 76(1):59-64.

Shah AH, Qureshi S, Ageel AM. 1991. Toxicity studies in mice of ethanol extracts of *Foeniculum vulgare* fruit and Ruta chalepensis aerial parts. *J Ethnopharmacol* Sep;34(2-3):167-172.

Shamaan NA, Kadir KA, et al. 1998. Vitamin C and *Aloe vera* supplementation protects from chemical hepatocarcinogenesis in the rat. *Nutrition.* Nov-Dec;14(11-12):846-52.

Shen CL, Hong KJ, Kim SW. 2003. Effects of ginger (*Zingiber officinale* Rosc.) on decreasing the production of inflammatory mediators in sow osteoarthrotic cartilage explants. *J Med Food.* Winter;6(4):323-8.

Shimpo K, Chikako T, et al. 2000. Inhibition of N-ethyl-N'-nitro-N-nitrosoguanidine-induced Duodenal Tumorigenesis in Mice by Whole-leaf *Aloe arborescens* Miller var. natalensis Berger. *Asian Pac J Cancer Prev.*;1(4):283-288.

Shimpo K, Ida C, et al. 2002. *Aloe arborescens* extract inhibits TPA-induced ear oedema, putrescine increase and tumour promotion in mouse skin. *Phytother Res.* Aug;16(5):491-3.

Shin TY, Kim SH, et al. 2000. Effect of *Vitex rotundifolia* on immediate-type allergic reaction. *J Ethnopharmacol.* Oct;72(3):443-50.

Shipochliev T. 1981. Uterotonic action of extracts from a group of medicinal plants. (article in Bulgarian) *Vet Med Nauki.*;18(4):94-

Shukla A, Rasik AM, Jain GK, et al. 1999. In vitro and in vivo wound healing activity of asiaticoside isolated from *Centella asiatica. J Ethnopharmacol.* Apr;65(1):1-11.

Shylesh BS, et al. 2000. In vitro cytotoxic and antitumor property of *Emilia sonchifolia* (L.) DC in mice. *J Ethnopharmacol* Dec;73(3):495-500.

Sicuteri, F., Fanciullacci, et al. (1990). Substance P theory: a unique focus on the painful and painless phenomena of cluster headache. Headache 30: 69-79.

Sidhu GS, Singh AK, et al. 1998. Enhancement of wound healing by curcumin in animals. *Wound Repair Regen* Mar-Apr;6(2):167-77

Singh A, Singh RG, et al. 1991. An experimental evaluation of possible teratogenic potential in *Boerhaavia diffusa* in Albino rats. *Planta Med.* Aug;57(4):315-6.

Singh B, et al. 2001. In vivo hepatoprotective activity of active fraction from ethanolic extract of *Eclipta alba* leaves. *Indian J Physiol Pharmacol.* Oct;45(4):435-41.

Singh S, Asad SF, Ahmad A, Khan NU, Hadi SM. 2001. Oxidative DNA damage by capsaicin and dihydrocapsaicin in the presence of Cu(II). *Cancer Lett.* Aug 28;169(2):139-46.

Singh YN. 1983. Effects of kava on neuromuscular transmission and muscle contractility. *J Ethnopharmacol*;7:267-276.

Sivarajan, V.V., and Indira Balachandran.1994. *Ayurvedic Drugs and their Plant Sources.* New Delhi: Oxford & IBH Publishing Company.

Sohni YR, Bhatt RM. 1996. Activity of a crude extract formulation in experimental hepatic amoebiasis and in immunomodulation studies. *J Ethnopharmacol.* Nov;54(2-3):119-24.

Somboonwong J, Thanamittramanee S, et al. 2000. Therapeutic effects of *Aloe vera* on cutaneous microcirculation and wound healing in second degree burn model in rats. *J Med Assoc Thai.* Apr;83(4):417-25.

Spingarn A, Sacks PG, et al. 1998. Synergistic effects of 13-cis retinoic acid and arachidonic acid cascade inhibitors on growth of head and neck squamous cell carcinoma in vitro. Otolaryngol Head Neck Surg. Feb;118(2):159-64.

Srivastava KC, Bordia A, Verma SK. 1995. Curcumin, a major component of food spice turmeric (*Curcuma longa*) inhibits aggregation and alters eicosanoid metabolism in human blood platelets. *Prostaglandins Leukot Essent Fatty Acids* Apr;52(4):223-7

Srivastava KC. 1984. Aqueous extracts of onion, garlic and ginger inhibit platelet aggregation and alter arachidonic acid metabolism. *Biomed Biochim Acta*; 43:S335-46.

Srivastava KC. 1986. Isolation and effects of some ginger components of platelet aggregation and eicosanoid biosynthesis. *Prostaglandins Leukot Med*; 25:187-98.

Stander, S., Luger, T. and Metze, D. 2001. Treatment of prurigo nodularis with topical capsaicin. *Journal of the American Academy of Dermatology* 44: 471-478.

Starley IF, et al. 1999. The treatment of paediatric burns using topical papaya. *Burns* 25(7):636-9

Steiner GG. 2000. The correlation between cancer incidence and kava consumption. *Hawaii Med J* Nov;59(11):420-2

Stewart JJ, Wood MJ, et al. 1991. Effects of ginger on motion sickness susceptibility and gastric function. *Pharmacology*;42(2):111-20.

Stone, Charles P. and Linda W. Pratt. 1994. *Hawai'i's Plants and Animals: Biological Sketches of Hawaii Volcanoes National Park.* Honolulu: University of Hawai'i Press.

Strehlow, Wighard and Gottfried Hertzka. 1988. *Hildegard of Bingen's Medicine.* Santa Fe: Bear & Company.

Suekawa M, Yuasa K, et al. 1986. Pharmacological studies on ginger. IV. Effect of (6)-shogaol on the arachadonic cascade (Article in Japanese) *Nippon Yakurigaku Zasshi.* Oct;88(4):263-9.

Suguna L, Sivakumar P, Chandrakasan G. 1996. Effects of *Centella asiatica* extract on dermal wound healing in rats. *Indian J Exp Biol.* Dec;34(12):1208-11.

Sui Z, Salto R, et al. 1993. Inhibition of the HIV-1 and HIV-2 proteases by curcumin and curcumin boron complexes. *Bioorg Med Chem* Dec;1(6):415-22

Sultana S, Perwaiz S, et al. 1995. Crude extracts of hepatoprotective plants, *Solanum nigrum* and *Cichorium intybus* inhibit free radical-mediated DNA damage. *J Ethnopharmacol* Mar;45(3):189-192

Sunilkumar, Parameshwaraiah S, Shivakumar HG. 1998. Evaluation of topical formulations of aqueous extract of *Centella asiatica* on open wounds in rats. *Indian J Exp Biol.* Jun;36(6):569-72.

Surh YJ, Ahn SH, Kim KC, Park JB, Sohn YW, Lee SS. 1995(c). Metabolism of capsaicinoids: evidence for aliphatic hydroxylation and its pharmacological implications. *Life Sci.* Mar 10;56(16):PL305-11.

Surh YJ, Han SS, Keum YS, Seo HJ, Lee SS. 2000. Inhibitory effects of curcumin and capsaicin on phorbol ester-induced activation of eukaryotic transcription factors, NF-kappaB and AP-1. *Biofactors.*;12(1-4):107-12.

Surh YJ, Lee E, Lee JM. 1998. Chemoprotective properties of some pungent ingredients present in red pepper and ginger. *Mutat Res.* Jun 18;402(1-2):259-67.

Surh YJ, Lee RC, Park KK, Mayne ST, Liem A, Miller JA. 1995(a). Chemoprotective effects of capsaicin and diallyl sulfide against mutagenesis or tumorigenesis by vinyl carbamate and N-nitrosodimethylamine. *Carcinogenesis.* Oct;16(10):2467-71.

Surh YJ, Lee SS. 1995(b). Capsaicin, a double-edged sword: toxicity, metabolism, and chemopreventive potential. *Life Sci.*;56(22):1845-55

Surh YJ, Lee SS. 1996. Capsaicin in hot chili pepper: carcinogen, co-carcinogen or anticarcinogen? *Food Chem Toxicol.* Mar;34(3):313-6.

Surh YJ, Park KK, et al. 1999. Anti-tumor-promoting activities of selected pungent phenolic substances present in ginger. *J Environ Pathol Toxicol Oncol.*;18(2):131-9.

Surh YJ. 2002. Anti-tumor promoting potential of selected spice ingredients with antioxidative and anti-inflammatory activities: a short review. *Food Chem Toxicol.* Aug;40(8):1091-7.

Szolcsanyi, J., Nemeth, J., Oroszi, G., Helyes, Z. and Pinter, E. (1998). Effect of capsaicin and resiniferatoxin on the release of sensory neuropeptides in the rat isolated trachea. *British Journal of Pharmacology* 124: 8P.

Takani M, Yajima T, Masuda H, Yamauchi O. 2002. Spectroscopic and structural characterization of copper (II) and palladium(II) complexes of a lichen substance usnic acid and its derivatives. Possible forms of environmental metals retained in lichens. *J Inorg Biochem.*

Jul 25;91(1):139-50.

Takasaki M, Konoshima T, et al. 1999(a). Anti-carcinogenic activity of *Taraxacum* plant. I. *Biol Pharm Bull.* Jun;22(6):602-5.

Takasaki M, Konoshima T, et al. 1999(b). Anti-carcinogenic activity of *Taraxacum* plant. II. *Biol Pharm Bull.* Jun;22(6):606-10.

Tamura Y, Nishibe S. 2002. Changes in the concentrations of bioactive compounds in plantain leaves. *J Agric Food Chem.* Apr 24;50(9):2514-8.

Tang X.Y., et al. 1994. Active constituents of *Commelina communis* L (Article in Chinese) *Zhongguo Zhong Yao Za Zhi* May; 19(5): 297-8.

Taniguchi M, Tsuru S, et al. 1984. Depression of protective mechanisms against ectromelia virus infection in tumor-bearing mice and its prevention by PSK. (Article in Japanese) *Gan To Kagaku Ryoho.* Dec;11(12 Pt 2):2760-5.

Taylor, Leslie. 1998. *Herbal Secrets of the Rainforest.* Rocklin, CA.: Prima Publishing.

Telefo PB, et al. 1998. Effects of an aqueous extract of *Aloe buettneri, Justicia insularis, Hibiscus macranthus, Dicliptera verticillata* on some physiological and biochemical parameters of reproduction in immature female rats. *J Ethnopharmacol.* Dec;63(3):193-200.

Tesoriere L, Butera D, et al. 2004. Supplementation with cactus pear (*Opuntia ficus-indica*) fruit decreases oxidative stress in healthy humans: a comparative study with vitamin C. *Am J Clin Nutr.* Aug;80(2):391-5.

Thomson B, Shaw I. 2002. A Comparison of Risk and Protective Factors for Colorectal Cancer in the Diet of New Zealand Maori and non-Maori. *Asian Pac J Cancer Prev.*;3(4):319-324.

Thomson M, Al-Qattan KK, et al. 2002. The use of ginger (*Zingiber officinale* Rosc.) as a potential anti-inflammatory and antithrombotic agent. *Prostaglandins Leukot Essent Fatty Acids.* Dec;67(6):475-8.

Thomson, William A. R., ed. 1983. *Medicines from the Earth. A Guide to Healing Plants.* San Francisco: Harper & Rowe

Tierra, Michael. 1987. *Planetary Herbology.* Published by Lotus Press

Tiwari KC, Majumder R, Bhattacharjee S. 1982. Folklore information from Assam for family planning and birth control. *Int J Crude Drug Res.* Nov;20(3):133-7.

Tjendraputra E, Tran VH, et al. 2001. Effect of ginger constituents and synthetic analogues on cyclooxygenase-2 enzyme in intact cells. *Bioorg Chem.* Jun;29(3):156-63.

Tolan I, et al. 2004. Isolation and purification of the hypoglycaemic principle present in *Capsicum frutescens. Phytother Res.*18(1):95-6.

Tona, L., et al. 1999(a). Antimalarial activity of 20 crude extracts from nine African medicinal plants used in Kinshasa, Congo. *J Ethnopharmacol* Dec 15;68(1-3):193-203

Tona, L., et al. 1999(b). Biological screening of traditional preparations from some medicinal plants used as antidiarrhoeal in Kinshasa, Congo. *Phytomedicine* Mar;6(1):59-66

Tona, L., et al. 2000. Antiamoebic and spasmolytic activities of extracts from some antidiarrhoeal traditional preparations used in Kinshasa, Congo. *Phytomedicine* Mar;7(1):31-8

Topics Entertainment. 2003. *Instant Immersion Hawaiian.* 8 Audio CD Deluxe Edition. Renton Washington: Topics Entertainment, Inc.

Torisu M, Hayashi Y, Ishimitsu T, Fujimura T, Iwasaki K, Katano M, Yamamoto H, Kimura Y, Takesue M, Kondo M, et al. 1990. Significant prolongation of disease-free period gained by oral polysaccharide K (PSK) administration after curative surgical operation of colorectal cancer. *Cancer Immunol Immunother.*31(5):261-8.

Tourles, Stephanie L. 1994. *Herbal Body Book: A Natural Approach to Healthier Skin, Hair, and Nails.* Storey Books.

Translation of A Barefoot Doctor's Manual 1977. Philadelphia: Running Press.

Tsanuo MK, et al. 2003. Isoflavanones from the allelopathic aqueous root exudate of *Desmodium uncinatum. Phytochemistry.* Sep;64(1):265-73.

Tsuchiya, H. (2001). Biphasic membrane effects of capsaicin, an active component in *Capsicum* species. *Journal of Ethnopharmacology* 75: 295-299.

Tsuru S, Nomoto K, et al. 1984(b). Depression of macrophage functions and T-cell-mediated immunity to listeria infection in tumor-bearing mice and its prevention by PSK. *Cancer Immunol Immunother.*;18(3):160-3.

Tsuru S, Taniguchi M, et al. 1984(a). Effect of PSK on the recovery of macrophage function and T cell-mediated immunity in tumor-bearing mice. (Article in Japanese) *Gan To Kagaku Ryoho.* Nov;11(11):2375-80.

Udoh P. et al. 1999. Studies on antifertility effect of pawpaw seeds (*Carica papaya*) on the gonads of male albino rats. *Phytother Res* 13(3):226-8.

Uebelhack R, Franke L, Schewe HJ. 1998. Inhibition of platelet MAO-B by kava pyrone-enriched extract from *Piper methysticum* Forster (kava-kava). *Pharmacopsychiatry.* Sep;31(5):187-92.

Uncle Butch Richards. 2004. The author's conversations with Uncle Butch Richards

USDA-NRCS. 2005. The PLANTS Database (http://plants.usda.gov). National Plant Data Center, Baton Rouge, LA 70874-4490 USA

Ushida J, Sugie S, et al. 2000. Chemopreventive effect of curcumin on N-nitrosomethylbenzylamine-induced esophageal carcinogenesis in rats. Jpn J *Cancer Res* Sep;91(9):893-8

Utasan Utjir Qollanaka by Jaime Zalles Asin and Manuel De Luca

Valier, Kathy. 1995. *Ferns of Hawai'i.* Honolulu: University of Hawai'i Press.

Vazquez B, Avila G, et al. 1996. Antiinflammatory activity of extracts from *Aloe vera* gel. *J Ethnopharmacol.* Dec;55(1):69-75.

Veerendra Kumar MH, Gupta YK. 2003. Effect of *Centella asiatica* on cognition and oxidative stress in an intracerebroventricular streptozotocin model of Alzheimer's disease in rats. *Clin Exp Pharmacol Physiol.* May-Jun;30(5-6):336-42.

Venkatesh S, Reddy YS, Suresh B, Reddy BM, Ramesh M. 1999. Antinociceptive and anti-inflammatory activity of *Sida rhomboidea* leaves. *J Ethnopharmacol.* Nov 1;67(2):229-32.

Veronin MA, Ramirez G. 2000. The validity of health claims on the World Wide Web: a systematic survey of the herbal remedy *Opuntia. Am J Health Promot.* Sep-Oct;15(1):21-8.

Vijaya, K., et al. 1995. Antibacterial effect of theaflavin, polyphenon 60 (*Camellia sinensis*) and *Euphorbia hirta* on *Shigella* spp.--a cell culture study. *J Ethnopharmaco* Dec 1;49(2):115-8

Vijayakumar CS, Viswanathan S, Reddy MK, Parvathavarthini S, Kundu AB, Sukumar E. 2000. Anti-inflammatory activity of (+)-usnic acid. *Fitoterapia.* Sep;71(5):564-6.

Vijayan P, Raghu C, Ashok G, Dhanaraj SA, Suresh B. 2004. Antiviral activity of medicinal plants of Nilgiris. *Indian J Med Res.* Jul;120(1):24-9.

Vimala S, Norhanom AW, Yadav M. 1999. Anti-tumour promoter activity in Malaysian ginger rhizobia used in traditional medicine. *Br J Cancer,* 80:110-6.

Visuthikosol V, Chowchuen B, et al. 1995. Effect of *Aloe vera* gel to healing of burn wound a clinical and histologic study. *J Med Assoc Thai.* Aug;78(8):403-9.

Vogel, Virgil J., 1970. *American Indian Medicine.* Norman and London: University of Oklahoma Press.

Volz HP, Kieser M. 1997. Kava-kava extract WS 1490 versus placebo in anxiety disorders. A randomized placebo-controlled 25-week outpatient trial. *Pharmacopsychiatry,*30:1-5.

Wagner H, et al. 1986. Coumestans as the Main Active Principles of the Liver Drugs *Eclipta alba* and *Wedelia calendulacea. Planta Medica*:5: 370-2

Wagner, Jill. *Yes, We Have Plenty Bananas.* Hawai'i Island Journal. May 16, 2004 p 25.

Wagner, Warren L., et al. 1999. *Manual of the Flowering Plants of Hawai'i.* Volumes 1 & 2. Revised ed. Honolulu: University of Hawai'i Press.

Walden J, von Wegerer J, Winter U, Berger M, Grunze H. 1997. Effects of kawain and dihydromethysticin on field potential changes in the hippocampus. *Prog Neuropsychopharmacol Biol Psychiatry.* May;21(4):697-706.

Walker, Bill. Kukui. *Hawai'i's Plants and Herbs.* Mana O Hawai'i. November 1, 1978 p 8.

Wang MY, Su C. 2001. Cancer preventive effect of *Morinda citrifolia* (Noni). *Ann N Y Acad Sci.* Dec;952:161-8.

Wang R, et al., 1999. Chemical and clinical investigations of ginseng: a survey, *International Journal of Oriental Medicine.* 24(2): 57-84.

Warnecke G. 1991. Psychosomatic dysfunctions in the female climacteric. Clinical effectiveness and tolerance of Kava Extract WS 1490. (Article in German) *Fortschr Med.* Feb 10;109(4):119-22.

Wasser SP, Weis AL. 1999. Therapeutic effects of substances occurring in higher Basidiomycetes mushrooms: a modern perspective. *Crit Rev Immunol.* 1999;19(1):65-96.

Wat CK, Biswas RK, et al. 1979. Ultraviolet-mediated cytotoxic activity of phenylheptatriyne from *Bidens pilosa* L. *J Nat Prod.* Jan-Feb 42(1):103-11

Wat CK, Johns T, Towers GH. 1980. Phototoxic and antibiotic activities of plants of the Asteraceae used in folk medicine. *J Ethnopharmacol.* Sep;2(3):279-90.

Watanabe K, Takada Y, et al. 1995 Rotundial, a new natural mosquito repellent from the leaves of *Vitex rotundifolia. Biosci Biotechnol Biochem.* Oct;59(10):1979-80.

Watanabe T, Kawada T, Kurosawa M, Sato A, Iwai K. 1988(a). Adrenal sympathetic efferent nerve and catecholamine secretion excitation caused by capsaicin in rats. *Am J Physiol.* Jul;255(1 Pt 1):E23-7.

Watanabe T, Kawada T, Yamamoto M, Iwai K. 1987. Capsaicin, a pungent principle of hot red pepper, evokes catecholamine secretion from the adrenal medulla of anesthetized rats. *Biochem Biophys Res Commun.* Jan 15;142(1):259-64.

Weenen H, et al. 1990. Antimalarial compounds containing an alpha,beta-unsaturated carbonyl moiety from Tanzanian medicinal plants. *Planta Med* Aug;56(4):371-3

Weidner MS, Sigwart K. 2001. Investigation of the teratogenic potential of a *Zingiber officinale* extract in the rat. *Reprod Toxicol.* Jan-Feb;15(1):75-80.

Whistler, W. Arthur. 1992(a). *Flowers of the Pacific Island Seashore.* Honolulu: Isle Botanica.

Whistler, W. Arthur. 1992(b). *Polynesian Herbal Medicine.* Lawai, HI.: National Tropical Botanical Garden.

Whistler, W. Arthur. 1992(c). *Tongan Herbal Medicine.* Honolulu: Isle Botanica.

Whistler, W. Arthur. 1995. *Wayside Plants of the Islands. A Guide to the Lowland Flora of the Pacific Islands.* Honolulu, HI: Isle Botanica.

Whistler, W. Arthur. 1996. *Samoan Herbal Medicine.* Honolulu: Isle Botanica.

Wiart C, et al. 2004. Antimicrobial screening of plants used for traditional medicine in the state of Perak, Peninsular Malaysia. *Fitoterapia.* Jan;75(1):68-73.

Wiart, Christophe. 2002. *Medicinal Plants of Southeast Asia.* Pearson Malaysia: Prentice Hall.

Widgerow AD, Chait LA, et al. 2000. New innovations in scar management. *Aesthetic Plast Surg.* May-Jun;24(3):227-34.

Wiese J, McPherson S, et al. 2004. Effect of *Opuntia ficus indica* on symptoms of the alcohol hangover. *Arch Intern Med.* Jun 28;164(12):1334-40.

Williams CA, Goldstone F, Greenham J. 1996. Flavonoids, cinnamic acids and coumarins from the different tissues and medicinal preparations of *Taraxacum officinale. Phytochemistry.* May;42(1):121-7.

Wolfram R, Budinsky A, et al. 2003. Daily prickly pear consumption improves platelet function. *Prostaglandins Leukot Essent Fatty Acids.* Jul;69(1):61-6.

Wolfram RM, Kritz H, et al. 2002. Effect of prickly pear (*Opuntia robusta*) on glucose- and lipid-metabolism in non-diabetics with hyperlipidemia--a pilot study. *Wien Klin Wochenschr.* Oct 31;114(19-20):840-6.

Womble D, Helderman JH. 1988. Enhancement of allo-responsiveness of human lymphocytes by acemannan (Carrisyn). *Int J Immunopharmacol.*;10(8):967-74.

World Health Organization. 1998. *Medicinal Plants in the South Pacific.* WHO Regional Publications. Western Pacific Series No. 19. ISBN 92 9061 119 7

Wrench A, Kock ND. et al. 1999. Investigation of selected plants as possible causes of flaccid trunk paralysis in free-ranging elephants (*Loxodonta africana*) in Zimbabwe. *Zimbabwe Veterinary Journal* 30:(3-4):93-97

Wu H, Shu W, et al. 1998. The experiment research of ginger detoxification to Rhizoma Pinelliae. (Article in Chinese) *Zhong Yao Cai.* Mar;21(3):137-40.

Wu H, Ye D, Bai Y, Zhao Y. 1990. Effect of dry ginger and roasted ginger on experimental gastric ulcers in rats. (Article in Chinese) *Zhongguo Zhong Yao Za Zhi.* May;15(5):278-80, 317-8.

Wu J, Zhang M, Ding D, Tan T, Yan B. 1995. Effect of *Cladonia alpestris* on *Trichomonas vaginalis* in vitro. (Article in Chinese) *Zhongguo Ji Sheng Chong Xue Yu Ji Sheng Chong Bing Za Zhi.*;13(2):126-9.

Xie Zong Wan and Yu You Qin, ed. 1996. *Quan Guo Zhong Cao Yao Ming Jian (A Compilation / Collection of Names of All of China's*

Herbal Medicines), 3 Volumes. Ren Min Wei Sheng Chu Ban She (People's Health Publishers). Translations by Robert Newman.

Xu Qun, et al. editors. 1993. *Zhong Yao Ci Hai (Oceanic Dictionary of Chinese Herbs)*, 3 Volumes. Beijing: Zhong Guo Yi Yao Ke Ji Chu Ban She" (Chinese Medical Technology Publishers). Translations by Robert Newman.

Xue JX, et al. 1993. Effects of the combination of *Astragalus membranaceus* (Fisch.) Bge. (AM), tail of *Angelica sinensis* (Oliv.) Diels. (TAS), *Cyperus rotundus* L. (CR), *Ligusticum chuanxiong* Hort. (LC) and *Paeonia veitchii* Lynch (PV) on the hemorrheological changes in normal rats. *Zhongguo Zhong Yao Za Zhi.* Oct;18(10):621-3, 640 [Article in Chinese].

Yagi A, Kabash A, et al. 2002. Antioxidant, free radical scavenging and anti-inflammatory effects of aloesin derivatives in *Aloe vera. Planta Med.* Nov;68(11):957-60.

Yamahara J, Hatakeyama S, et al. 1992. Stomachic principles in ginger. II. Pungent and anti-ulcer effects of low polar constituents isolated from ginger, the dried rhizoma of *Zingiber officinale* Roscoe cultivated in Taiwan. The absolute stereostructure of a new diarylheptanoid. Article in Japanese. *Yakugaku Zasshi.* Sep;112(9):645-55.

Yamahara J, Miki K, et al. 1985. Cholagogic effect of ginger and its active constituents. *J Ethnopharmacol.* May;13(2):217-25.

Yamahara J, Mochizuki M, Rong HQ, 1988. Matsuda H, Fujimura H. The anti-ulcer effect in rats of ginger constituents. *J Ethnopharmacol*; 23:299-304.

Yamamoto Y, Miura Y, Kinoshita Y, Higuchi M, Yamada Y, Murakami A, Ohigashi H, Koshimizu K. 1995. Screening of tissue cultures and thalli of lichens and some of their active constituents for inhibition of tumor promoter-induced Epstein-Barr virus activation. *Chem Pharm Bull* (Tokyo). Aug;43(8):1388-90.

Yang MS, Ha YL et al. 1995. Screening of domestic plants with antibacterial activity. (Article in Korean) *Agricultural Chemistry and Biotechnology* v.38, n.6: 584-589.

Yeoh KG, Kang JY, et al. 1995. Chili protects against aspirin-induced gastroduodenal mucosal injury in humans. *Dig Dis Sci.* Mar;40(3):580-3.

Yoshikawa M, Yamaguchi S, et al. 1994. Stomachic principles in ginger. III. An anti-ulcer principle, 6-gingesulfonic acid, and three monoacyldigalactosylglycerols, gingerglycolipids A, B, and C, from Zingiberis Rhizoma originating in Taiwan. *Chem Pharm Bull* (Tokyo). Jun;42(6):1226-30.

You KM, Son KH, et al. 1998 Vitexicarpin, a flavonoid from the fruits of *Vitex rotundifolia*, inhibits mouse lymphocyte proliferation and growth of cell lines in vitro. *Planta Med.* Aug;64(6):546-50.

Younos C, Rolland A, et al. 1990. Analgesic and behavioural effects of *Morinda citrifolia. Planta Med.* Oct;56(5):430-4.

Yuan Z, He P, Takeuchi H. 1998. Ameliorating effects of water-soluble polysaccharides from woody ear (*Auricularia auricula-judae* Quel.) in genetically diabetic KK-Ay mice. *J Nutr Sci Vitaminol* (Tokyo). Dec;44(6):829-40.

Yuen, Jeffrey C. 1993-1996. Lectures by Jeffrey C. Yuen.

Yun SI, Cho HR, Choi HS. 2002. Anticoagulant from *Taraxacum platycarpum. Biosci Biotechnol Biochem.* Sep;66(9):1859-64.

Zalles, Jaime, and Manuel De Lucca. *Utasan Utjir Qollanaka: Medicinas Que Hay En Nuestro Jardin.*

Zava D.T., et al. 1998. Estrogen and progestin bioactivity of foods, herbs, and spices. *Proc Soc Exp Biol Med.* Mar;217(3):369-78.

Zhang JS, et al. 2001. Studies on the chemical constituents of *Eclipta prostrata* (L.). (article in Chinese) *Yao Xue Xue Bao.* Jan;36(1):34-7.

Zheng M. 1990. Experimental study of 472 herbs with antiviral action against the herpes simplex virus. (Article in Chinese) *Zhong Xi Yi Jie He Za Zhi.* Jan;10(1):39-41, 6.

Zheng MS. 1989 An experimental study of the anti-HSV-II action of 500 herbal drugs. *J Tradit Chin Med.* 9(2):113-6.

Zhong Yao Da Ci Dian (Big Chinese Herb Dictionary), 4 Volumes, 2nd ed. 1993. Shanghai: Shanghai Ke Xue Ji Shu Chu Ban She (Shanghai Science and Technology Publishing Co) Translations by Robert Newman.

Zhu M, Wong PY, Li RC. 1999. Effects of taraxacum mongolicum on the bioavailability and disposition of ciprofloxacin in rats. *J Pharm Sci.* Jun;88(6):632-4.

Zhu, Liangfeng. 1993. *Aromatic Plants and Essential Constituents.* Hong Kong: South China Institute of Botany.

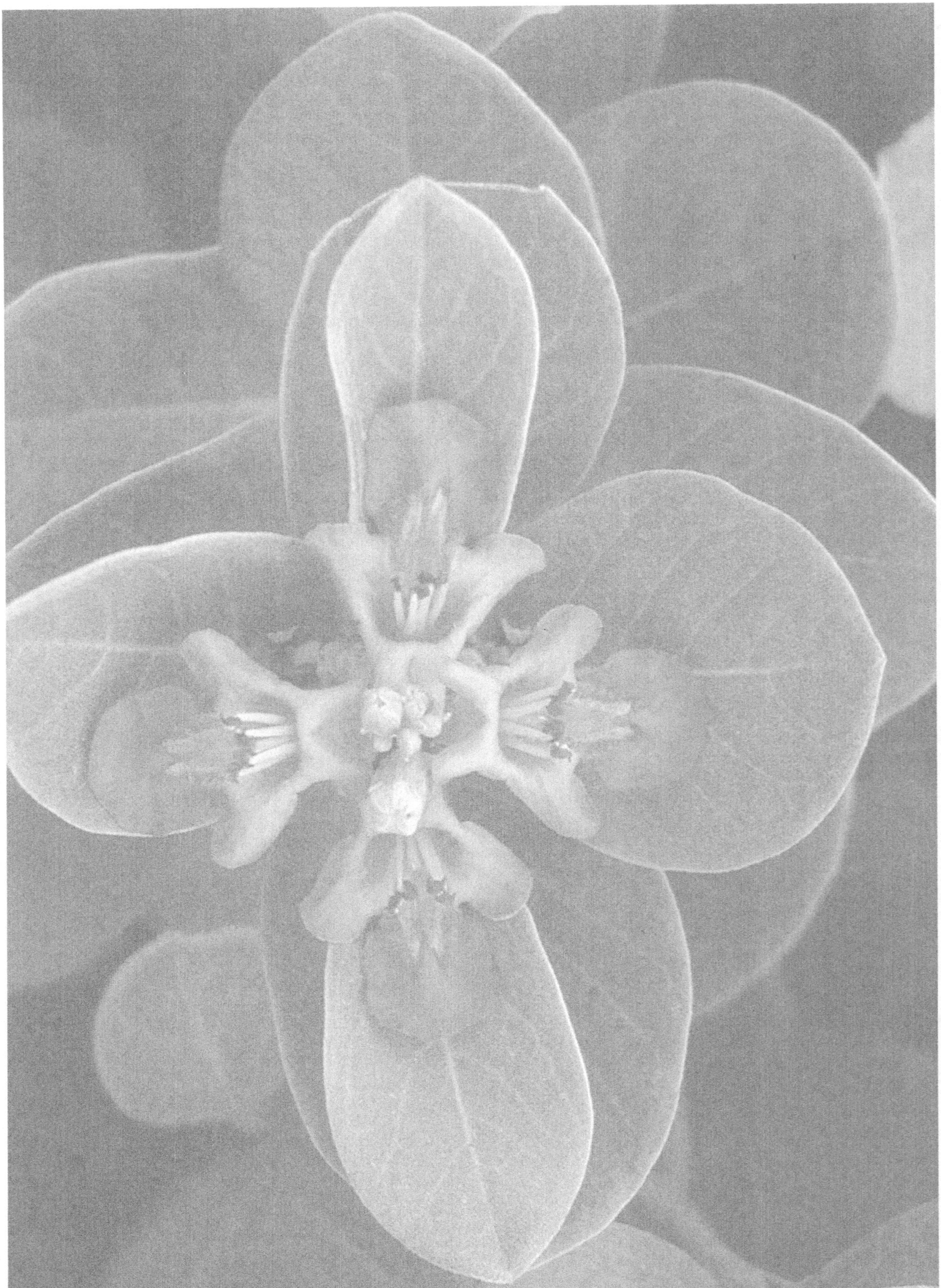

A

B

C

D

E

F

G

H

I

J

K

L

M

N

R

S

T

U

V

W

X

Y

Z

Printed in Dunstable, United Kingdom

91335472R00152